STRENGTH TRAINING

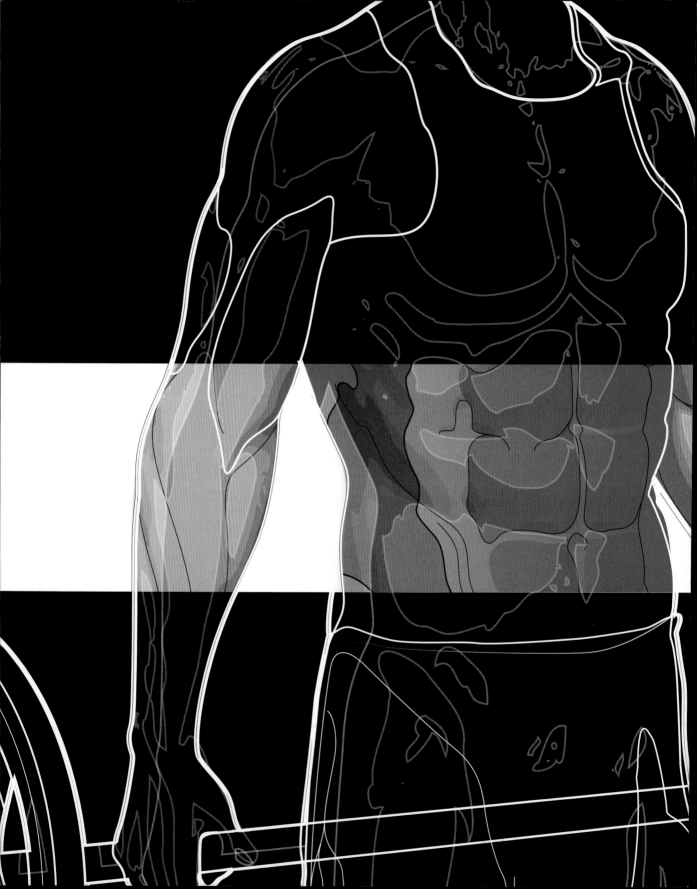

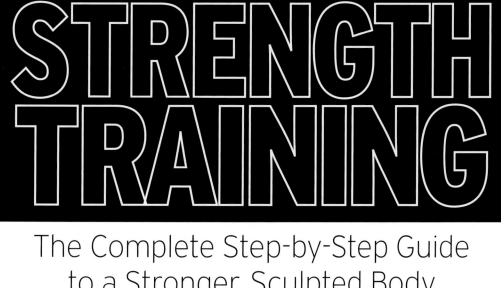

STRENGTH TRAINING

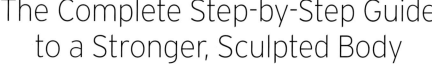

The Complete Step-by-Step Guide to a Stronger, Sculpted Body

DK

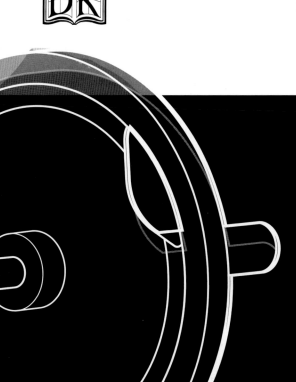

LONDON, NEW YORK, MUNICH,
MELBOURNE, and DELHI

Senior Editor	Gareth Jones
Senior Art Editor	Gillian Andrews
US Editor	Margaret Parrish
Managing Editor	Stephanie Farrow
Managing Art Editor	Lee Griffiths
Production Controller	Tony Phipps
Creative Technical Support	Adam Brackenbury
Jacket Designer	Mark Cavanagh
Art Director	Bryn Walls
Publisher	Jonathan Metcalf
Illustrators	Mike Garland, Mark Walker, Darren R. Awuah, Debajyoti Dutta, Richard Tibbitts, Jon Rogers, Phil Gamble

Produced for Dorling Kindersley by

cobaltid

The Stables, Wood Farm, Deopham Road,
Attleborough, Norfolk NR17 1AJ
www.cobaltid.co.uk

Editors
Marek Walisiewicz, Maddy King

Art Editors
Rebecca Johns, Paul Reid, Darren Bland,
Claire Dale, Lloyd Tilbury, Annika Skoog

First American Edition, 2009

Published in the United States by
DK Publishing
375 Hudson Street
New York, New York 10014

09 10 11 12 13   10 9 8 7 6 5 4 3 2 1

TD444–December/2009

Published in Great Britain by
Dorling Kindersley Limited.

A catalog record for this book is available
from the Library of Congress

ISBN 978-0-7566-5447-4

Printed and bound in Singapore by
Tien Wah Press Ltd.

Discover more at www.dk.com

CONTENTS

INTRODUCTION

Strength training is an increasingly popular activity among men and women of all ages, and offers you a wealth of health benefits—from bigger muscles to stronger bones to increased confidence. With so much conflicting information available, however, how can you be sure that you are getting the best out of your training?

This authoritative, comprehensive, and beautifully illustrated guide, written in conjunction with the BWLA (British Weight Lifters' Association) by strength training experts with more than thirty years' experience of coaching, contains everything you need to know to get the very best from your regimen, whether you want to develop your strength, or build your physique, or are training for specific gains within a chosen sport or activity.

The first chapter, Principles, provides you with all the basic nuts-and-bolts information about how strength training works, and the best ways to achieve your goals, whether you are an experienced gym user, or a complete novice.

The main section of the book covers more than 125 exercises in detail, working through the whole body systematically, providing a section on dynamic lifts for those with more experience. The exercises feature detailed anatomical artworks to show you

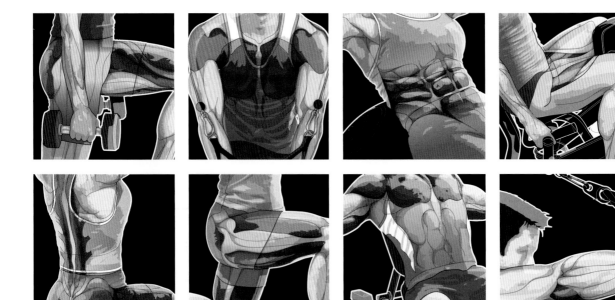

exactly which muscles you are working, and clear step-by-step artworks to guide you through each movement. You are shown how to perform the exercise with optimum technique, and offered a range of helpful features such as variations, or tips on avoiding common mistakes to keep you safe and maximize the effectiveness of your training. And should you know what a particular exercise looks like but not what it's called, you can locate it at a glance using the Exercise Gallery on page 8–11.

The final section offers a pragmatic, no-nonsense approach to the subject of training programs, and includes a range of specially commissioned goal-based examples to suit your needs, whatever your aims or experience, along with useful information on the key exercises for specific sports, to help you tailor your training to suit a particular activity.

Clear, user-friendly, and packed with extremely useful advice, *Strength Training* is the ultimate resource for anyone engaged in strength training.

WARNING

All sport and physical activity involves some risk of injury. Please check the safety information on page 256 before embarking on any of the exercises or programs shown in this book.

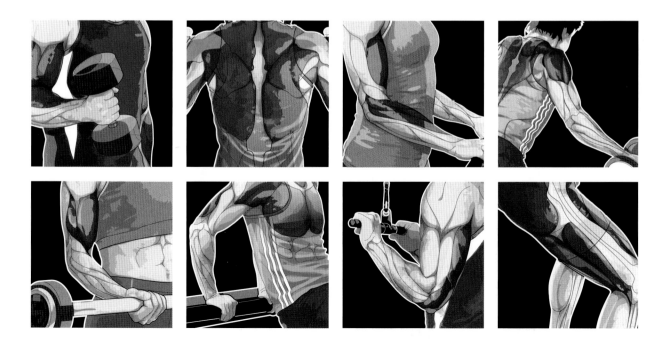

EXERCISE **GALLERY**

LEGS

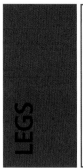

Back Squat
p.64

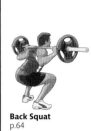

Front Barbell Squat
p.66

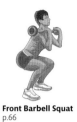

Barbell Hack Squat
p.67

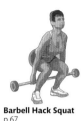

Dumbbell Split Squat
p.68

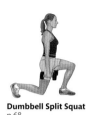

Overhead Split Squat
p.69

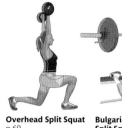

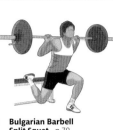

Bulgarian Barbell Split Squat p.70

Machine Leg Curl
p.80

Machine Leg Extension p.80

Hip Abductor
p.82

Hip Adductor
p.82

Calf Raise
p.84

Straight Leg Deadlift
p.85

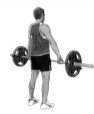

Barbell Deadlift
p.86

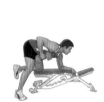

One Arm Row
p.98

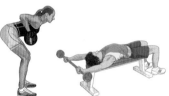

Bent-Over Row
p.100

Barbell Pull-Over
p.102

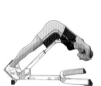

Good Morning Barbell p.104

Back Extension
p.104

Prone Row
p.106

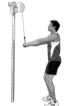

Straight-Arm Pull-Down p.106

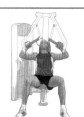

Machine Bench Press p.118

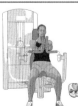

Machine Fly
p.118

Press-Up
p.120

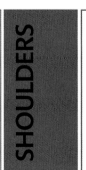

Frame-Supported Press-Up p.121

SHOULDERS

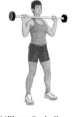

Military Barbell Press p.124

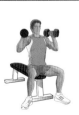

Dumbbell Shoulder Press p.125

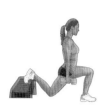
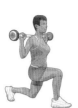
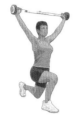
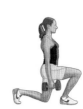

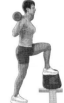

Bulgarian Dumbbell Split Squat p.71

Barbell Lunge p.72

Overhead Barbell Lunge p.73

Forward Lunge p.74

Lateral Lunge p.75

Barbell Step-Up p.76

45-Degree Leg Press p.78

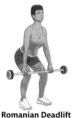
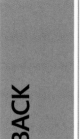
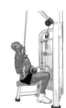
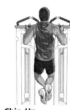
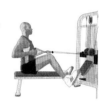

Romanian Deadlift p.88

BACK

Assisted Chin-Up p.92

Lat Pull-Down p.93

Chin-Up p.94

Seated Pulley Row p.96

Standing Pulley Row p.98

CHEST

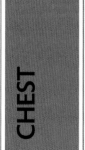

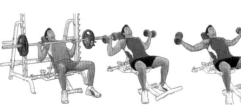
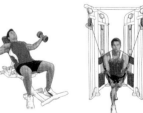

Barbell Bench Press p.110

Dumbbell Bench Press p.110

Incline Barbell Bench Press p.112

Incline Dumbbell Bench Press p.113

Incline Fly p.114

Cable Cross-Over p.116

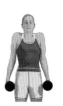
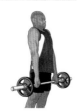
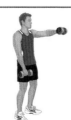
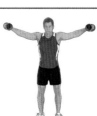
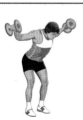
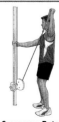

Upright Row p.126

Dumbbell Shoulder Shrug p.128

Shoulder Shrug From Hang p.129

Front Dumbbell Raise p.130

Lateral Dumbbell Raise p.131

Rear Lateral Raise p.132

Scarecrow Rotation p.134

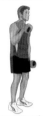
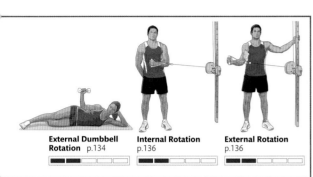
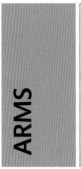

External Dumbbell Rotation p.134

Internal Rotation p.136

External Rotation p.136

ARMS

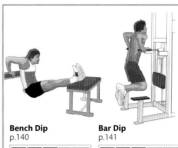
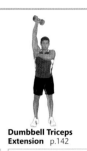

Bench Dip p.140

Bar Dip p.141

Dumbbell Triceps Extension p.142

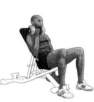

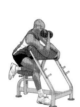
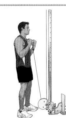
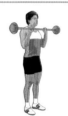
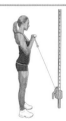

Hammer Dumbbell Curl p.150

Incline Dumbbell Curl p.152

Concentration Curl p.152

Preacher Curl p.154

Pulley Curl p.154

Reverse Barbell Curl p.156

Reverse Pulley Curl p.156

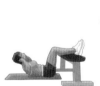

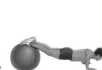
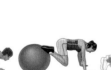

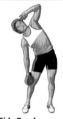

90-90 Crunch p.166

Ball Crunch p.166

Ball Twist p.168

Ball Press-Up p.169

Ball Jack Knife p.170

Ball Back Extension p.171

Side Bend p.172

DYNAMIC LIFTS

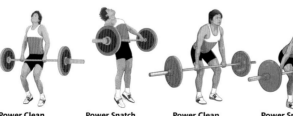

Power Clean p.182

Power Snatch p.184

Power Clean From Hang p.186

Power Snatch From Hang p.188

Squat Clean p.190

Heavy Front Squat p.192

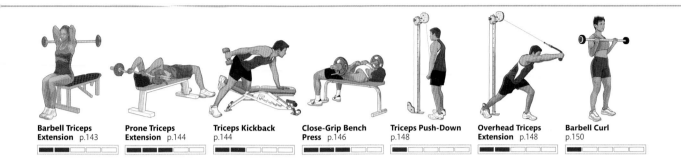

Barbell Triceps Extension p.143

Prone Triceps Extension p.144

Triceps Kickback p.144

Close-Grip Bench Press p.146

Triceps Push-Down p.148

Overhead Triceps Extension p.148

Barbell Curl p.150

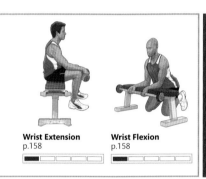

Wrist Extension p.158

Wrist Flexion p.158

CORE AND ABS

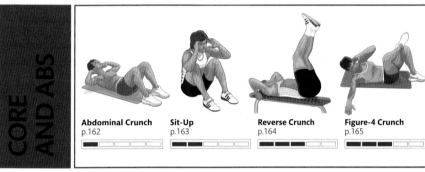

Abdominal Crunch p.162

Sit-Up p.163

Reverse Crunch p.164

Figure-4 Crunch p.165

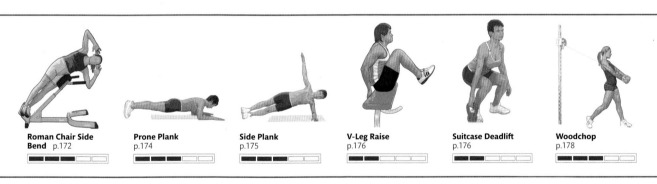

Roman Chair Side Bend p.172

Prone Plank p.174

Side Plank p.175

V-Leg Raise p.176

Suitcase Deadlift p.176

Woodchop p.178

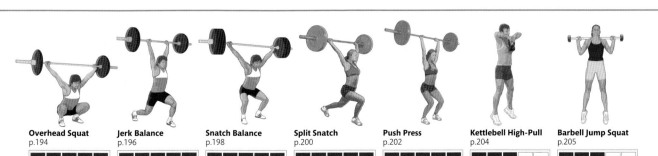

Overhead Squat p.194

Jerk Balance p.196

Snatch Balance p.198

Split Snatch p.200

Push Press p.202

Kettlebell High-Pull p.204

Barbell Jump Squat p.205

ANATOMICAL CHART

ANTERIOR MUSCLES

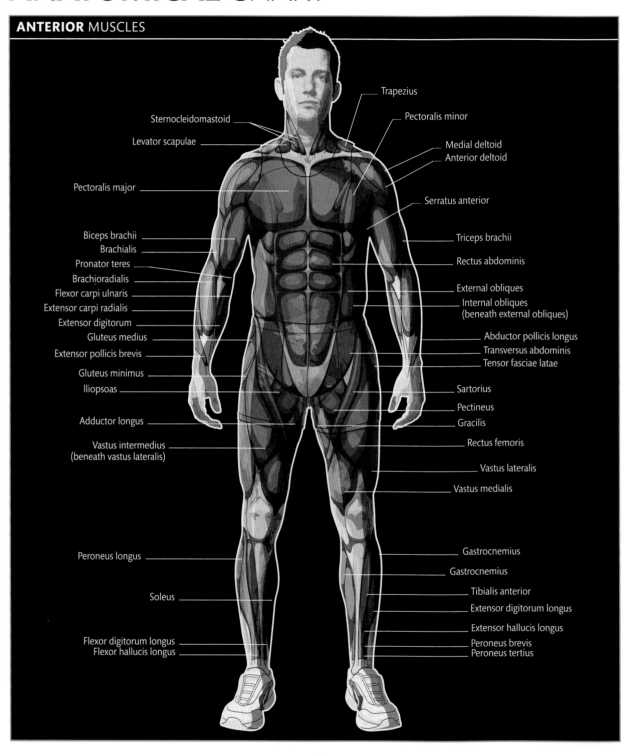

Trapezius

Sternocleidomastoid

Pectoralis minor

Levator scapulae

Medial deltoid
Anterior deltoid

Pectoralis major

Serratus anterior

Biceps brachii
Brachialis
Pronator teres
Brachioradialis
Flexor carpi ulnaris
Extensor carpi radialis
Extensor digitorum
Gluteus medius
Extensor pollicis brevis
Gluteus minimus
Iliopsoas

Triceps brachii
Rectus abdominis

External obliques
Internal obliques
(beneath external obliques)

Abductor pollicis longus
Transversus abdominis
Tensor fasciae latae

Adductor longus

Sartorius
Pectineus
Gracilis

Vastus intermedius
(beneath vastus lateralis)

Rectus femoris

Vastus lateralis

Vastus medialis

Peroneus longus

Gastrocnemius
Gastrocnemius

Soleus

Tibialis anterior
Extensor digitorum longus

Extensor hallucis longus

Flexor digitorum longus
Flexor hallucis longus

Peroneus brevis
Peroneus tertius

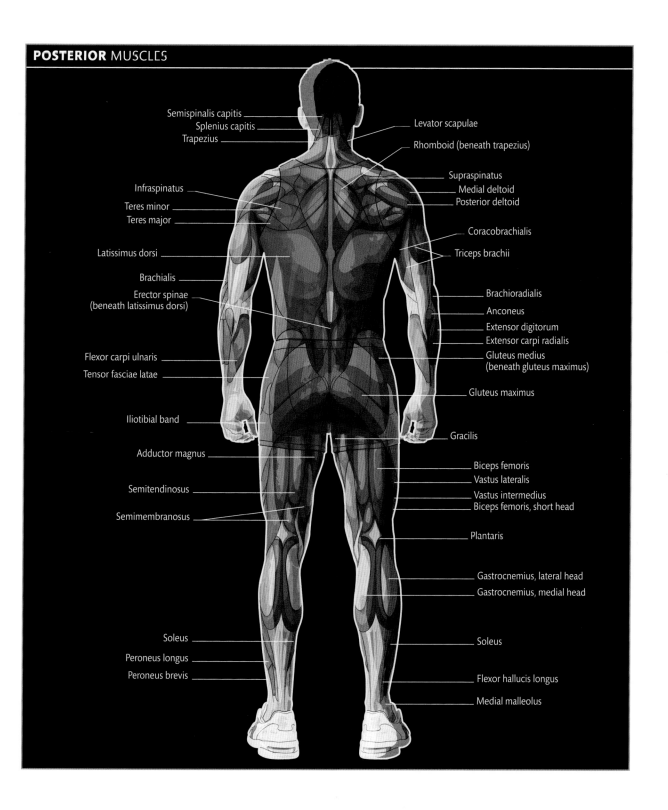

POSTERIOR MUSCLES

Semispinalis capitis
Splenius capitis
Trapezius

Levator scapulae
Rhomboid (beneath trapezius)

Supraspinatus
Medial deltoid
Posterior deltoid

Infraspinatus
Teres minor
Teres major

Coracobrachialis
Triceps brachii

Latissimus dorsi

Brachialis
Erector spinae
(beneath latissimus dorsi)

Brachioradialis
Anconeus
Extensor digitorum
Extensor carpi radialis
Gluteus medius
(beneath gluteus maximus)

Flexor carpi ulnaris
Tensor fasciae latae

Gluteus maximus

Iliotibial band

Gracilis

Adductor magnus

Biceps femoris
Vastus lateralis
Vastus intermedius
Biceps femoris, short head

Semitendinosus

Semimembranosus

Plantaris

Gastrocnemius, lateral head
Gastrocnemius, medial head

Soleus
Peroneus longus
Peroneus brevis

Soleus

Flexor hallucis longus
Medial malleolus

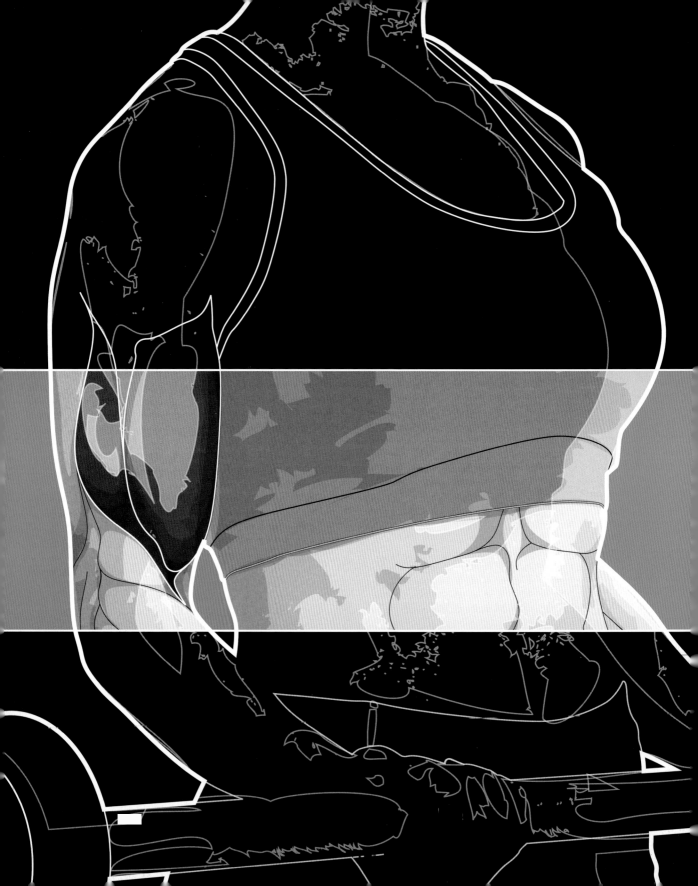

1

PRINCIPLES

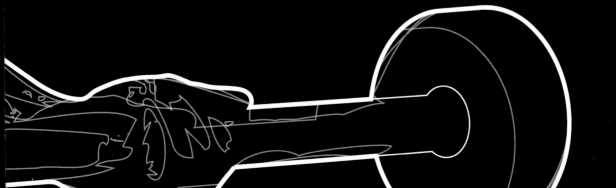

UNDERSTANDING YOUR GOALS

Some of you will have picked up this book because you want greater strength and physical power, perhaps to boost self-confidence, to ease day-to-day activities, to prevent injury, or to improve your posture. It may be that you are not happy with your appearance and desire a more muscular, defined body—that elusive concept of looking more "toned." Your primary goal may be to improve your performance in a particular sport, or you may be intrigued by the challenges of the strength sports—weightlifting and powerlifting.

Your progress toward all of these goals can be aided—to a greater or lesser degree—by strength training. There are other benefits, too, whether intended or incidental. Strength training helps build bone density and can offset the effects of conditions like osteoporosis; it raises your metabolic rate (the amount of energy your body uses at rest) and so can help keep your weight under control; it builds muscle mass, and so can counteract the muscle loss that accompanies aging beyond the age of 30.

Bodybuilding and strength training

The sport—or art—of bodybuilding differs from strength training in that its primary goals are to maximize muscle mass (promote hypertrophy) while reducing body fat, so sculpting your physique. It is a cosmetic activity, in which any gain in strength or power is a by-product.

On the positive side, bodybuilding has undoubtedly inspired many people to get involved in strength training and to think about improving their fitness. The sport certainly provides some spectacular visuals, especially at the highest competitive levels. However, for every person who is

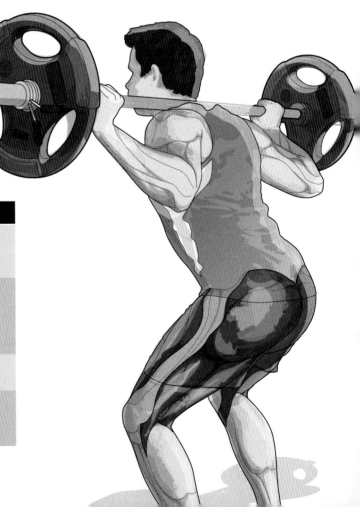

WHAT IS STRENGTH TRAINING?

The term "strength training" is often used interchangeably with "resistance training" and "weight training," but they are not synonymous.

Resistance training is any form of exercise that causes muscles to contract against an external resistance. Weights are just one tool: you can use elastic bands, your own bodyweight, cables, hydraulics, water, a partner, or even a vibration platform to provide resistance.

Strength training is any form of resistance training engaged in to enhance muscle strength.

Weight training is any form of resistance training where weights are used to provide resistance and challenge your strength.

enthralled at the prospect of huge biceps and rippling abs, there is another who finds such displays unappealing, and whose primary goal is simply to keep his or her body healthy and in optimum condition for everyday life.

Training for the sport of life

You may not want to be a bodybuilder, weightlifter, or powerlifter. Instead, you may simply want to look a bit better, increase your muscle mass a small amount, and reduce your body fat levels. Perhaps you want to be able to cope better with the demands of daily life and be able to continue to do this effectively well into old age. Resistance training can assist you in achieving any or all of these goals.

Training for sports

It is widely accepted today that athletes need to engage in strength and power training to enhance their sporting performance. Sport-specific conditioning may include aspects of general strength training (including those with a physiotherapy slant), weightlifting, powerlifting, and even bodybuilding (in sports where gains in bodyweight and muscle mass may be of benefit). The huge subject of training for sports is addressed further on pages 40–45.

Strength sports

Another aspect of strength training is participation in the two strength sports of weightlifting and powerlifting. The object in both is to lift as much weight as physically possible, in particular styles of lift, for one repetition.

Weightlifting features two lifts; the snatch, and the clean and jerk. In the snatch, the objective is to lift as much weight overhead, as quickly as possible and in one movement; in the clean and jerk, two movements are utilized. Both these lifts are very technical and are performed powerfully and explosively. Weightlifting is an Olympic sport and weightlifters are arguably the most powerful athletes competing at an Olympic games. The abilities required by the weightlifter include technique, power, speed, strength, flexibility, and courage. Although weightlifting is a sport in its own right, the techniques of the clean and jerk and the snatch are used extensively within sport-specific

ONE SIZE DOESN'T FIT ALL

To succeed in any training program, you should have a clear idea of what you want to achieve, where you are starting from, and who you are. The responses of two people to the same training program are likely to be very different depending on the following factors:

Chronological age: age in years.

Biological age: age in relation to physical maturity—especially important for trainees in their early- to mid-teens.

Training age: age in relation to the number of years of experience of training with weights and of sport in general.

Emotional maturity: ability to concentrate during training and handle the fact that results may sometimes be elusive.

Gender: men and women respond differently to strength training in both physiological and psychological terms.

Physical capability: affected by both heredity (see below) and training history (degree of skill and fitness developed).

Heredity: some people have innate strength, or can add bone and muscle mass more quickly than others; the preponderance of fast- and slow-twitch muscle fibers (see page 19) and some aspects of personality are also genetically determined.

Lifestyle: the degree to which training programs can be fit into life outside the gym.

Having a firm grip on your goals is vital to developing an effective resistance training program that will, in the long run, leave you feeling satisfied with your achievements.

strength training and conditioning, as well as in more general strength training, due to their unparalleled ability to develop an individual's power.

Powerlifting comprises the lifts of the bench press, squat, and deadlift. Ironically, powerlifting requires a large amount of pure strength but little explosive power, because the lifts are completed with incredibly heavy weights that can be moved only very slowly. Elite powerlifters are arguably the strongest athletes in the world.

TRAINING PHYSIOLOGY

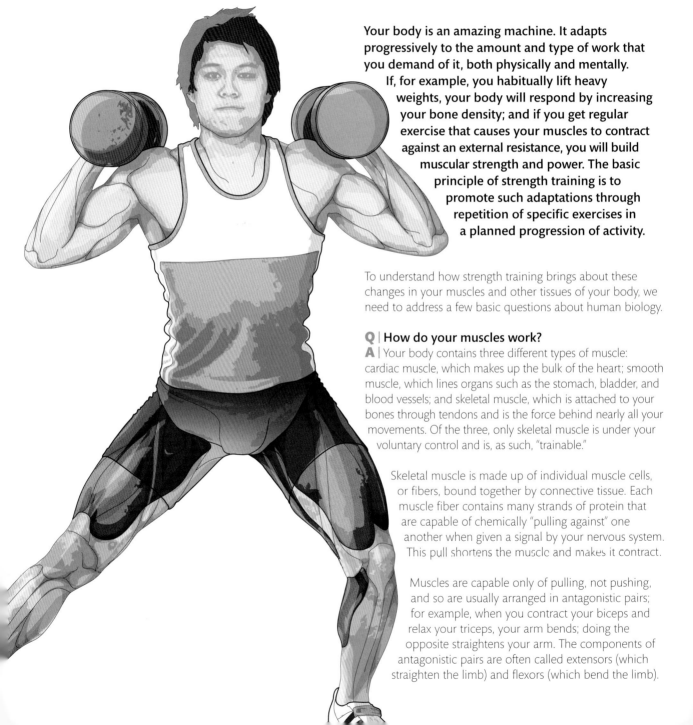

Your body is an amazing machine. It adapts progressively to the amount and type of work that you demand of it, both physically and mentally. If, for example, you habitually lift heavy weights, your body will respond by increasing your bone density; and if you get regular exercise that causes your muscles to contract against an external resistance, you will build muscular strength and power. The basic principle of strength training is to promote such adaptations through repetition of specific exercises in a planned progression of activity.

To understand how strength training brings about these changes in your muscles and other tissues of your body, we need to address a few basic questions about human biology.

Q | How do your muscles work?

A | Your body contains three different types of muscle: cardiac muscle, which makes up the bulk of the heart; smooth muscle, which lines organs such as the stomach, bladder, and blood vessels; and skeletal muscle, which is attached to your bones through tendons and is the force behind nearly all your movements. Of the three, only skeletal muscle is under your voluntary control and is, as such, "trainable."

Skeletal muscle is made up of individual muscle cells, or fibers, bound together by connective tissue. Each muscle fiber contains many strands of protein that are capable of chemically "pulling against" one another when given a signal by your nervous system. This pull shortens the muscle and makes it contract.

Muscles are capable only of pulling, not pushing, and so are usually arranged in antagonistic pairs; for example, when you contract your biceps and relax your triceps, your arm bends; doing the opposite straightens your arm. The components of antagonistic pairs are often called extensors (which straighten the limb) and flexors (which bend the limb).

66 Strength training works by overloading muscles, allowing them to adapt, and overloading them again 99

Q | How does strength training work?

A | Strength training works by overloading muscles, or groups of muscles, then allowing the muscle tissue to adapt, and then overloading the muscle again. On the cellular level, this works because overloading causes microscopic tears to the muscle cells. The damage is rapidly repaired by your body and the affected muscles regenerate and grow stronger. After you work out, testosterone, insulinlike growth factor, growth hormone, proteins, and other nutrients rush to your muscles to help repair them and make them stronger.

Q | How does your body respond to training?

A | Your body responds to training in several ways. The first of these is typically adaptation of the central nervous system—what physiologists call neural adaptation. Put simply, you become more efficient and coordinated when performing a given movement. The gains in strength that occur during this skill-learning process can be quick and significant, but they tend to taper off after a fairly short time.

As you continue to train, your muscles grow in size because individual muscle fibers enlarge, or the fluid sac surrounding them increases in size, or both. You do not grow new muscle fibers. Changes also occur in the type of fiber in your muscles (see feature box, right). Most of your muscles contain both Type 1 and Type 2 fibers—the balance of which is partly determined by genetics. Training can change one type of fiber into another, or at least alter the way in which some muscle fibers work. The muscular changes are accompanied by shifts in enzyme and hormone levels, and changes in the way that your body stores the fuel needed to power muscle action.

It is not just your skeletal muscles that change in response to training. Your heart becomes larger, beats more slowly, and it pumps more blood with each beat. The length of time taken for your heart to return to its normal rate after exercise decreases; the volume of blood plasma increases; and the efficiency of your capillaries to deliver oxygen-rich blood to your tissues rises.

Another key training adaptation is psychological. You learn how to train and listen to your body (see overleaf). This comes with experience, but a good coach will give you guidance.

MUSCLE FIBERS

The fibers in your skeletal muscles are not all the same. Physiologists distinguish between two main types—Type 1, or slow-twitch fibers, and Type 2, or fast-twitch fibers.

Type 1 fibers
- Are responsible for long-duration, low-intensity activity because they are efficient at using oxygen to "burn" the body's fuel resources for repeated contractions over long periods (aerobic activity).
- Are slow to fatigue and are brought into play during activities requiring endurance.

Type 2 fibers
- Produce powerful bursts of contraction at high rates.
- Are ideally suited to brief, high-intensity activity in strength training or powerlifting.
- Work without the need for oxygen (anaerobically) and fatigue quickly.
- Can be further divided into 2a, 2b, and 2x fibers.
- The 2a fiber is a fast-twitch muscle fiber that has endurance properties. It can be trained to act like a Type 1 or 2b fiber.
- The 2b fiber is the classic fast-twitch fiber—explosive, powerful, and strong.
- The 2x fiber is uncommitted and capable of developing into a Type 1 or 2a fiber.

Most of our muscles contain both types of fibers, but some people are genetically gifted with a preponderance of Type 2 fibers, giving them a natural aptitude for high-intensity explosive activities, such as weightlifting or sprinting. Others have genetic weighting toward the slow-twitch Type 1 fibers; most long-distance runners and cyclists fall into this category.

TRAINING PSYCHOLOGY

To make the most of your precious training time, it is important to understand how your body responds to physical demands. You also need to appreciate how you learn new skills and respond mentally to the challenges of training, both for peak performance and for fun. That's where training psychology comes in.

LEARNING MOVEMENT PATTERNS

Research suggests that a new trainee goes through a series of stages in learning new patterns of movement.

Unconscious incompetent	You don't yet know what you don't know and are unaware of your deficiencies. You may even deny the relevance of a particular skill or think that you "know better." You need to understand the usefulness of the new skills you are learning.
Conscious incompetent	You can see what the skills are that you need to learn, and recognize that you are not yet capable of performing them. This stage of learning is dangerous because your frustrations can lead you to select strategies hastily and without due consideration.
Conscious competent	You understand and can perform the movements needed for effective training, but you do so self-consciously and require too much "thinking time" about the moves and positions you need to adopt. This is less of an issue in recreational training, but becomes far more important when performing under pressure or in competition.
Unconscious competent	You are highly skilled and mature, and so well versed in a wide variety of techniques that you can tailor a response to what is needed. You are able to "listen" to your body about what is appropriate on any given training day and respond with a correct choice of movement patterns.

Progressive movement through these stages of development requires may hours of practice, patience, high levels of motivation, and the use of techniques such as visualization.

Positive motivation

To succeed in your training objectives, you have to WANT to train and, for those drawn to competitive sport, to compete. Without the right motivation, it is unlikely that you will hit the volume and intensity of training (see page 32) that you need to achieve difficult goals. Getting to the gym regularly can itself become a chore, and what motivates you to start an exercise program may not be what motivates you to carry on through adversity.

Psychologists talk about two kinds of motivation. Extrinsic motivation is where the drivers come from outside—for example, the input of a coach, the opinion of your peer group or training partner, or the award of trophies and certificates. In intrinsic motivation, the drivers spring from within—for example, the personal satisfaction of mastering a skill, such as being able to move from machine-based to free weight exercises, and the satisfaction of feeling more in charge of your life and increasing your self esteem. Extrinsic motivation will only take you so far; intrinsic motivation is what will keep you going through adversity, such as injury or periods of limited progress.

Your motivation needs to be positive, predominantly about wanting to succeed, rather than about the fear of failure to make progress. For this reason, you must set yourself realistic goals and this demands an honest assessment of those goals relative to your potential.

Don't forget that training should also be fun and suit your individual character: it is in this area that a good coach or instructor can make the difference between continuing with a program and losing momentum.

Too highly motivated?

Motivation can be a destructive as well as a constructive force in training and in competition. Put simply, it is possible to want something too much. Psychologists have shown that there are increasing degrees of motivation that help you achieve peak performance, but when your motivation to succeed becomes too great and you try too hard, your hard-learned skills may, in fact, break down and you may forget your tactics.

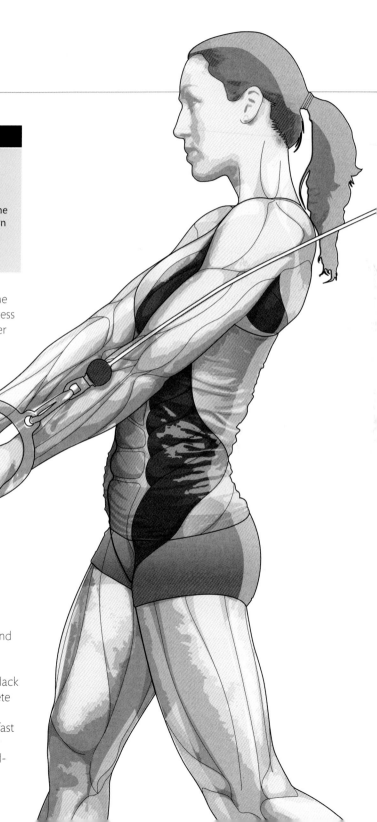

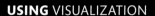

USING VISUALIZATION

Visualization is a technique developed by psychologists in which an athlete creates mental images of actions that he or she performs—visualizing a perfect run up to a long jump, for example, or the ideal throw of a javelin. During this mental process, the athlete's brain directs the muscles required for the move to work in the desired way, laying down a neural pattern that is identical to that created by the actual performance of the movements.

In high-level sport, where the ability to perform under the most severe pressure makes the difference between success and failure, you need to find the most appropriate—rather than just the highest—level of motivation in order to succeed. This is the art of coaching.

Even if you don't compete at a high level, too much motivation may still become a problem. You may be tempted to shorten or even eliminate the crucial rest and recovery phases of training and start to feel the symptoms of overtraining (see page 34). You should never forget that more training is not necessarily better, just as practice does not necessarily make perfect. Bad practice hampers performance and overtraining can result in both physical and psychological damage.

Not wanting it enough

Just as it is possible to want something too much it is also possible—often more likely—not to want something enough to be prepared to put in the considerable time and effort to achieve it.

Many people drop out of strength training because they lack the motivation to train hard enough to be able to compete successfully or to achieve their goals. This issue becomes critical when the rate of progress, which may have been fast and motivating at first, starts to slow. Progress can stall or seem to stop altogether. Self-motivation and realistic goal-setting are the keys to avoiding these pitfalls.

SMARTER GOALS ARE:

SPECIFIC	MEASURABLE	ADJUSTABLE	REALISTIC	TIME-BASED	EXCITING	RECORDED
Identify exactly what you want to achieve. Is it strength, power, muscularity, or fat loss?	How will you measure your progress? Weight loss per week? Changes in BMI? Or the ability to do more reps with heavier weights?	Can you adapt to changing circumstances? For example, what would you do if you were unable to spend as much time in the gym as you originally planned?	Are your goals really achievable? Don't expect to gain a body-builder type physique in four weeks.	Try to set short-term goals and use them as milestones in the journey to achieving your long-term goals.	You are much more likely to stick to a program if it provides some excitement. Training should be fun, though not at the expense of serious work.	Keep a record of the weights you have lifted and the time you have spent in the gym. This can be can be very motivating.

Constructive goal setting

Volumes have been written on the role of goal setting in providing motivation in almost every field of human activity—from dieting to business management. Strength training is no exception, and the usual rules of setting SMART or SMARTER goals (see above) apply to gym work.

Getting good guidance

Many newcomers to strength training will enter a gym, watch others perform marathon two-hour workouts, and reach the conclusion that time on the gym floor and the number of exercises performed is critical to progress. The truth is that many people you observe in gyms are not great role models. Always think about the nature of the work being done, not just its volume and intensity, and consider whether it is consistent with your goals. The sample programs in this book (see Chapter 10) give a broad indication of how to manipulate the training variables to achieve a variety of objectives.

TAKING ADVICE

A major source of confusion for the novice trainee is the information published in some of the popular fitness and bodybuilding magazines. These programs can be quite advanced and will be unsuitable for a new trainee—by trying to emulate them you risk disappointment and even injury. Be realistic about your goals, physical potential, and lifestyle and seek the advice of a certified and impartial coach or trainer.

> **66 You need to find the most appropriate—not just the highest—level of motivation if you are to succeed in your goals 99**

Motivation through coaching

Your coach or instructor must also be motivated—whether or not they are getting paid. They should be able to identify with you and understand your circumstances and the motivating factors that drive you. They should work with you to set mutually agreed to, realistic objectives. If you train primarily to please your coach (or, even worse, to avoid their wrath), or to justify your investment in a gym membership, you are very unlikely to achieve your potential.

The power of partnership

Working out with others—especially a trusted training partner—is a great motivator. Having a partner introduces welcome elements of competition, aspiration, and emulation to your training. Your training partner may be more gifted than you physically, but you may be more focused mentally; ideally, choose a partner whose strengths complement your own.

USING A TRAINING PARTNER

Choose your training partner carefully and reassess your compatibility with your current partner after each phase of training. Things can go wrong if your partner picks up poor exercise habits or takes bad training advice. Radically different physical types can also be a limiting factor in the success of the training partnership—even if the goals of both people are similar. Exercises that might suit one physical type with a slender build and long bones might be counterproductive for a short, stocky type, and vice versa.

Personality factors

Your personality type has a strong effect on what will motivate you in training. The ways in which different personality factors come together in training situations are complicated and are influenced by both genetics and experience, and their intricacies are beyond the scope of this book. However, it is helpful to recognize two broad personality types and how they may respond to the challenges of training.

Extroverts

■ Are outgoing, sociable, and confident personalities.
■ Don't spend too much time reflecting upon or planning their workouts in advance.
■ May have short attention spans and can be easily distracted if not immediately rewarded by success.

If you recognize yourself in this description, you may respond better to extrinsic motivators and to directive approaches to coaching.

Introverts

■ Tend to be quiet, reflective personalities.
■ Avoid pushing themselves forward in a group or drawing attention to themselves.
■ May possess great mental strength in both training and competition.
■ Will take a relatively long-term view of where they are and where they want to be.

If you recognize yourself in this description, you will probably respond better to intrinsic motivators and to a nondirective approach to training.

NUTRITION: THE BASICS

Eating well and staying hydrated are just as important to your training plan as doing the right exercises at the right intensity and volume. The objective of a nutrition program for strength training is to develop and maintain a body with appropriate lean muscle that has the reserves of strength, power, and endurance to meet the demands of daily life, training, and competition. The human body is a complex machine, but research has given us a good understanding of the role played by the various elements of nutrition in staying healthy, getting fit, and gaining and losing weight.

Foods, calories, and body weight

The weight of your body is made up principally of your skeleton, organs, and the muscle, fat, and water that the body carries. Muscular development (though not the number of muscle fibers), body fat, bone density, and the amount of water can all be changed by training and diet.

The basic facts about weight loss and gain are simple. You gain weight if you take on board more calories than you burn; and you lose weight if you eat fewer calories than you need to fuel your basic body functions and exercise regimen.

Some foods contain many calories for a given weight (they are energy-dense, see below), while others, such as dietary fiber or roughage (see page 30), minerals, and vitamins, contain few or no calories but are still a necessary component of your diet.

PROPORTIONS OF MAIN NUTRIENTS

Carbohydrates (carbs)
Carbohydrates are our main source of energy. Nutritionists once distinguished between simple carbohydrates—those found in table sugar, cookies, fruits, and fruit juices—and complex carbohydrates, found in bread, pasta, potatoes, rice, and whole-grain foods. The advice was to eat more complex and fewer simple carbohydrates because complex carbohydrates took longer to break down and absorb and so led to fewer peaks and troughs in levels of blood sugar.

However, the relationship between carbohydrate intake and the effect on blood sugar turned out to be a little more complex. Today, it is more common to refer to foods as having a high or low glycemic index (GI). GI is a measure of the effect that a particular carbohydrate has on blood sugar levels. Low GI foods release their energy more slowly (preventing the feeling of "sugar rush") and are believed to have other health benefits (see pages 30–31).

Fats
Dietary fat is a rich source of energy as well as an essential nutrient. It enables your body to absorb some vitamins and is important for proper growth, development, and health. Fat gives food much of its taste and helps you feel "full."

Not all fats are the same and most foods contain a combination of several fats. Unsaturated fats, such as those found in oily fish and some vegetable and nut oils, are more beneficial than the saturated fats found in meat and animal products, such as butter. Saturated fat in large quantities is implicated in the development of coronary heart disease and needs to be kept to a minimum in a healthy diet. Eating too much fat of any kind will lead to an increase in weight.

ENERGY DENSITY

Carbohydrate	113 calories per ounce (4 calories per gram)
Protein	113 calories per ounce (4 calories per gram)
Fat	255 calories per ounce (9 calories per gram)
Water, vitamins, and minerals	Zero calorific value

Proteins

The building blocks of the human body, proteins are essential to the growth and repair of muscles and other body tissues. We all need protein, and competing athletes may need a little more than sedentary people because intense training places demands on the ability of the body to repair itself. Proteins are made up of chemical units called amino acids, and foods such as fish, meat, and eggs provide a complete source of the essential amino acids. Fruit, vegetables, and nuts contain protein, but on their own may not supply all the amino acids needed by an athlete in training. For this reason, vegetarian and vegan athletes should get nutritional advice before embarking on high-level training.

Protein needs to be taken in regularly because it is not readily stored by the body. However, the daily amount of protein needed—even by a competing athlete—may be within the range of a "normal" healthy diet.

Vitamins

Vitamins are biologically active compounds used in the chemical processes that make the human body function. Vitamins are needed only in tiny amounts and come in two types—those soluble in fat and those soluble in water (which needs to be replenished regularly).

Minerals

Minerals such as potassium, sodium, calcium, zinc, and iron are involved in many biochemical processes that maintain life and fuel growth. Mineral deficiency is rare in a balanced diet.

Water

Water is crucial in maintaining health. The human body is composed largely of water and it is the medium in which most of the body's chemistry is played out. Dehydration is potentially a very serious condition and in extreme cases can lead to death.

PROPORTIONS OF MAIN NUTRIENTS IN THE DIET

There is no universally "correct" balance of daily nutrient intake; the proportions of the main nutrients you need depends on your individual characteristics and lifestyle. However, the following figures are a useful reference point:

60% carbohydrate

25% fat

15% protein

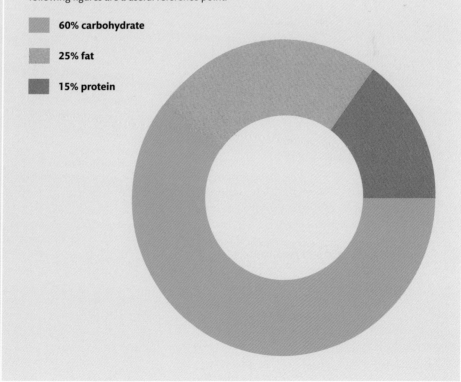

Your energy requirements

Your Basic Energy Requirement (BER) is the amount of energy you need to maintain your basic life processes, such as breathing and circulation, when at rest. In addition to your BER, you need energy to live your lifestyle and sustain your personal work patterns. The nature of your job is important. If you do a lot of manual work, you will have a different energy requirement from someone who works at a desk all day. You can calculate your approximate daily energy requirement by using the table below.

CALCULATING ENERGY REQUIREMENTS

Find your age range and enter your weight into the appropriate equation to find your BER. Then, multiply this figure by the factor associated with your type of lifestyle—sedentary, moderately active, or very active. The figure you arrive at is the level of calorie intake that will allow you to maintain your present bodyweight.

SEX			
Male	10–17 years	8 x weight in lb (17.5 x weight in kg)	+ 651
	18–29 years	7 x weight in lb (15.3 x weight in kg)	+ 679
	30–59 years	5.2 x weight in lb (11.6 x weight in kg)	+ 879
Female	10–17 years	5.5 x weight in lb (12.2 x weight in kg)	+ 746
	18–29 years	6.7 x weight in lb (14.7 x weight in kg)	+ 496
	30–59 years	5.5 x weight in lb (8.7 x weight in kg)	+ 829
Sedentary		multiply by 1.5	
Moderately active		multiply by 1.6	
Very active		multiply by 1.7	

If you take in more calories than your daily energy requirement (including the exercise you get), you will gain weight. If you take in fewer calories than your daily energy requirement (including training), you will lose weight.

Q | How do I lose weight and gain muscle?

A | The common goals of most strength training programs are a reduction in body fat (which involves weight loss) combined with a gain in muscle mass (which involves weight gain). Neither a weight training nor a nutrition program on its own will have the desired effect, but in combination they will achieve the goal. Planning your training program without considering your diet will slow your progress, or even make you sick.

Q | How do I add muscular bodyweight?

A | To build lean muscle, you will need to combine your exercise regimen with extra calories in your diet. Scientists calculate that an excess of 300 calories per day will provide enough fuel for muscle growth. Regardless of how much you eat and exercise, you should not expect to put on huge amounts of muscle in a short period—there are genetic limits to muscle growth. The maximum lean muscle mass that it is possible to gain per year is somewhere between 7¾ and 18 lb (3.5 and 8 kg).

There's little to be gained by consuming large amounts of protein or protein supplements to build muscle because, depending your weight and constitution, your body can absorb only ⅞–1¼ oz (25–35 g) of protein at one sitting. So, if you drink a protein shake containing ½ oz (40 g) of protein, the excess protein will just be excreted in your urine, while the extra calories within the drink will be laid down as fat. Stick to a well balanced diet with frequent small meals (every 3–4 hours) and good natural protein sources from whole grains, beans and legumes, lean meat, fish, eggs, and low-fat dairy products. This diet will give you all the protein you need for muscle growth.

Q | How do I control fat?

A | Fat is produced by your body when you take in more calories than you need to fuel body maintenance and support your current level of physical activity. There is some scientific evidence that we are genetically programmed to stay within about 26 lb (12 kg) of our optimal bodyweight. If you drop below 26 lb (12 kg) of your optimal weight, you will trigger the desire to eat; if you go 26 lb (12 kg) above your optimal weight, food will become unappealing.

Your body does not like change. It is programmed for what physiologists call "homeostasis"—maintaining its internal conditions at a steady level. This helps the body to protect itself by staying on an even keel. So, for example, if your body temperature is low you shiver to generate body heat, and if it's too hot you sweat to cool down. You don't choose to do these things; they happen automatically under control of your central nervous system.

Homeostasis also applies to body weight; the more drastic the changes you try to impose, the more your body will fight against them. So when you try to lose a large amount of weight over a short period, your body will respond by "slowing down"; your basic metabolic rate (BMR), which is the amount of energy that you use while at rest, will fall.

> **" Planning your training program without considering your diet will slow your progress, or even make you sick "**

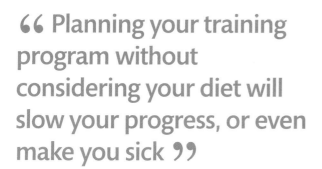

WHAT IS THE RIGHT LEVEL OF BODY FAT?

Average person
It is generally accepted that men should have less than 18 percent of their bodyweight as fat and women 23 percent or less. A certain amount of body fat is essential to good health. There is plenty of evidence to indicate that carrying less than 5 percent body fat compromises your immune system, making you prone to illnesses and infections.

Less than 23% fat   **Less than 18% fat**

Athletes
Athletes in training, especially at the elite level, will have significantly less body fat; around 8–10 percent for men and 10–12 percent for women. High levels of fat in relative terms are a serious disadvantage to most athletes, especially in disciplines where "making weight" for a specific competitive weight class is a priority.

10–12% fat   **8–10% fat**

Hazardous
Carrying more fat than the average person is not particularly hazardous to health until you accumulate 35 percent (men) or 40 percent (women) of total bodyweight as fat. Such levels constitute obesity and have a detrimental effect on health. Too low a level of body fat can also be hazardous, because fat is an important store of energy for aerobic activity.

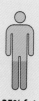 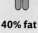

40% fat   **35% fat**

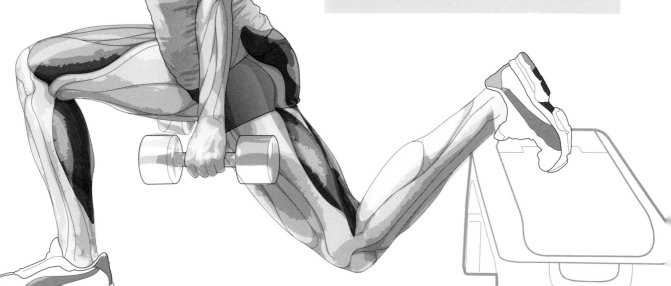

This has the effect of reducing your performance in training and makes it harder to lose weight in the long run. Science also tells us that weight losses of more than 2¼ lb (1 kg) per week will result in a far greater percentage of the loss coming from lean muscle tissue than from fat. This means that useless fat is retained at the expense of muscle. You should therefore limit weight loss to less than 2¼ lb (1 kg) per week in order to remain healthy and capable of training at high intensity.

There are numerous methods of assessing your body fat level. You may be familiar with the term BMI (Body Mass Index), which is a relationship of height to weight and is often used to determine obesity. BMI can be calculated using the following equation:

$$BMI = \frac{weight\ (in\ kg)}{height^2\ (in\ m^2)} \quad or \quad \frac{(in\ lbs)}{703 \times height^2\ (in\ inches^2)}$$

The problem is that BMI does not distinguish between the weight of muscle and that of fat; indeed, most bodybuilders and muscular athletes are deemed to be obese according to BMI only. So, while it is a useful gauge for the general public, BMI needs to be interpreted with caution by anyone with significant muscle mass.

A far more useful gauge is actual body fat percentage, which can be measured in a number of ways, including bio-electrical impedance, skinfold callipers, hydrostatic weighing, and so on. Many health clubs and gyms offer such body fat testing.

Q | What type of exercise will help me lose fat?
A | Getting regular exercise will burn calories; the more active you are, the more calories you burn. How much fat you burn depends on the quantity and quality of the exercise: to lose 2¼ lb (1 kg) of fat, you need to expend approximately 8,000 calories, but there is much debate surrounding the type of exercise that is most effective at burning fat. It is true that when performing cardiovascular exercise at lower

intensities—from 68-79 percent of maximum heart rate— a greater percentage of energy is provided by the breakdown of fat. On the other hand, at higher intensities during anaerobic exercise, while a smaller percentage of energy may be derived from fat metabolism, the total energy burned (from fat and other fuel sources) may be so much higher. So even if fat metabolism forms a smaller percentage of the proverbial pie, the total pie may be so much larger as to make the fat slice of the pie (the contribution from fat in real terms) much greater. Some argue that training the fat-burning systems through low-intensity exercise on occasion may be of benefit because it "trains" your body to become a more efficient fat-burning machine.

Gaining muscle through resistance training is another way of losing fat. As your muscle bulk increases, so does your metabolic rate: muscle is living tissue and it is the furnace of your body. The more muscle mass you have, the more calories you'll burn just to maintain it. Simply being more muscular means you are burning many more calories at all times, whether at rest or at play. So, you should not discount strength training as a calorie burner in its own right.

YOUR WEIGHT LOSS STRATEGY

Your own weight loss plan needs to be tailored to your particular needs, taking into account age, physiology, lifestyle, and training patterns. We are all individuals, and our metabolic rates vary—so one size definitely does not fit all.

■ Whatever strategy you adopt, you should monitor your weight and body fat percentage.
■ Assess your weight and body fat percentage regularly against your food intake and exercise routines.
■ Don't get obsessed—weigh yourself no more than once a week.
■ Don't get overly worried if your weight fluctuates by a few pounds.

THE BODY'S ENERGY SYSTEMS

Different types of activity are fueled by one of three principal energy systems, or biochemical pathways, within the body. These are the aerobic system, the anaerobic system, and the creatine phosphate system.

In practice, the three systems work at the same time, but one or another will predominate, depending on the intensity and the duration of the activity.

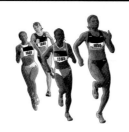

Aerobic
The aerobic system comes into play when you exercise constantly and rhythmically for a period of at least 30 minutes, while keeping your heart rate at around 60–80 percent of its maximum. Aerobic activity is long in duration but low in intensity and includes activities such as jogging, cycling, working on a cross-trainer, and swimming.

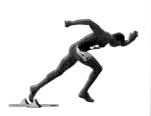

Anaerobic
The anaerobic system is used during short-duration, high-intensity activity, where your body's demand for oxygen exceeds the supply available. Anaerobic exercise relies on energy sources that are stored in the muscles in the form of glycogen and, unlike aerobic exercise, is not dependent on oxygen from the air (breathing). Anaerobic activities include sprinting and interval training.

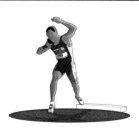

Explosive
Very explosive anaerobic activity, such as weightlifting, shot putting, and short distance sprinting of up to 10 seconds' duration, is fueled by the creatine phosphate system. Creatine phosphate is a substance stored in muscle, which is broken down in a chemical reaction to liberate energy to facilitate very high intensity activity.

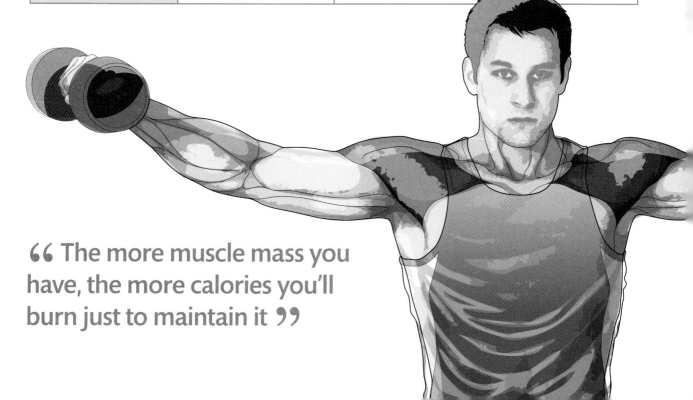

66 The more muscle mass you have, the more calories you'll burn just to maintain it **99**

NUTRITION AND FAT: FAQS

Q | Can I target a specific part of my body for fat loss?
A | No. It is not possible to "spot reduce"—target fat loss to a particular part of the body. If you exercise a particular part of your body, the muscle tissue beneath the fat will become firmer and improve the appearance of that region. However, the exercise will not specifically reduce the fat in the area; fat deposits will diminish with appropriate nutrition and training wherever they are on the body. So if you do 300 abs crunches every day but maintain your fatty diet, you will develop strong abs, but they will be hidden under a layer of fat.

Q | Will my muscle turn to fat if I stop exercising?
A | Muscle does not turn into fat and, conversely, no amount of exercise will turn fat into muscle. The two are completely different types of tissue. When you stop a program of hard training but still eat in the way you did to fuel the regimen, you are taking in more calories than you are burning off and so a gain in body fat is inevitable. If you stop your healthy diet and start to eat junk then the problems get even worse and the fat builds up faster still.

Q | Can I "sweat off" fat in the sauna?
A | Unfortunately not. The small weight loss you experience when you sit in a sauna or steam room comes from losing water, not fat. The weight returns immediately after you consume fluid.

Q | What is dietary fiber?
A | Dietary fiber, also sometimes known as "roughage" is the edible parts of plants that cannot be digested in the human intestines. Taking in enough fiber—around ⅝ oz (18 g) per day for the average adult—is important because it helps prevent constipation and intestinal diseases, as well as lowering cholesterol levels and regulating blood sugar. Fiber is abundant in foods such as fruit, vegetables, beans, and whole-grain cereals.

Q | I've heard people use the terms "essential fat" and "storage fat." What's the difference?
A | There are two types of body fat. Essential fat is needed for normal body function, especially of the hormone and immune systems. It is present in the heart, lungs, spleen, kidneys, and other organs. Women carry more essential fat than men. This gender-specific fat is important for child bearing and other hormone-related functions. Storage fat is the fat that you lose or put on as your weight changes; it is laid down by your body in various areas, especially your hips, thighs, and abdomen in times of plenty, to be used in times of need.

Q | Are all dietary fats created equal?
A | No. The sort of fats you get from oily fish (Omega 3 fats) are important in a healthy diet. Saturated fats, which are found in foods like full-fat milk and in the skin of grilled chicken, are best avoided as much as possible.

Q | What are high and low GI foods?
A | Low GI (glycemic index) foods are those that release their energy slowly. They are an excellent basic fuel for sports—and for life—because they increase blood sugar levels slowly for ready use and so provide a boost of energy without the big "surge" that typifies high GI foods. High GI foods are very quickly absorbed and will typically give you a "sugar rush" or spike, followed by a trough when your energy levels drop below where they were before you ate. The result is that you may feel lethargic and sleepy—not a desirable feeling before or during a training session. You can replenish after your session by eating small quantities of high GI foods along with a little protein. Typical GI values for different foods are given opposite (see box).

GI SCORES

The GI of a food is given on a scale of 0–100, with 100 being pure sugar. Here are some examples of foods and their GIs :

Typical energy drink	95 GI
Orange juice	52 GI
White bread	78 GI
Whole-grain bread	51 GI
Cornflakes	80 GI
Bran cereal	30 GI
Spaghetti (white)	61 GI
Spaghetti (wholemeal)	32 GI
Ice cream	61 GI

A GI of 55 or less is considered low and 70+ high.

Q | How frequently should I eat every day?

A | Begin with a good breakfast of low GI foods, then try to eat at three-hour intervals so that your body always has fuel to burn. Try not to skip meals; go for lower-calorie alternatives instead—try snacking on fruits and yogurt and lean sources of protein. Skipping meals and feeling hungry puts the body on "red alert" and it starts to conserve fat.

Q | What is glycogen?

A | Glycogen is one of the body's major fuel sources. It is basically the substance in which the body stores carbohydrate for the long term. The majority is stored in the muscles and the liver.

Q | Does the right mix of vitamins and minerals matter for healthy body function?

A | Yes. A lack of minerals can cause serious problems. At one end of the scale, you may experience muscular cramp after severe sweating, but in the most serious cases mineral deficiency combined with dehydration can cause heart malfunction and even death. Vitamins are crucial to the chemical processes on which the healthy body depends. Some vitamins are fat soluble and so require some fat in the diet if they are to be absorbed.

Q | Should I eat anything special after my workout?

A | If your training is recreational and of reasonable intensity and volume, the answer is "nothing special"; you should get everything you need from a healthy, balanced diet. However, if you are engaged in intense training with heavy weights, the period 30 minutes after finishing is a crucial window of opportunity when you should take in high GI foods (about 50 g/1¾ oz) to replenish your glycogen stores. Combine this with protein to repair the tissues stressed during the workout.

Q | How big is a "portion"?

A | You will often see references in nutritional articles to "portions." In practice, a portion is a serving of food about the size of a pack of playing cards, which can be held in the palm of the average person's hand.

Finally

This book can provide only a very basic introduction to the complex issues of nutrition, where research into various foods and their effects, and into the body's mode of functioning under a variety of conditions, is ongoing. The conclusion has to be, however, that most people's lifestyles and sporting goals can be achieved by eating a "balanced" diet—one made up of natural, unprocessed foods, taken in moderate quantities. There is little need for supplements or tablets for the majority of non-elite, recreational athletes.

PLANNING YOUR TRAINING

Elite athletes work with their coaches to develop sophisticated training programs that run over months or years, manipulating intensities and loading patterns so that the athlete reaches peak performance at just the right time. But even if you are a recreational trainee, some degree of planning is highly desirable. Your body will respond optimally to training only if it is subjected to progressive overload at the right volume, intensity, and frequency, allowing sufficient periods for recovery between your sessions.

The world of strength training has its own jargon, so before considering the subject of planning, let's introduce some key concepts and terms that are used in this area.

KEY TERMS

Weight/mass: the weight to be lifted.

Repetition (or "rep"): each time a weight is lifted is termed a repetition, or a rep for short.

Set: groups of repetitions are organized into sets. You could, for example, perform three sets of ten repetitions.

1RM (one repetition maximum): the maximum amount of weight you can lift in a single repetition of a given exercise.

%1RM: the percentage of your 1RM that a weight represents: if the maximum weight you can lift in one repetition is 220 lb (100 kg), a weight of 175 lb (80 kg) represents 80% of 1RM.

Inter-set rest period/interval: the time spent recovering between sets—usually seconds or minutes.

Inter-session rest period/interval: the amount of time spent recovering between sessions. Usually hours or days.

Work-to-rest ratio: the ratio of the time spent active during a set to the time spent recovering between sets. For example, if a set takes 20 seconds and you recover for 3 minutes, that is a work-to-rest ratio of 1:9. Basically, the lower the %1RM lifted, the lower the inter-set rest period required.

> 66 Training at a high volume with lots of reps and sets is an excellent way to learn movements 99

Training intensity

The greater the load lifted, the greater is your training intensity. Intensity is commonly expressed as a percentage of your one repetition maximum (see box, left). Opinions vary, but it is generally assumed that an intensity of more than 70–80% 1RM is required to enhance strength.

Often you will see programs described in terms of %1RM (see box, left), although you will also see terms such as 3RM and 10RM; your 3RM is the weight you can lift a maximum of three times and your 10RM is the weight you can lift a maximum of ten times before your muscles fail: these are often a more useful measure than the 1RM.

To measure your 1RM for a particular exercise, first warm up, then choose and lift a weight that is achievable. After a rest of at least a few minutes, increase the weight and try again. Repeat until you arrive at the heaviest weight that you can lift while still maintaining good technique. This is your 1RM. Be sure to progress to the maximum weight without prior fatigue to your muscles.

Training volume and recovery

Training volume is the total amount of weight shifted in a workout—the load multiplied by the number of reps and sets performed. The relationship between intensity and volume is not straightforward. Typically, as you increase intensity, you will decrease volume, and vice versa. Training at a high volume, with lots of reps and sets performed with comfortable weights, is an excellent way to learn movements, but if you avoid more challenging loads you will not develop power and strength. Conversely, performing high-intensity training for too many weeks can be detrimental.

TRAINING PRINCIPLES

Your training program should be appropriate to your goals, effective in achieving them, and take into account your particular needs and personal circumstances (for safety information see page 256). Before starting to plan a program, it helps to explore some of the key principles of strength training.

Specificity
If your desire is to gain muscle bulk, it makes little sense to do long sessions of aerobic training on the treadmill or exercise bike. Similarly, if you want to enhance your explosive power there's little benefit in working with very heavy weights that you can only move incredibly slowly. Specificity means tailoring your training to your goals. It is a simple concept, but one that is generally given insufficient thought, especially by beginners in strength training.

If you are training for a particular sport, specificity gets a little more involved: the exercises you perform should in some way mimic the sporting movements and reflect the loads and speeds relevant to the sport. Sports specificity relates to selecting the correct muscles, joint angles, and postural positions to utilize during strength training. The exercise need not be identical to the sport, but it should include the same movements, in the same order, and be performed at the same speeds.

Overload
This means subjecting yourself to a greater demand in training than you experience in everyday life. In other words, your training session should challenge you physically. Opinions about what constitutes overload do vary, but it is generally assumed that an intensity of around 70–80% 1RM (see box, opposite) is required to enhance strength.

Progression
The point of training is to overload your body, for your body to feel challenged by the demand, and for adaptation to occur. If you lift a 100 lb (45 kg) dumbbell today and find it challenging, your body will adapt. Next time you lift the same weight, it will be less difficult. After a few sessions your body will have largely adapted to that weight. Continuing to lift it for the same number of sets and repetitions will promote little or no further response; you will stagnate. The weight, or the number of times you repeat the movement, must increase to stimulate further development. Progression does not have to happen on every single training session—sometimes taking a step back for a session can allow you to take two steps forward in the long run.

Recovery
An often overlooked, yet absolutely vital, element of any training program is recovery time. Your body adapts and strengthens after a training session while it is in recovery. If you don't provide adequate rest you will, at best, stagnate and, at worst, suffer from overtraining and deteriorate (see page 34).

Continuous training is not necessarily better training, and many recreational gym-goers train intensely far too often and do not take enough advantage of the greatest training aid of all—sleep!

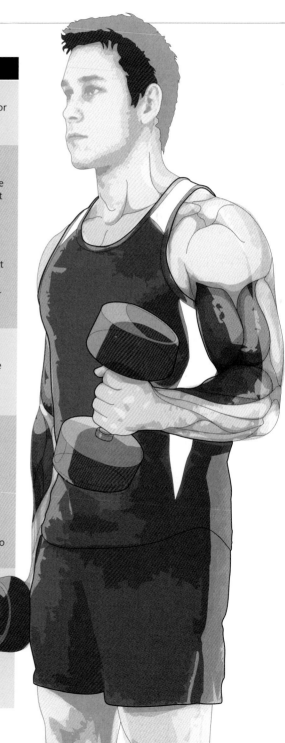

Recovery is as important an aspect of building strength as the training itself. If your recovery period between sessions is inadequate or excessive, you will simply not develop. It is often suggested that a muscle requires 48 hours to recover following a strength training session, which means that a training frequency of 2–3 times per week is optimal. While this is a good starting point, recovery capacity differs greatly between individuals: some people can train daily and still recover and adapt, while others can manage just one session a week. Working out your optimum training frequency is largely a process of trial and error, in which the best advice is to begin with less training volume and more recovery time.

Your body needs rest to repair its tissues and replace energy stores. If your training frequency, volume, and intensity are too high and your recovery phase too short, your body will suffer a progressive physical breakdown resulting in lower levels of performance. This "overtraining syndrome" may also result in poor sleeping patterns, an elevated resting heart rate, susceptibility to colds and other viral infections, aching limbs, reduced stamina, and a lack of explosive power. Ample recovery time is also vital to your psychological state. You need to switch off from time to time—especially after

66 You grow while you are resting—time in the gym just provides the impetus for growth 99

heavy training or intense competition—in order to maintain your enthusiasm and prevent the mental staleness that can result from repetitious training programs. Good exercise habits such as performing "cool down" exercises (see page 47) are critical because your body's recovery from the stress of training and competition starts at this point.

Keep it simple

When you are starting out in strength training, and even as you reach an intermediate level, the easiest program is usually the best. The worst mistake you can make is to adopt the training programs of the elite bodybuilder, often touted in magazines. You have to remember that these people are exceptional, endowed with genes that enable them to develop and perform at phenomenal rates. So swallow your pride, admit that you are probably genetically average, and become comfortable with this concept.

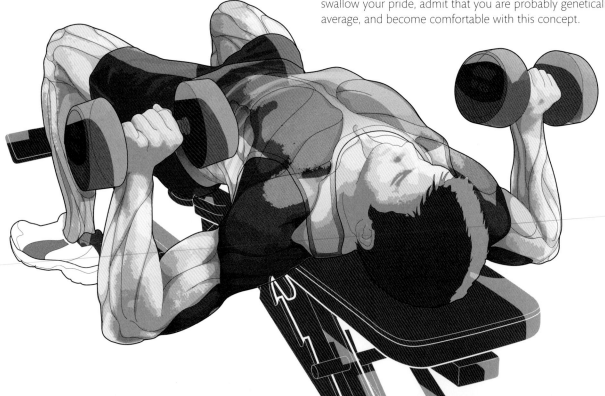

Many people begin strength training with a simple program that employs relatively low volumes, few exercises, and simple loading patterns. They achieve great results and start to think that they must adopt a more complex program in order to progress. More often than not, though, "complex" doesn't equal better, and progress stagnates or even goes into reverse. Rather than admit that the "beginner" program was working for them, they increase the number of sets and exercises, spend more time in the gym and less time recovering, and wonder why they see little progress or, even worse, get injured.

This misconception is often compounded by a fitness industry that emphasizes the importance of changing exercises far too often. There may well be a benefit to altering the exercise composition of your program but such change should be for a reason, not because of some assumption that altering exercises is a panacea to progress. Variation is important to long-term development, but the variation should be more in terms of alterations to the reps, sets, and loads you use, rather than changing the nature of the exercises themselves.

Basic planning principles
Here are five basic pieces of advice to follow when you plan your strength training program.

Select a small number of highly effective exercises: put large, multijoint, compound exercises at the core of your workout. Exercises such as squats, deadlifts, bench presses, chin-ups and pull-ups, bent-over rows, and standing shoulder presses work the largest amounts of muscle mass and are associated with a hormone response that is key to muscle growth. Avoid doing three, four, or five separate exercises that target one body part; such multiple exercises will batter your muscles into submission, rather than stimulating them into more growth.

KEY EXERCISES FOR A SIMPLE PROGRAM	
Chest and triceps	Bench presses
Back and biceps	Pull-ups or bent-over rows
Legs and lower back	Squats or deadlifts
Shoulders	Standing shoulder presses
Biceps	Standing biceps curls
Triceps	Close-grip bench presses

Rest more than you train: don't get caught up in the macho mindset of feeling you have to live in the gym. If you do the above key exercises (see box) a couple of times a week, you will get great results. In fact, you will get far better results than doing it four times a week or doing a routine that has you in the gym almost every day, performing multiple exercises per body part. Remember that you grow while you are resting—time you spend in the gym just provides the impetus for growth.

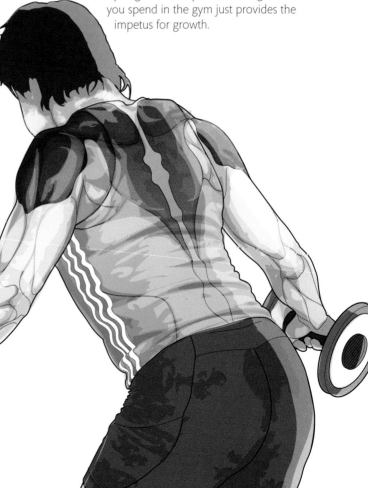

Don't overdo the sets: for the everyman or woman, performing many sets per exercise or body part is counterproductive. Your goal should be to stimulate growth, then put the barbell down and step away from it. You should do a couple of warm-up sets, followed by two, or at most three, actual work sets.

Alternate training: alternate periods of training to muscular failure with periods of working within your comfort zone. Muscular failure is the point at which you are no longer able to perform another repetition with the weight you are lifting. Training to failure is believed to deliver greater muscle mass but is less than optimal in developing strength, and when done to excess it may actually become detrimental to your strength. In strength training, the point at which your movement becomes shaky and irregular is called "being on the nerve." To develop strength you should try to be just shy of this point.

Progress loads slowly: progressive overloading of your muscles is key to developing strength. However, when working at high intensities, you will not be able to add large amounts of weight at every workout. The smallest plate in most gyms weighs 2½ lb (1.25 kg),

" Put large, multi-joint, compound exercises like the squat and deadlift at the core of your workout "

which means the smallest jump you can make on a barbell is 5 lb (2.5 kg). If you are able to bench press 165 lb (75 kg) for 10 repetitions, an addition of 5 lb (2.5 kg) equates to a load increase of about 3 percent. If you could add this amount to your bench press every session, for two sessions per week and for one year, you would be bench pressing well over 700 lb (330 kg) for 10 repetitions, making you one of the strongest people in the world! Smaller jumps are more sustainable. If you can find them, invest in some small, fractional plates. For a standard-diameter weight training bar it is easy to find 1¼ lb (0.5 kg) plates, but they are also available for Olympic-sized bars. Even a gradual increase of just 1¼–2½ lb (0.5–1 kg) per week on your lifts will result in a gain of between 57 and 115 lb (26 and 52 kg) per year. That is immense.

If you cannot find small plates, there is another technique for progression that works well. Imagine you can perform ten repetitions of a shoulder press with 35 lb (16 kg) dumbbells and you decide to progress the weight to 40 lb (18 kg)—a total jump of 12.5 percent. You are very unlikely to be able to perform 10 repetitions with the new weight right away. Instead, try progressing loads slowly (see box, below). If your rate of adaptation outstrips the weekly weight increase, then try jumping by two reps per week instead of one. Remember, there is no rush. It's a marathon, not a sprint.

PROGRESSING LOADS SLOWLY	
Week 1	1 rep with 40 lb (18 kg) immediately followed by 9 reps with 35 lb (16 kg)
Week 2	2 reps with 40 lb (18 kg) immediately followed 8 reps with 35 lb (16 kg)
	and so weekly on until
Week 10	10 reps with 40 lb (18 kg)

Putting it all together

By taking all of these factors into account, you should be well on your way to creating your own tailored training program, which may resemble the one set out here (see box, right), based on visiting the gym twice a week. There are also some excellent programs outlined later in this book (see Programs, page 214). Above all, your program should reflect your individual objectives and your limitations.

Loading and progression

To maximize the effects of your training, try the following plan for loading.

For the first 6-8 weeks of training:

■ Select a weight for each exercise that allows you to perform 12-14 reps before muscle failure, but perform only 10 reps.
■ With each session, add around 3-5 lb (1.5-2 kg) to the lift.
■ Rest for around 3-5 minutes between sets, and try to complete 3 sets of each exercise. In these weeks you will enhance strength in the 12-14 repetition range. With this more manageable weight, focus on performing each exercise with a perfect technique to maximize neural adaptation (see page 19).

For the next 4-8 weeks of training:

■ Devote at least one session per week to training the lift to failure on each set. Failure on the first set should be on the 11th attempted rep, but on the second it will probably occur earlier.
■ Use small progressions from week to week, perhaps 2½ lb (1 kg) on larger lifts and 1¼ lb (0.5 kg) on more isolated ones.
■ Take shorter rest periods of 1-2 minutes between sets. Perform just 2 sets to failure—this should be enough to stimulate muscular growth. In these weeks you are effectively taking advantage of the strength you built up in the first 6-8 weeks, so you can work to failure with heavier weights than you could have previously managed.

EXERCISES, REPETITIONS, AND SETS	
Chest and triceps	Bench press: 2-3 sets of 10 reps
Back and biceps	Bent over row: 2-3 sets of 10 reps
Legs and lower back	Back squat: 2-3 sets of 10 reps
Shoulders	Standing shoulder press: 2-3 sets of 10 reps
Biceps	Standing biceps curl: 2-3 sets of 10 reps
Triceps	Close-grip bench press: 2-3 sets of 10 reps

Working to failure is what produces real results in building strength; however, it is very challenging and overtraining is a distinct possibility if you continuously work at your limit.

After this 4-8 week period, in which you should have accumulated significant muscle mass, go back to the beginning of the cycle and work in the 12-14 reps zone, but with heavier weights, and so on.

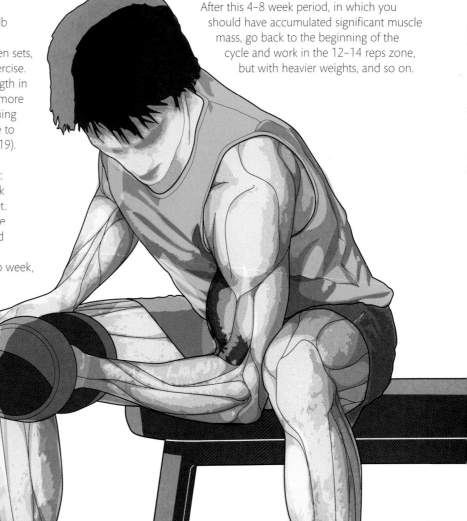

MACHINES OR FREE WEIGHTS?

Most gyms today contain different types of resistance training equipment. These broadly fall into two categories—machines and free weights. Often you will find the free weights in their own area of the gym, which is usually populated by some pretty large people, while the machines occupy most of the floor space and appear more accessible and somehow "friendlier". So which equipment should you use to make best use of the precious time you spend in the gym? Here are some of the pros and cons.

MACHINES	FREE WEIGHTS
Machines require less effort to use than free weights. You sit on the machine, select the weight you want to lift with a pin, and perform an easily learnt movement. It's simple to change the weight on the stack (making machines very good for drop sets, see opposite) and there are usually illustrated instructions on the side of the machine to guide you through the movement.	**Working with free weights** takes some learning. Seemingly subtle variations in movements carried out with identical weights may produce very different results in terms of muscular development, and you need to invest time to learn the correct movement paths for different exercises.
Machines often place you in a seated position; however, very few real-world physical activities or sports are performed while sitting. Seated machines do little to improve the balance and stabilization you need for real-life strength.	**In the majority of sports and day-to-day movements**, forces are transferred through your entire body while you are upright. These natural types of movements are far better reflected in exercises that use free weights than those using machines.
Machines dictate the exact direction and range of your movement in a particular exercise. If you apply any force in the general direction required by the machine, it will move along its dictated path.	**Free weights can** and will deviate from the "ideal" movement path, forcing you to correct and stabilize the deviation. If you do not perform a movement correctly, the weight will deviate from its path and you may not complete the lift.
Machines train only the main muscles involved in a movement: this has implications on real-life performance and, vitally, to injury risk. Continually lifting through a restricted range of motion may lead to long-term reductions in flexibility.	**Free weights train** not just your main muscles, but also the many muscle groups that stabilize a joint. There is little more hazardous than a joint with incredible strength in its prime movers but little or no strength in the stabilizing muscle groups around it.
Machines are designed and hinged to fit an "average" person. However, no-one is really average; machines that are not specifically designed to fit your body can generate dangerous shearing forces at your working joints.	**Using free weights** allows for natural movements that are not constrained by the design of a machine. Carried out with good form, free-weight exercises are not only more effective but arguably safer than machine exercises.
Machine weights make you stronger at using machine weights.	**Free weights** make you stronger in real life.

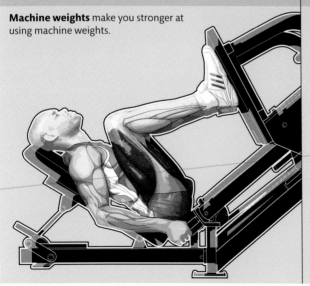

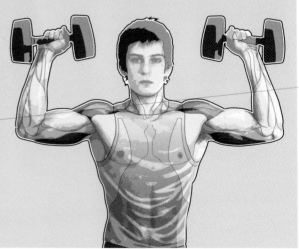

The simple, uncomplicated type of program described on page 37 is considered by many to be the most effective for developing strength. However, training lore is full of complex training methods that, supposedly, enhance the process. You will almost certainly come across some of these concepts at your gym, so it pays to know what they are, and understand their strengths and limitations.

Split routines

Here you do not train your whole body in one session, but split your training between sessions. This division could involve, for example, training the upper and lower body in different sessions or performing different types of movements, such as pulling and pushing, in different sessions.

Split routines are not damaging if implemented cautiously. Their danger lies in the fact that they make it all too tempting to increase the total volume of training above the optimal. So, if you split your twice-weekly routine of six exercises into four routines of three exercises, you may be tempted to add another exercise on each session. Your exercise volume has just risen by a massive 33 percent! You should remember that fatigue and recovery are not only local processes affecting just the muscle(s) trained—your system as a whole becomes fatigued and needs recovery time.

Supersetting

Here you perform one set of an exercise, immediately followed by a set of another exercise that targets the same muscle group. Examples include: bench press followed by dumbbell fly; bent-over row followed by chin-up; and squat followed by leg extension. Theoretically, this type of training is more intense and, as such, may force adaptation, yet there is little evidence to support this.

Pre-exhaustion training

In this form of supersetting, you perform an isolation exercise for a muscle group, immediately followed by a compound exercise for the same area. For example, in the bench press the pre-exhaustion argument goes that your triceps become fatigued before your pectorals; the result is that you cannot work your pectorals maximally, resulting in "undertraining" of these muscles. Thus it is recommended that you perform dumbbell flys to failure and only then move on to the bench press with your pectorals already fatigued.

This technique may have some merit, but there is a far simpler alternative: just stick with the bench press to bring your triceps quickly up to speed with your pectorals. From that point they will gain strength and size together.

Drop sets

In a drop set, you work a muscle to failure, then reduce the load a little and immediately take it to failure once again. In theory, you could do this until the load is zero and the muscle is at "total muscular failure". The idea is that by training the muscle to complete failure, every single muscle fiber is trained, exhausted, and stimulated, resulting in full growth. In reality, the endurance fibers of your muscles have very limited capacity for growth. Also, ask yourself if you really wish to train your muscles for this type of endurance rather than for strength and size.

Do these more complex programs have any real merit? The answer is equivocal. Sporadic use may provide some extra interest and perhaps some more stimulus for growth, yet there is little hard evidence to back this up. Using them in every session is likely to be fatiguing in the long run. As with most things in training, outside of the core fundamentals trial and error and a well kept training diary will play a key role in developing an optimum approach for you.

SPORTS-SPECIFIC TRAINING

It is widely accepted today that athletes need to engage in some form of strength training to enhance their sports performance. However, the needs of a football player are obviously different from those of a swimmer, and a cyclist will not benefit from a program designed for a baseball player. The key point is that strength training for athletes must be specific to the demands of their sport.

STRENGTH TRAINING ATTRIBUTES

Athletes will need to develop some of the following attributes through strength training:

Explosive power: think of a sprinter or a tennis player. Success in these and many other sports depends more on explosive power than it does upon pure, slow strength.

Muscular endurance: think of a rower or a cyclist. In sports like these, the ability to generate a moderate force over a prolonged period is far more important than being able to exert a huge force for a short period of time.

Maximal strength: think of a powerlifter, who needs to exert an enormous amount of force for one repetition. Here, pure strength is the key determinant of success. Similarly, members of the defensive line of a football team also require high levels of pure strength.

- You should also not neglect the importance of pure strength to power output. Power (P) is a product of the force applied (F) and the velocity (V), or speed, at which it is applied: $P = F \times V$. If the force applied is low, power will always be low, regardless of how much speed you can generate. For this reason, weightlifters wishing to develop their power will train for a high level of pure strength.

- Maximal strength is also very relevant to muscular endurance. The more weight you can lift in a single repetition, the less challenging any given force will be. So if your 1RM for the bench press is 660 lb (300 kg), you will be able to perform many more repetitions with 220 lb (100 kg) than someone with a 265 lb (120 kg) 1RM.

Hypertrophy: think of a football player or a rugby player. For these athletes, sheer muscular bulk is required to counter aggressive body contact. However, for athletes in other sports, too much bulk can be a hindrance.

Train movements, not muscles

If you have trained in a gym it is likely that you will have heard someone say something like: "I train my chest and biceps on Monday, my back and triceps on Wednesday, and my legs on Friday." For bodybuilding, and even recreational training, such a muscle-centered approach may make some sense, but from the point of view of enhancing sports performance, who cares how developed your biceps are? What relevance is it to anyone how much weight you can lift in a leg extension? When will any athlete rely on specific, isolated strength in these exact movements in a sports environment? The answer is never.

Sport is all about movement, and your training should address your ability to perform movements more effectively, efficiently, and powerfully. Simply maximizing strength in the muscles involved in a movement, but in an isolated fashion, does not maximize strength development in that movement. To become stronger in squatting movements, you need to squat. To become more powerful in rotation, you need to rotate powerfully. It is common sense.

The reason for this is that the development of coordination (both within and between muscles), skill learning, and the adaptation of your nervous system to the movement patterns trained plays huge roles in the development of strength in movements. Unless you give your body many opportunities to do a movement, it has only limited ability to become better at performing it. All of this should lead you to the inevitable conclusion: train movements, not muscles.

General sports movements

Although each sport has its own specific movements, different sports have similarities in terms of the movements they require. Most team games, for example, involve triple extension through the hip, knee, and ankle (the motion required for jumping and straight-line acceleration), single leg strength and power (for running, changing direction, etc.), strength and stability through the core and pillar, trunk rotation, and so on. This means that sports can be broken down into the types of general movement that need to be trained (see box, opposite), as opposed to treating each sport as totally unique.

KEY SPORTING MOVEMENT PATTERNS

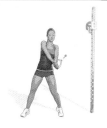

Rotation

This is a common sports movement pattern, but is often neglected in training. Rotational sports include shot putt, hammer and discus throws, boxing, and golf, although there are few sports that require no rotation. There are two types of rotation that require targeted training. In trunk rotation, you rotate your shoulders through your trunk with little or no movement of your hips; an example is golf. In full pillar rotation, you rotate your body around your foot; a good example is tennis.

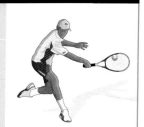

Triple extension

One of the key buzz-phrases in athletic conditioning, this term describes the way in which your ankle, knee, and hip joints go through near-simultaneous extension in jumping, running, lifting, and some throwing actions. In some sports, you will see this triple extension take place off two legs and in others, just one. In either case, it is usually executed explosively. Athletes also use the single leg triple extension in a much less exaggerated, reactive fashion, when changing direction.

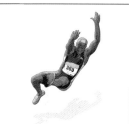

Push

Many sports, for example, football or rowing, involve pushing actions, mostly with one arm, but sometimes two, and it makes sense to train these movements. However, the way in which you train a pushing action in the gym (for example, in a bench press) does not really replicate the way you may push in a sport, where your push may be combined with a rotation. As such, it may make sense to train the two together so that you do not neglect the muscles that fight to control torque.

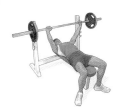

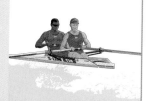

Pull

Many sports, including martial arts and kayaking, involve variations of pull movements. In traditional strength training exercises, the movement is often in just one plane (backward and forward, while in sports the movements are typically multiplanar—adding side-to-side and rotational moves. Training the pull in the context of a sport should also involve elements of balance—keeping your body stable while pulling.

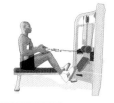

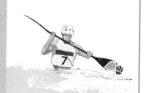

Weight shifting, acceleration, and deceleration

Weight shifting is a key skill in sports such as boxing, golf, and fencing. Acceleration and deceleration—getting the body moving and changing direction as quickly as possible (or "cutting")—is key to activities such as sprinting, jumping, throwing, and lifting. While many athletes will consciously train their ability to accelerate, they will neglect their ability to decelerate. It is also common to see athletes struggle with deceleration as they enter a "cut"; injuries are a real risk at this point.

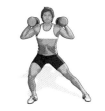

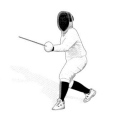

Squat

This movement pattern occurs in the vast majority of sports, including cycling, running, and rowing. It can occur in exaggerated or less exaggerated forms, on one or two legs, to accelerate or decelerate the body or to bring about change of direction. Squatting is also a core component of triple extension (see above), so training this movement is vital to the development of peak performance.

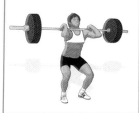

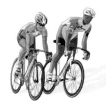

" Strength training for athletes must be specific to the demands of their sport: you should train movements, not muscles "

Sports movements and physical demands

Understanding the training regimen most appropriate to your sport means appreciating the basic movement patterns you will perform (see page 41), and analyzing how those movements are done.

Rate: many people overlook the rate or speed of a movement that they perform in their sport, and so train that movement inappropriately. Boxers, for example, often train too much like powerlifters or bodybuilders, utilizing slow lifting speeds. Given that a boxer's success relies upon rapid, explosive movement, does this make any sense? There is an argument that boxers should develop some pure strength, but it is vital that they focus much of their strength training upon explosive movement, using weightlifting techniques or the ballistic propulsion of implements, such as shot putts or kettlebells, in specific movement patterns.

On the other hand, a rugby prop in a scrum has to apply large forces very slowly and sometimes even statically (isometrically), so high-intensity or isometric (working against an immovable force) training is more appropriate. That said, in the modern game the prop also has to be able to run with the ball explosively and get back into position to defend as quickly as possible. Changes in the prop's role have been reflected in the training regimens used.

The above account seems to indicate a clear distinction between quick vs. slow, or power vs. strength. Yet it may not be so straightforward. In some of the classic Eastern bloc texts on strength training there is no single translation of the word "power." Instead, two distinct phrases are used, the closest approximations of which are "strength–speed" and "speed–strength." Strength–speed relates to movements involving large loads being accelerated moderately quickly, whereas speed–strength describes lighter objects being accelerated very rapidly. It is evident that the type of power

exhibited in the clean and jerk in weightlifting is very different from that of throwing a baseball. This is should be reflected in the way you train for each of these sports.

Frequency: certain sports, such as weightlifting, powerlifting, throwing sports, and golf require a single isolated effort; others, including racket sports, boxing, and rowing demand a more frequent application of force. As soon as more than one expression of force is required there is an endurance element to the sport, which needs to be addressed in your strength training.

It is possible to talk about pure strength vs. strength endurance, or pure power vs. power endurance. The boxer, for example, requires pure power but also needs to be able to reproduce that pure power with as little weakening as possible for the duration of a fight: this is power endurance. The rower, on the other hand, relies upon the capacity to exert relatively high force continuously for the entire race: this is strength endurance.

There is a trend in modern athletic conditioning to develop the pure strength of endurance athletes in the gym and let their muscular endurance develop through their training for

STRENGTH AND ENDURANCE	
Athlete A	can squat 550 lb (250 kg) for one repetition.
Athlete B	can squat 330 lb (150 kg) for one repetition.
Both athletes	are asked to perform as many squats as possible with a 265 lb (120 kg) weight.
For athlete A	this weight is only 48 percent of the one repetition maximum (1RM).
For athlete B	this is 80 percent of the 1RM, a challenging weight that will greatly limit how many repetitions they can perform; that is, their muscular endurance.

running, cycling, rowing, or whatever sport. Consider the advantages of this approach through the example above (see box). For an endurance cyclist, every application of force to the pedal is like performing a mini-squat. If each one of these mini-squats is a smaller percentage of the cyclist's maximum squat then it will be less fatiguing and will enhance cycling economy and muscular endurance.

Direction of force and the impact of gravity: if a golfer wants to enhance driving power, should he train by swinging a club with a really heavy head? If a boxer wants to build straight punching power, should he train by throwing straight punches while holding heavy dumbbells? Both are forms of resistance training but neither is appropriate to its sport. To understand why, try to visualize the direction in which gravity acts upon the weight and then ask the question: "is this the direction in which force is applied in this sports movement?"

Returning to the golf example, you can see that force is applied through the swinging arc; at the point of contact with the ball, the direction of the force applied is parallel to the ground. If you train with a heavy club head, gravity acts vertically upon the head, making it more challenging to lift from the floor but not to swing, so it does not build horizontal strength. At best, this has no positive outcome, but, at worst, it could damage your swing.

Functional training

For anyone involved with health and fitness or sports preparation it has been impossible to escape the recent boom in the concept of "functional training." This is training performed to make your body better at performing those movements that you will use in a particular sport or in daily life. Functional training is today at the cutting edge of preparing athletes for competition.

It is easy to start making huge distinctions between bodybuilding and athletic conditioning along the lines of nonfunctional vs. functional, but that certainly doesn't tell the full story. Yes, most bodybuilders will

use exercises that isolate a muscle in a way in which it would never be used in sports performance, but many also utilize exercises, such as squats and bent-over rows, that fit into the "movements, not muscles" philosophy. The key to functional strength training is to think carefully about how applicable a particular exercise—including its rate, frequency, and direction—is to the movements you perform on the field or on court. Sometimes this means questioning exercise orthodoxy.

Consider, for example, the abdominal crunch, which has for years had a place in almost every athlete's training program. Think about the way in which gravity loads the upper body when you perform this movement from a lying position. Then consider how dramatically this changes as soon as you are on your feet, where hip and spinal flexion require no effort at all. Unless you take part in a sport where you spend a great deal of time horizontal, such as wrestling, jiu-jitsu, and gymnastics, the crunch is of questionable functional benefit. That is not to say it is a bad exercise, but you should question its blanket use as an means of strengthening your trunk.

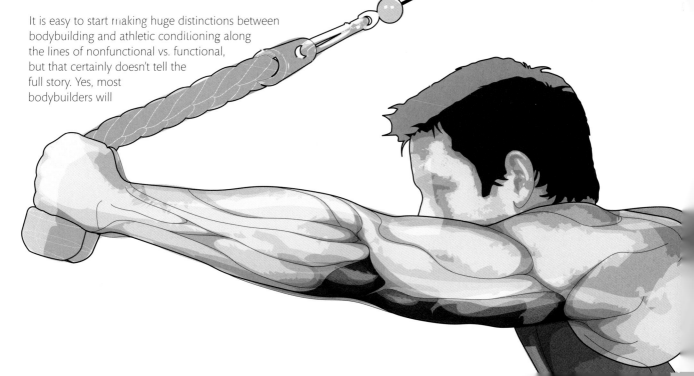

Planning sports-specific training

Developing a program for sports-specific conditioning can be more challenging than planning a general strength training program. Even at its best, it is a far from precise science and requires a great deal of personal interpretation, careful monitoring, and trial and error. The skill of sports-specific training lies in the planning of the training year—manipulating intensities and loading patterns, judging how and when to focus on, for example, power more than strength, or agility more than endurance, and building in rest and regeneration at the correct time. Planning acknowledges that it is impossible for any athlete effectively to train power, strength, strength endurance, power endurance, speed, speed endurance, aerobic endurance, anaerobic endurance, agility, and flexibility to their maximum every single week. It also recognizes that athletes in most sports need to reach their peak performance at a particular time of year, or in a particular season.

Linear/classical periodization

You may have heard the term "periodization" used interchangeably with training planning, but this is somewhat erroneous—periodization is the process of structuring training into phases and as such is simply one form of training planning.

The idea of linear periodization originated in the Eastern bloc in the 1950s, and today most high-level athletes use some form of the technique. Imagine a boxer. He will train hard for three months prior to a fight and then, following the fight, build in a transition phase, doing little or no training. Then he will return to some light, general training before embarking on his next prefight buildup. Similarly, a baseball player will do most of his conditioning work during the off/pre-season period.

How linear/classical periodization works: linear/classical periodization is in essence the splitting up of the training year into numerous blocks, or cycles, each with a different focus, which may be power, strength, endurance, and so on, by stressing different modalities, training loads, lifts, speeds of contraction, intensities, etc.

During the off-season, the focus is typically placed on generalized training designed to redress imbalances that will have inevitably developed during the season, and on developing pure strength, which is essential for maximum power.

Later in the cycle, the volume of pure strength training is significantly reduced as focus on power increases (see diagram, opposite). A simple approach—applicable to all athletes—may be to maintain a ratio of two strength sessions to one power session early in the cycle, and then to reverse this toward competition. As the season or competition approaches, sports-specific training sessions—in the boat, on the bike, or in the ring—are used to build specific muscular endurance and sports-specific speed. It goes without saying that a poorly planned program will result in poor performance, and programs should always be developed with qualified coaches.

Conjugate/undulating planning

Classical/linear approaches work exceptionally well in sports where the athlete is training for one, important competition—training to compete in the Olympic games, for example. However, in many sports, simply peaking for one meet, game, or competition is inappropriate. A soccer or football season may last for up to forty games, each as important as the last. This type of sport demands a method of

LINEAR PERIODIZATION

The basic concept of linear periodization is demonstrated in the diagram below. Note the progressive increase in intensity (and therefore focus on building power over pure strength) every four weeks in the buildup to competition.

week 01 week 02 week 03 week 04	**STRENGTH**
week 05 week 06 week 07 week 08	
week 09 week 10 week 11 week 12	
week 13 week 14 week 15 week 16	
week 17 week 18 week 19 week 20	**POWER**
	COMPETITION DATE

A SAMPLE UNDULATING PROGRAM

This basic example of a wave program shows how workouts undulate from light to moderate to heavy over the course of one week; in the first session you work with weights that allow 12–15 reps before muscle failure, and so on. If you miss a workout one day, just do it on the next day and resume the cycle.

WORKOUT	INTENSITY
Session 1	12–15 RM
Session 2	8–10 RM
Session 3	4–6 RM

planning that maintains good—if not peak—levels of strength, power, strength endurance, power endurance, speed, agility, etc. Conjugate planning is exactly this: the simultaneous training of each of these components of fitness, with equal or similar focus placed on all. A "wave" type or undulating variation may be used in conjugate planning, in which different maximum repetition ranges and intensities are used in the same training week (see box, above right).

Unplanned and instinctive planning

Unplanned planning does not mean following no training plan: it simply recognizes that an athlete will sometimes not be in a fit state to engage in the training session programmed for that day. Often, following a brief warm-up,

the athlete will complete a maximal vertical jump test. If they fail to get within 90 percent of their personal best jump they will not engage in a high-intensity or power-based session. Instead, they may elect to do a higher volume, lower-intensity session.

Instinctive planning means that the athlete does what he or she feels like on the day. The problem is that subjective feelings may not reflect true physical state: it is not uncommon for an athlete to set a personal best when they report feeling lethargic, or to perform poorly when feeling great!

Combining planning methods

It is not unusual for athletes to combine different forms of planning. In many team games, the off- and pre-seasons are perfect opportunities to utilize a form of linear periodization to get to the season in top condition. Then, when the season begins, and each weekly game requires good levels of fitness in multiple areas, conjugate methods may be employed. Within each of these phases, unplanned and perhaps even instinctive forms of planning can also play their own roles.

In conclusion, training for a sport is very different from general fitness training. The goal in athletic strength and conditioning is to maximize sports performance specific to an athlete's sport, while minimizing injury risk, and then strive to push on to higher and higher levels. Sport is organized into competitive calendars and while winning is always great, who remembers who won the race before the Olympics? One of the true arts in athletic conditioning, therefore, is peaking perfectly for the big competition or game.

WARM UP, COOL DOWN

Warming up and cooling down are too often overlooked in many training programs. Time pressures make it tempting to skip a warm-up, but you do so at your peril. Warming up is essential—it gets your body ready for intense work, while minimizing the risk of injury and maximizing your potential to learn and improve.

A warm-up need take no longer than 20 minutes; begin by skipping, jogging, or working on a cross-trainer for 10 minutes, and then perform 10 minutes of mobilization exercises (see opposite page). Consistently warming up will improve your level of performance.

BENEFITS OF WARMING UP

- Increased heart rate to prepare you for work.

- Increased blood flow through active tissues, which leads to increased metabolism.

- Increased speed of contraction and relaxation of warmed muscles.

- Reduction in pre-workout muscle stiffness.

- Better use of oxygen by warmed muscles.

- Better quality and fluency of movement from warmed muscles.

- Higher temperatures, which help nerve transmission and metabolism in muscles.

- Specific warm-ups can help with what physiologists call "motor unit recruitment." A motor unit consists of a nerve fiber together with all its associated muscle fibers. Warming up will increase both the number of motor units brought into play and the rate at which they fire (contract).

- Increased mental focus on the training and competition.

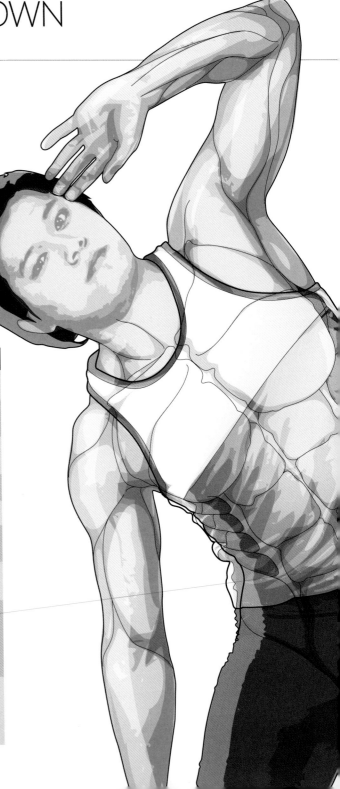

Mobilization exercises

Sometimes called dynamic stretching, or movement preparation, mobilization exercises are controlled movements, where you go through a full range of motion without stopping (see pages 50–61).

They are an ideal way to prepare for a workout because they reduce muscle stiffness and help reduce the chance of injury. As you become more advanced and flexible, you can add a controlled swing to push a body part past its usual range of movement. The force of the swing may be gradually increased but should never become too extreme.

Warm-up is not the time for static stretches (see pages 208–13)—those in which you put your body into a position where the target muscles are under tension. Indeed, using static stretches before a workout may reduce your capacity to release power and does little or nothing to minimize the chances of injury.

Cooling down and recovery techniques

When you have finished your workout, you should bring your body back down to its pre-exercise state in a controlled manner. During a workout, your body is under stress: muscles get damaged and waste products build up. A good cool-down will help your body to repair itself.

Cooling down need not be a lengthy process: start with 5–10 minutes of gentle jogging or walking, which decreases your body temperature and allows the waste products to be removed from your working muscles. Follow this with 5–10 minutes of static stretches, which help your muscles to relax and the muscle fibers to realign and reestablish their normal range of movement. To perform a static stretch (many are described on pages 208–13), extend the target muscle(s) as far as it can comfortably go, easing into the stretch, and then hold that position for around 10 seconds.

66 Warming up gets your body ready for intense work, while minimizing the risk of injury 99

Post-exercise static stretching is controversial. Some suggest the cool-down phase of the workout is an ideal time for "developmental stretching," which is designed to increase muscle flexibility and your range of movement. Developmental stretches have the same form as simple static stretches: you first hold the static stretch for around 10 seconds, then take the stretch a little farther— ½ in (1–2 cm) will do—and hold for another 20–30 seconds.

Others propose that stretching a muscle after exercise may actually increase muscle damage and delay recovery. Picture a muscle like a pair of panty hose. Following intense exercise the muscle is full of small micro-tears that are akin to small runs in the hose. Stretching a muscle at this point is like stretching the hose; possibly not good news. A happy medium may be some light, gentle developmental stretching after your workout for muscles that feel particularly tight. Don't compare yourself to others in the gym—some people have great mobility and you could be in trouble if you try to match their range of movement.

BENEFITS OF COOLING DOWN

- Allows the heart rate to recover to its resting rate.

- Reduces the level of adrenaline in the blood.

- Potentially reduces Delayed Onset Muscle Soreness (DOMS), pain that is sometimes experienced one to three days after intense muscle activity.

- Aids in the reduction of waste products in the blood, including lactic acid.

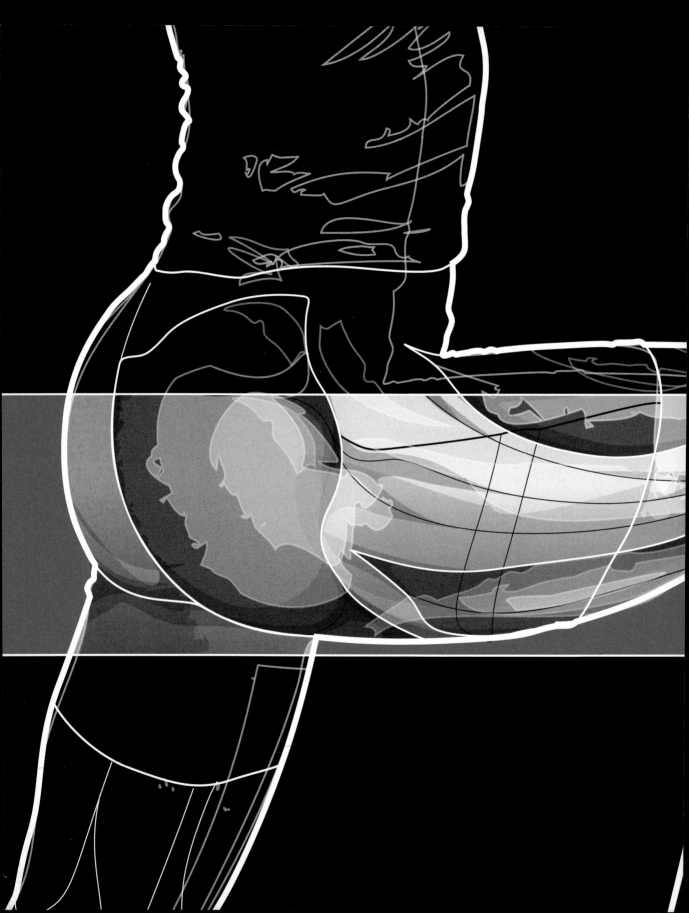

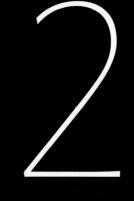

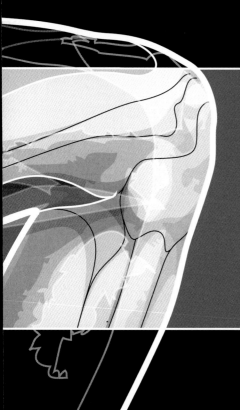

MOBILITY
EXERCISES

NECK EXTENSION AND FLEXION

This easy movement, which can be carried out standing or seated, will help prevent general neck stiffness and give you an advantage in sports in which head position and movement are important—for example, where you need to follow a fast-moving ball or other object.

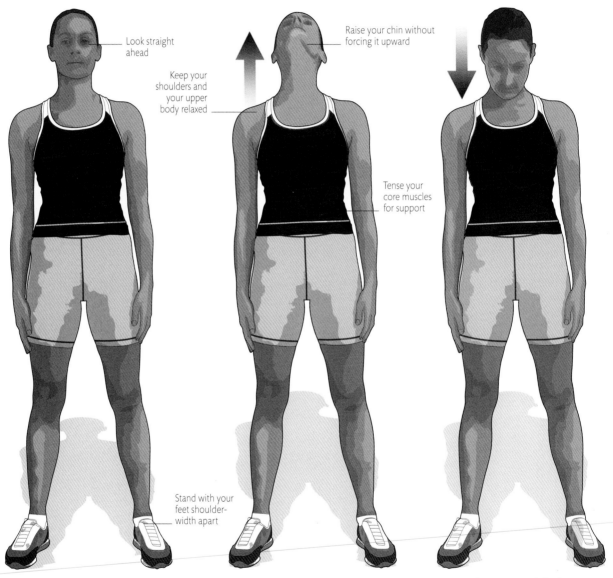

Look straight ahead

Keep your shoulders and your upper body relaxed

Stand with your feet shoulder-width apart

Raise your chin without forcing it upward

Tense your core muscles for support

1 Stand upright with your arms by your sides in a relaxed posture or clasp your hands together to prevent your shoulders from rising. Look straight ahead and keep your spine in a neutral position.

2 Extend your neck by slowly raising your chin so you are looking up at the ceiling. Hold for a few seconds. Do not force the movement beyond a position that feels comfortable.

3 Flex your neck by letting your head drop forward without straining. Return your head to the start position and repeat the process slowly and with a gentle rhythm.

NECK ROTATION

This very simple movement can help ease neck aches. It helps to maintain neck flexibility and delays or prevents age-related stiffening. You should be able to rotate your neck through at least 70 degrees to each side without feeling "pulls" or hearing cracking sounds.

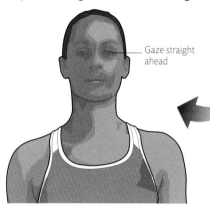

Gaze straight ahead

Hold your chin level throughout the movement

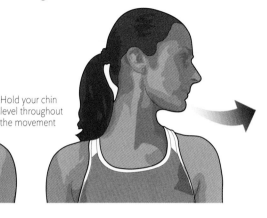

1 Begin by looking straight ahead, holding your spine in a neutral position. Keep your upper body relaxed and your arms loose by your sides.

2 Move your head slowly to the side to look over your right shoulder. Turn as far as you can comfortably go, then hold for a few seconds.

3 Move your head back through the midline, until you are looking over your left shoulder, without straining. Return to the start position.

NECK SIDE FLEXION

Imbalances in the muscles of the neck and shoulders can arise from a poor sleeping position or bad posture; they may cause pain or even headaches, especially in sedentary office workers. This useful mobility exercise is ideal for those suffering from aching muscles in the upper back and neck.

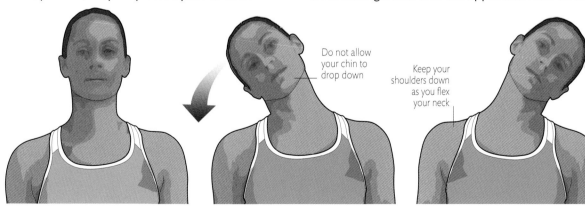

Do not allow your chin to drop down

Keep your shoulders down as you flex your neck

1 Stand upright, holding your body in a relaxed posture, with your shoulders loose and your eyes looking straight ahead.

2 Tilt your head so that your right ear moves toward your right shoulder as far as comfortable. Hold for a few seconds.

3 Flex your neck in the opposite direction, passing through the start position to the limit of flexion. Hold and return.

ARM CIRCLE

Many strength training exercises involve your arms and shoulders, so it makes good sense to warm them up thoroughly. Get your blood flowing, your muscles warmed up, and your joints moving fluently by circling your arms in a continuous smooth motion.

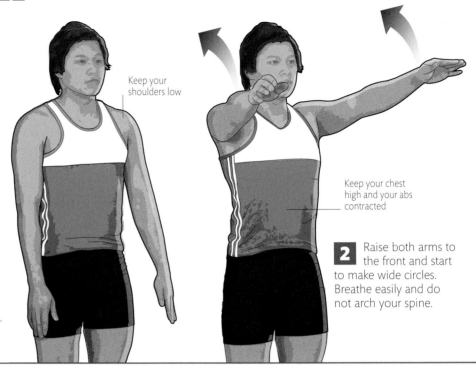

Keep your shoulders low

Keep your chest high and your abs contracted

1 Let your arms hang loose by your sides. Keep your shoulders down and relaxed. Look straight ahead and concentrate on maintaining a neutral spine.

2 Raise both arms to the front and start to make wide circles. Breathe easily and do not arch your spine.

SHOULDER ROTATION

The stability of your shoulder joints comes from the muscles and ligaments around them, rather than from your skeletal system. This exercise provides an excellent way of freeing up your shoulder joints, and also warming your trapezius muscles, before beginning a resistance training session.

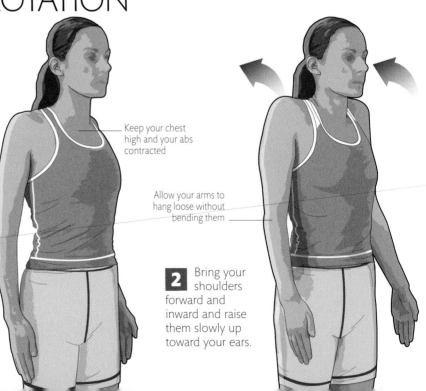

Keep your chest high and your abs contracted

Allow your arms to hang loose without bending them

1 Let your arms hang loose by your sides and keep your shoulders relaxed. Keep your head level and your spine in a neutral position.

2 Bring your shoulders forward and inward and raise them slowly up toward your ears.

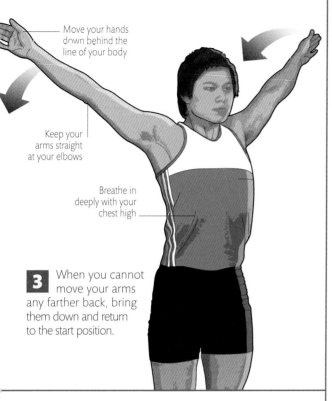

Move your hands down behind the line of your body

Keep your arms straight at your elbows

Breathe in deeply with your chest high

3 When you cannot move your arms any farther back, bring them down and return to the start position.

WRIST ROTATION

Good grip is fundamental to performing many upper body exercises. This movement will help ensure that your wrist joints are mobile and ready for work. It also helps to prevent wrist injuries like carpal tunnel syndrome that commonly affect desk workers.

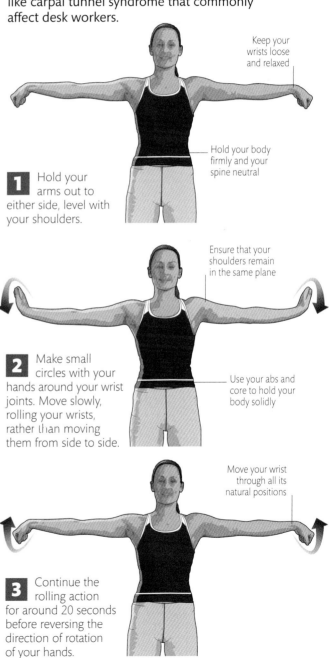

Keep your wrists loose and relaxed

Hold your body firmly and your spine neutral

1 Hold your arms out to either side, level with your shoulders.

Ensure that your shoulders remain in the same plane

Use your abs and core to hold your body solidly

2 Make small circles with your hands around your wrist joints. Move slowly, rolling your wrists, rather than moving them from side to side.

Move your wrist through all its natural positions

3 Continue the rolling action for around 20 seconds before reversing the direction of rotation of your hands.

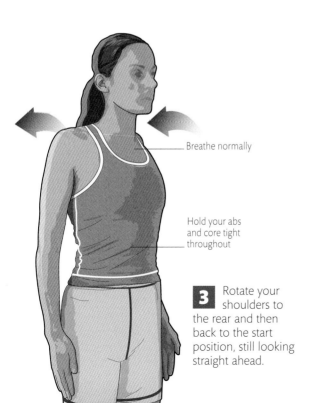

Breathe normally

Hold your abs and core tight throughout

3 Rotate your shoulders to the rear and then back to the start position, still looking straight ahead.

HIP CIRCLE

The core muscles of your torso are involved in many strength training movements, especially those performed standing up. This exercise, in which you rotate your hips as if swinging a hula-hoop around your body, helps to mobilize your core muscles.

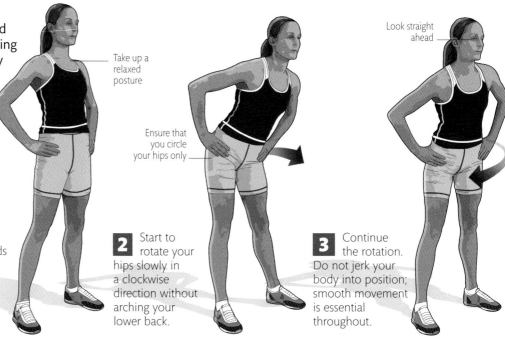

Take up a relaxed posture

Ensure that you circle your hips only

Look straight ahead

1 Stand upright with your hands on your hips, your legs straight, and your feet shoulder-width—or slightly more—apart.

2 Start to rotate your hips slowly in a clockwise direction without arching your lower back.

3 Continue the rotation. Do not jerk your body into position; smooth movement is essential throughout.

TORSO ROTATION

This exercise complements the hip circle (above) in mobilizing your core muscles, but here your upper body moves while your hips remain stationary.

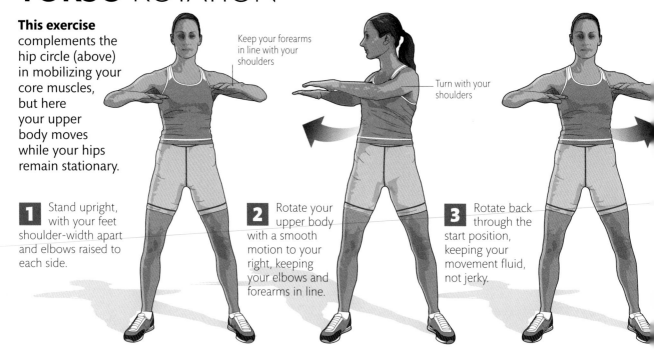

Keep your forearms in line with your shoulders

Turn with your shoulders

1 Stand upright, with your feet shoulder-width apart and elbows raised to each side.

2 Rotate your upper body with a smooth motion to your right, keeping your elbows and forearms in line.

3 Rotate back through the start position, keeping your movement fluid, not jerky.

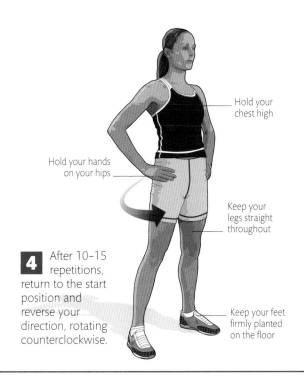

Hold your chest high

Hold your hands on your hips

Keep your legs straight throughout

4 After 10–15 repetitions, return to the start position and reverse your direction, rotating counterclockwise.

Keep your feet firmly planted on the floor

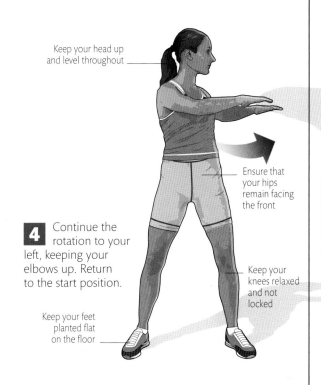

Keep your head up and level throughout

Ensure that your hips remain facing the front

4 Continue the rotation to your left, keeping your elbows up. Return to the start position.

Keep your feet planted flat on the floor

Keep your knees relaxed and not locked

TRUNK FLEXION

After performing the hip circle and torso rotation (left) you should mobilize your upper body by flexing from side to side. This engages your core muscles at a different angle.

1 Stand upright, with your arms by your sides and close to your body. Keep your shoulders relaxed.

Move only your upper body

Keep your feet planted on the floor

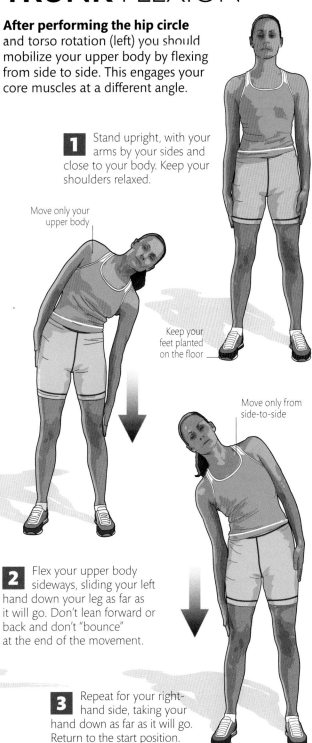

Move only from side-to-side

2 Flex your upper body sideways, sliding your left hand down your leg as far as it will go. Don't lean forward or back and don't "bounce" at the end of the movement.

3 Repeat for your right-hand side, taking your hand down as far as it will go. Return to the start position.

FRANKENSTEIN WALK

This exercise mobilizes your hips and hamstrings. You can perform it standing in one spot or walking. It is important to keep a steady tempo and extend your front leg under tight control rather than swinging too enthusiastically.

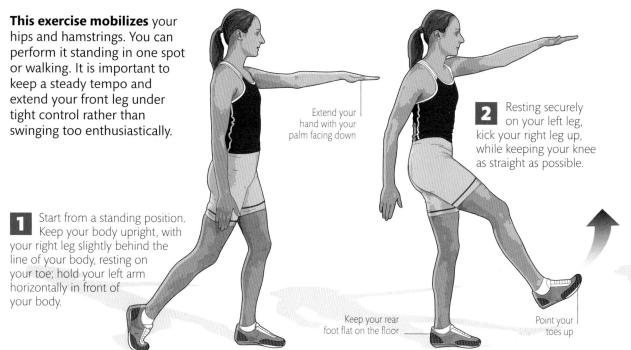

Extend your hand with your palm facing down

2 Resting securely on your left leg, kick your right leg up, while keeping your knee as straight as possible.

1 Start from a standing position. Keep your body upright, with your right leg slightly behind the line of your body, resting on your toe; hold your left arm horizontally in front of your body.

Keep your rear foot flat on the floor

Point your toes up

PIKE WALK

This challenging mobilizer works your calves, hamstrings, and the core muscles of your lower back. With practice, some people can bend almost in half, but persevere if your movement is more limited.

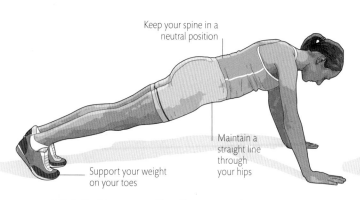

Keep your spine in a neutral position

Maintain a straight line through your hips

Support your weight on your toes

1 Position yourself as if you were about to perform a push-up, with your hands shoulder-width apart and flat on the floor, and your arms straight.

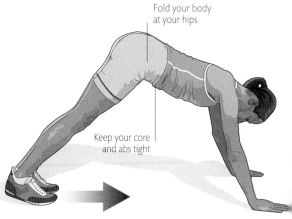

Fold your body at your hips

Keep your core and abs tight

2 "Walk" your hands into a position in front of your head. Then keeping your legs straight, slowly walk your feet up toward your hands.

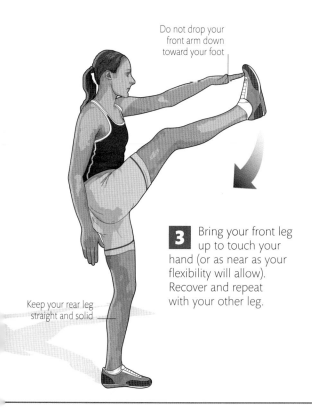

Do not drop your front arm down toward your foot

3 Bring your front leg up to touch your hand (or as near as your flexibility will allow). Recover and repeat with your other leg.

Keep your rear leg straight and solid

HIP WALK

Good hip mobility helps keep your body steady, upright, and well balanced. This simple but effective mobilizer targets your hips and glutes and can be used as a developmental stretch (see page 57) as well as a warm-up exercise.

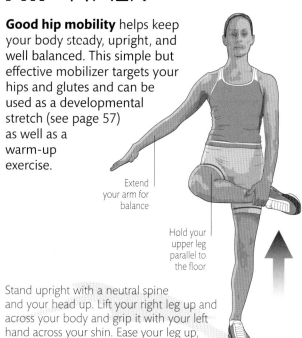

Extend your arm for balance

Hold your upper leg parallel to the floor

Stand upright with a neutral spine and your head up. Lift your right leg up and across your body and grip it with your left hand across your shin. Ease your leg up, hold, and repeat with your left leg.

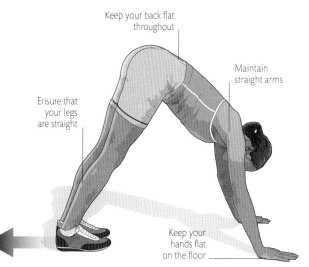

Keep your back flat throughout

Maintain straight arms

Ensure that your legs are straight

Keep your hands flat on the floor

3 When you reach the point at which you cannot continue walking forward and your body is piked, start to walk your feet back to the start position.

QUAD STRETCH

This stretch works the muscles at the front of your thigh, the function of which is to straighten your knee. Because you perform it in a standing position, the stretch emphasizes good posture and balance.

Keep your head forward and your spine neutral

Grasp your ankle firmly

Keep your knee just behind the line of your body

Stand upright. Bring your right leg back so your knee points straight down. Grasp your ankle and ease your leg back, balancing with your opposite arm. Repeat on your left leg.

SQUAT

This is the fundamental mobilizer for your lower body and core, and an essential warm-up for the squatting movement around which so much strength training and power work is based. Maintaining good form is key: go as low as possible to improve your range of motion and do not "bounce" at the bottom of the squat.

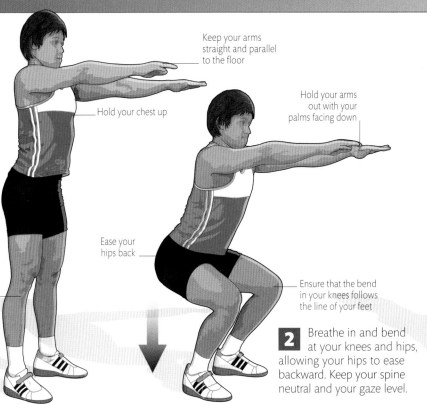

Keep your arms straight and parallel to the floor

Hold your chest up

Hold your arms out with your palms facing down

Ease your hips back

Keep your legs straight and your feet slightly turned out

Ensure that the bend in your knees follows the line of your feet

1 Start from a position in which your body is upright, your spine is neutral, and your are feet slightly wider than shoulder-width.

2 Breathe in and bend at your knees and hips, allowing your hips to ease backward. Keep your spine neutral and your gaze level.

LEG FLEXION

Your hips and hamstrings are the targets for this mobilizer. Like the more difficult Frankenstein walk (see page 56) this exercise involves moving one leg at a time; however, here both your moving leg and your stabilizing limb are worked at once.

1 Stand on your left leg with your right leg slightly behind the line of your body. Rest your right foot on tiptoe. Place your left palm lightly against a wall or piece of apparatus to help maintain your balance.

2 Keep your left foot firm and flat on the floor, and raise your right leg, stretching it out in front of you. Keep your right knee as straight as possible.

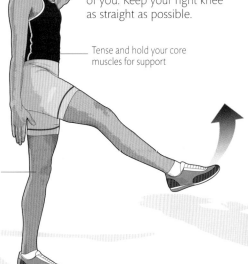

Tense and hold your core muscles for support

Keep your trailing leg as straight as possible

Bend your knee very slightly for balance

Hold your torso upright throughout the exercise

Keep your head level and your gaze forward

3 Squat down until your thighs are parallel to the floor (or farther if you have the mobility). Return to the start position.

LEG ABDUCTION

In this hip mobilizer you move your leg in a different arc to that in the leg flexion (left). It works to free up your glutes and the muscles in your groin area.

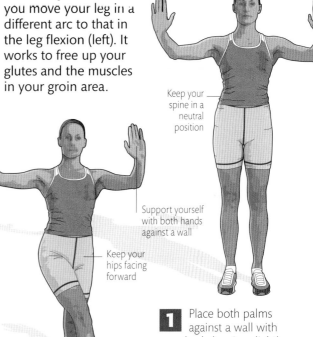

Keep your spine in a neutral position

Support yourself with both hands against a wall

Keep your hips facing forward

Move your leg across your body

1 Place both palms against a wall with your body leaning slightly forward. Shift your weight on to your left leg.

2 In a slow and controlled manner, swing your right leg across your body, pointing your toes out at the end of the swing.

Point your foot outward

3 Swing your right leg across your body to full extension. Do the required reps and repeat on your left leg.

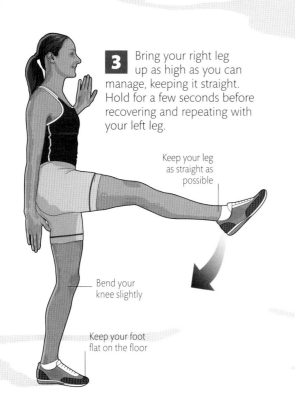

3 Bring your right leg up as high as you can manage, keeping it straight. Hold for a few seconds before recovering and repeating with your left leg.

Keep your leg as straight as possible

Bend your knee slightly

Keep your foot flat on the floor

LUNGE

This is an excellent way to mobilize your hips and thighs. You can perform the exercise either in one fixed position (like a split squat, see pages 68–69) or with alternate legs, stepping forward. The lunge tests both your balance and coordination, making it an excellent mobility exercise for all sports.

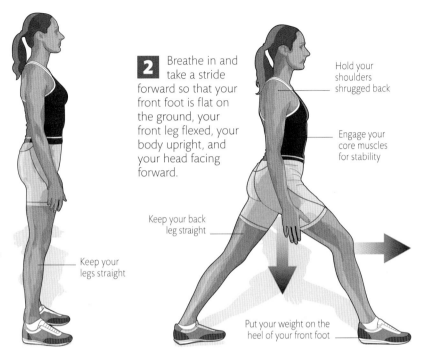

2 Breathe in and take a stride forward so that your front foot is flat on the ground, your front leg flexed, your body upright, and your head facing forward.

Hold your shoulders shrugged back

Engage your core muscles for stability

Keep your back leg straight

Put your weight on the heel of your front foot

1 Begin upright with your feet shoulder-width apart, your arms relaxed by your sides, your feet flat on the floor, your chest high, and your spine neutral.

Keep your legs straight

ROTATIONAL LUNGE

This is another good mobilizer for your hips and thighs. You should feel it stretching the hip flexor of your back leg and the glute of your front leg. The movement also engages your torso, which rotates as you turn your head, first to one side and then to the other.

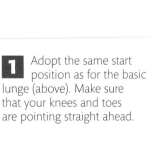

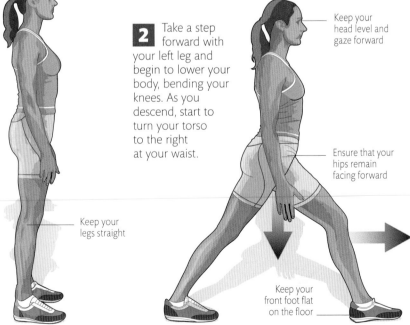

2 Take a step forward with your left leg and begin to lower your body, bending your knees. As you descend, start to turn your torso to the right at your waist.

Keep your head level and gaze forward

Ensure that your hips remain facing forward

Keep your front foot flat on the floor

1 Adopt the same start position as for the basic lunge (above). Make sure that your knees and toes are pointing straight ahead.

Keep your legs straight

3 Bend your front and back legs so that your rear knee drops close to the floor. Push back up with your front heel and return to the standing position.

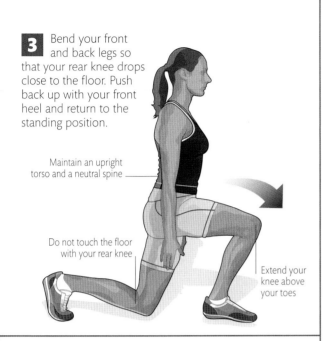

Maintain an upright torso and a neutral spine

Do not touch the floor with your rear knee

Extend your knee above your toes

3 Turn your head, extend your left arm across your body, and twist at your waist. Recover to the start position; repeat the movement on your right leg.

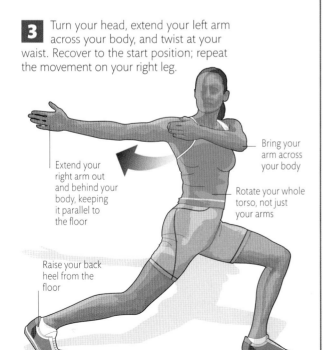

Extend your right arm out and behind your body, keeping it parallel to the floor

Bring your arm across your body

Rotate your whole torso, not just your arms

Raise your back heel from the floor

OVERHEAD LUNGE

This more demanding version of the lunge movement mobilizes your hips and thighs. Adding a light weight overhead works the stabilizers in your shoulders and puts emphasis on the mobility of your hips and lower back.

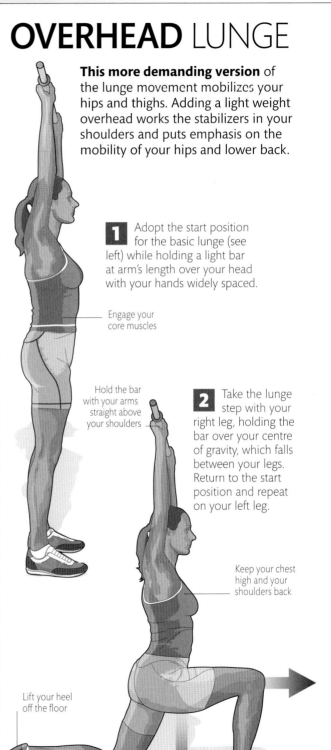

1 Adopt the start position for the basic lunge (see left) while holding a light bar at arm's length over your head with your hands widely spaced.

Engage your core muscles

Hold the bar with your arms straight above your shoulders

2 Take the lunge step with your right leg, holding the bar over your centre of gravity, which falls between your legs. Return to the start position and repeat on your left leg.

Keep your chest high and your shoulders back

Lift your heel off the floor

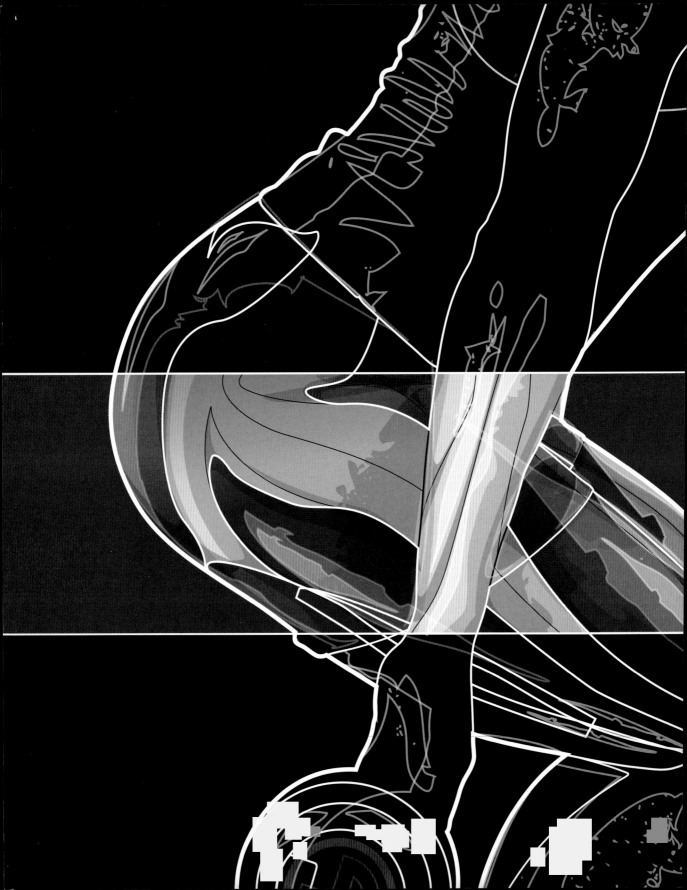

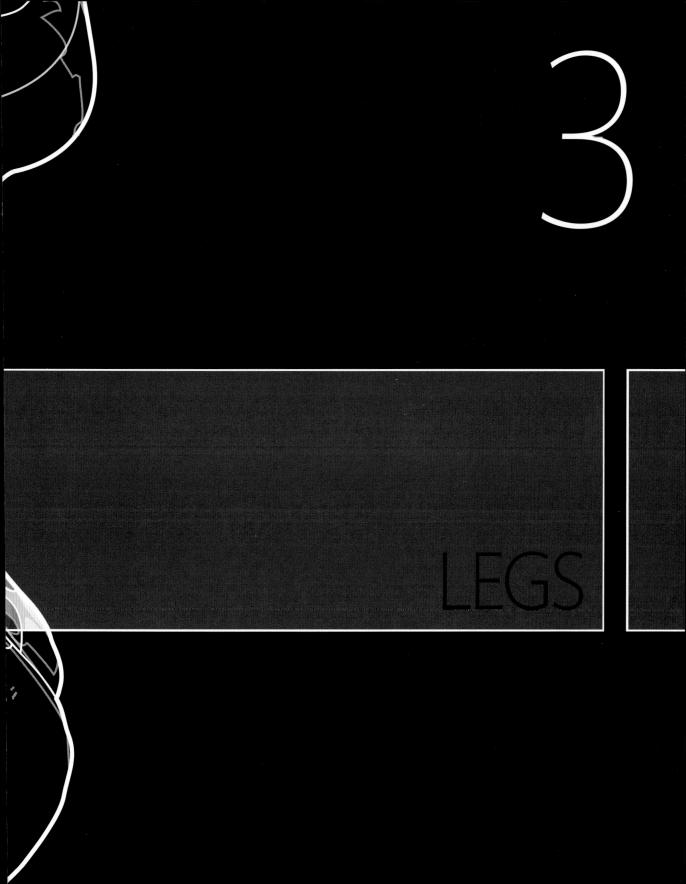

3

LEGS

BACK SQUAT

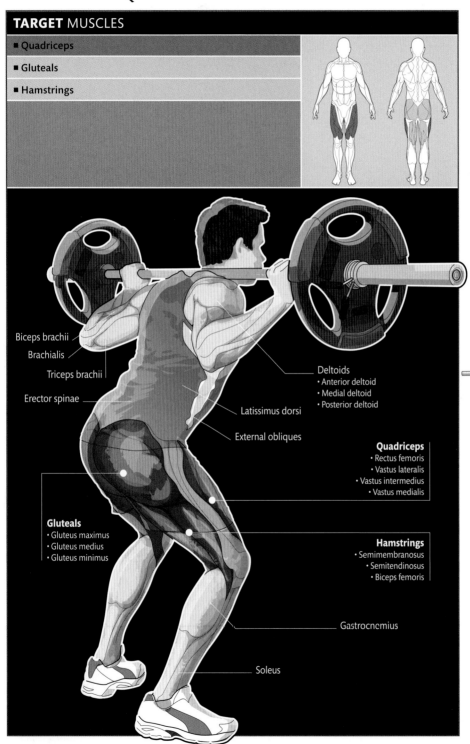

TARGET MUSCLES

- Quadriceps
- Gluteals
- Hamstrings

This multijoint exercise is extremely effective at developing the muscles of your legs. It is a great foundation exercise for building overall power and strength, but must be performed correctly.

Biceps brachii
Brachialis
Triceps brachii
Erector spinae

Deltoids
· Anterior deltoid
· Medial deltoid
· Posterior deltoid

Latissimus dorsi

External obliques

Quadriceps
· Rectus femoris
· Vastus lateralis
· Vastus intermedius
· Vastus medialis

Gluteals
· Gluteus maximus
· Gluteus medius
· Gluteus minimus

Hamstrings
· Semimembranosus
· Semitendinosus
· Biceps femoris

Gastrocnemius

Soleus

VARIATION

Some competitive powerlifters use a "Sumo" position for the back squat. Here, you place your feet much wider than shoulder-width apart, with your feet and knees turned slightly outward. The Sumo squat puts additional emphasis on the muscles of the inner thigh; however, it demands great hip mobility, and so is not suitable for beginners.

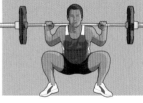

WARNING!

Don't "round" your back or lean forward when performing the squat; this places too much stress on the lower back and can lead to injury. Concentrate on keeping your gaze level: don't allow your head to look down or your knees to turn in.

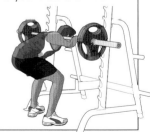

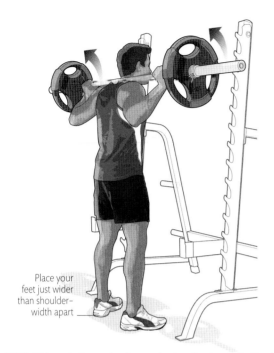

Place your feet just wider than shoulder-width apart

1 Take a balanced grip on the bar in the rack. Duck beneath it and stand up with your feet directly under the bar. Step back and stand upright with the bar resting on the upper part of your back.

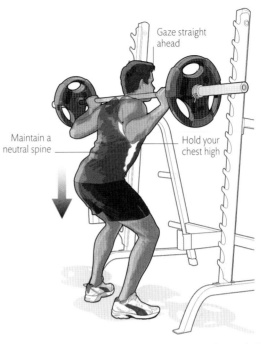

Gaze straight ahead

Maintain a neutral spine

Hold your chest high

2 Breathe deeply, and tensing your abs and glutes, start the descent. Keep your feet pointing slightly outward and ensure that your knees follow the angle of your feet as you bend your knees and ease your hips back.

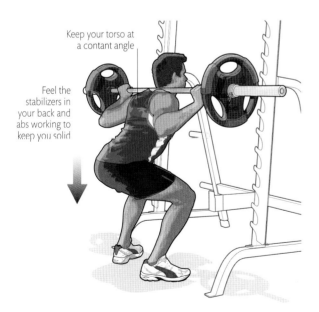

Keep your torso at a contant angle

Feel the stabilizers in your back and abs working to keep you solid

3 Keep bending at your knees with your spine in neutral position. Lower your body slowly and under tight control as you ease your hips farther back. Keep your knees over your toes.

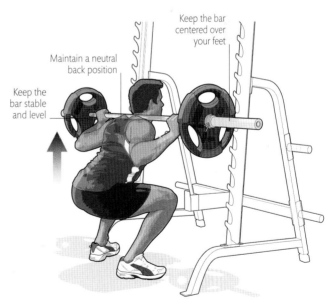

Keep the bar centered over your feet

Maintain a neutral back position

Keep the bar stable and level

4 Continue bending at your knees, easing your hips back until your thighs are parallel to the floor. Your body should now be at a 45-degree angle. Return to the start position, breathing out as you stand up.

FRONT BARBELL SQUAT

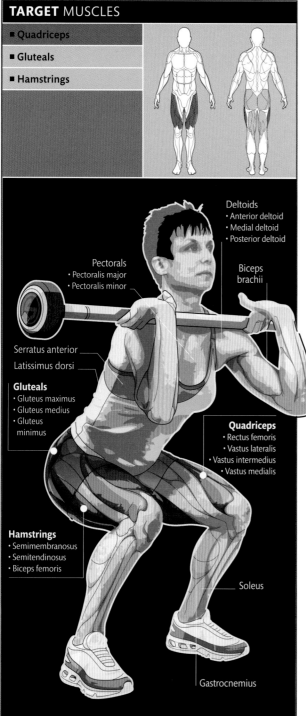

TARGET MUSCLES

- Quadriceps
- Gluteals
- Hamstrings

In this key multijoint exercise you position the weight on the front of your shoulders. It demands a more upright body posture than the back squat and places more emphasis on your quads and core.

Deltoids
- Anterior deltoid
- Medial deltoid
- Posterior deltoid

Pectorals
- Pectoralis major
- Pectoralis minor

Biceps brachii

Serratus anterior

Latissimus dorsi

Gluteals
- Gluteus maximus
- Gluteus medius
- Gluteus minimus

Quadriceps
- Rectus femoris
- Vastus lateralis
- Vastus intermedius
- Vastus medialis

Hamstrings
- Semimembranosus
- Semitendinosus
- Biceps femoris

Soleus

Gastrocnemius

Brace your hips and engage your core muscles

Hold the bar across your collar bone and deltoids

Point your elbows forward

1 Take the bar from a rack with your hands outside your shoulders, or clean it (see page 182) to your shoulders. Stand upright with your feet a little more than shoulder-width apart and slightly out-turned.

Bend your knees in line with your outturned feet

2 With your chest held high, take a deep breath and start to bend at the knees, easing your hips back and keeping your elbows pointing forward.

Keep a relatively upright body position

Gaze straight ahead

Ease your hips back as you flex at your knees

WARNING!

Keep your body at the same upright angle throughout the movement and do not allow your heels to lift off the floor. Ensure that you do not drop your elbows or let them touch your knees at the bottom of the lift. Never sacrifice good technique by overloading the bar with weight.

3 Keep your head level and your chest high, squatting down until your thighs are parallel to the floor, or as close as possible. Return to the start position, breathing out as you stand.

BARBELL HACK SQUAT

TARGET MUSCLES

- Quadriceps
- Gluteals
- Hamstrings

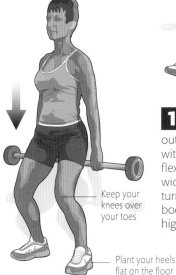

This squat variation really works your quads. It is a great development exercise because it fosters the good back position and the correct angle at the hip joint that you need to perform the front squat.

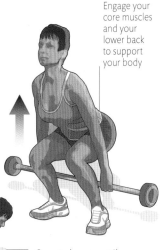

Grip the bar with your hands outside your hips

1 Hold the bar with an overhand grip outside your thighs. Start with your knees slightly flexed, your feet shoulder-width apart, and your feet turned slightly out. Keep your body upright and your chest high, and look straight ahead.

Keep your knees over your toes

Plant your heels flat on the floor

2 Keeping your chest high and your heels flat on the floor, take a deep breath and flex at your knees, allowing the bar to hang straight down.

Engage your core muscles and your lower back to support your body

WARNING!

Avoid rounding your back or bending at the waist when performing this action. Keep your hips low, your body as upright as possible, and the bar as close to your calves as you can.

3 Squat down until your thighs are parallel to the floor and then return to the start position, breathing out as you stand.

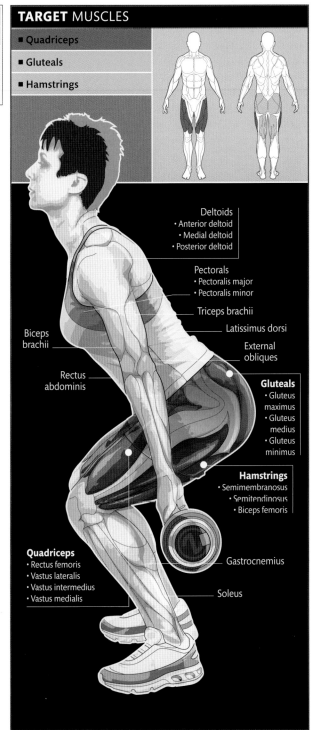

Deltoids
- Anterior deltoid
- Medial deltoid
- Posterior deltoid

Pectorals
- Pectoralis major
- Pectoralis minor

Triceps brachii

Latissimus dorsi

Biceps brachii

External obliques

Rectus abdominis

Gluteals
- Gluteus maximus
- Gluteus medius
- Gluteus minimus

Hamstrings
- Semimembranosus
- Semitendinosus
- Biceps femoris

Quadriceps
- Rectus femoris
- Vastus lateralis
- Vastus intermedius
- Vastus medialis

Gastrocnemius

Soleus

DUMBBELL SPLIT SQUAT

TARGET MUSCLES

- Quadriceps
- Gluteals
- Hamstrings

This exercise builds on the basic lunge movement (see pages 60–61) but allows you to lift more weight. It is valuable for developing hip mobility and good shoulder posture as well as strength in your quads.

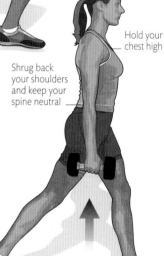

Rise up on your toes on the rear foot and keep your front foot flat

Hold the dumbbells between your feet

1 From a standing position with your feet shoulder-width apart and your arms hanging by your sides, take a stride forward keeping your chest high and looking straight ahead.

Keep your body upright throughout the movement

Use your lead leg to carry most of your weight

2 Flex at your knee and hip and drop slowly into a split position. Your front knee should not move beyond your toes and your rear knee should not touch the ground.

Hold your chest high

Shrug back your shoulders and keep your spine neutral

3 Return to the start position and perform the required number of reps on one leg before switching to the other and repeating the sequence.

Keep your rear foot on tiptoe

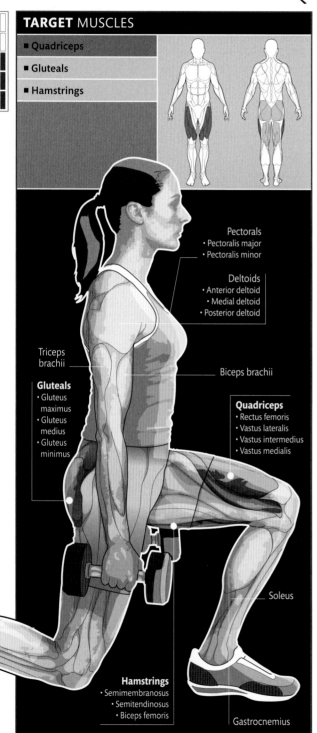

Pectorals
• Pectoralis major
• Pectoralis minor

Deltoids
• Anterior deltoid
• Medial deltoid
• Posterior deltoid

Triceps brachii

Biceps brachii

Gluteals
• Gluteus maximus
• Gluteus medius
• Gluteus minimus

Quadriceps
• Rectus femoris
• Vastus lateralis
• Vastus intermedius
• Vastus medialis

Soleus

Hamstrings
• Semimembranosus
• Semitendinosus
• Biceps femoris

Gastrocnemius

OVERHEAD SPLIT SQUAT

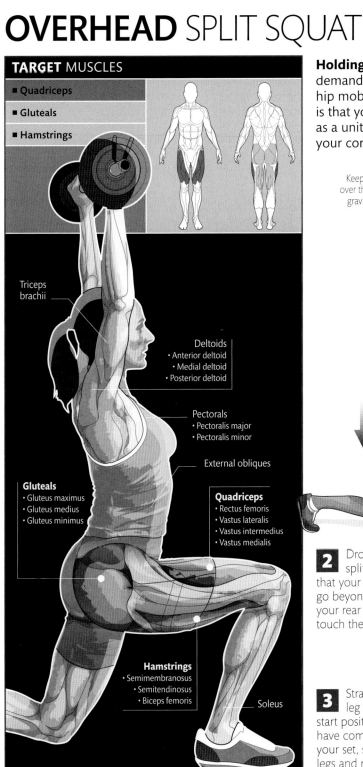

TARGET MUSCLES

- Quadriceps
- Gluteals
- Hamstrings

Triceps brachii

Deltoids
- Anterior deltoid
- Medial deltoid
- Posterior deltoid

Pectorals
- Pectoralis major
- Pectoralis minor

External obliques

Gluteals
- Gluteus maximus
- Gluteus medius
- Gluteus minimus

Quadriceps
- Rectus femoris
- Vastus lateralis
- Vastus intermedius
- Vastus medialis

Hamstrings
- Semimembranosus
- Semitendinosus
- Biceps femoris

Soleus

Holding a barbell overhead demands good shoulder and hip mobility but the payoff is that your body functions as a unit and you strengthen your core as well as your legs.

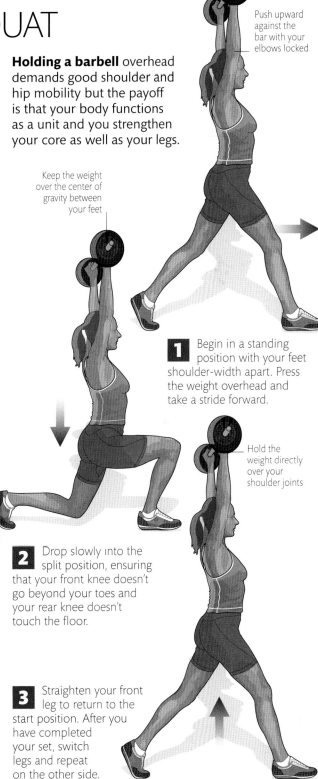

Push upward against the bar with your elbows locked

Keep the weight over the center of gravity between your feet

1 Begin in a standing position with your feet shoulder-width apart. Press the weight overhead and take a stride forward.

Hold the weight directly over your shoulder joints

2 Drop slowly into the split position, ensuring that your front knee doesn't go beyond your toes and your rear knee doesn't touch the floor.

3 Straighten your front leg to return to the start position. After you have completed your set, switch legs and repeat on the other side.

BULGARIAN BARBELL SPLIT SQUAT

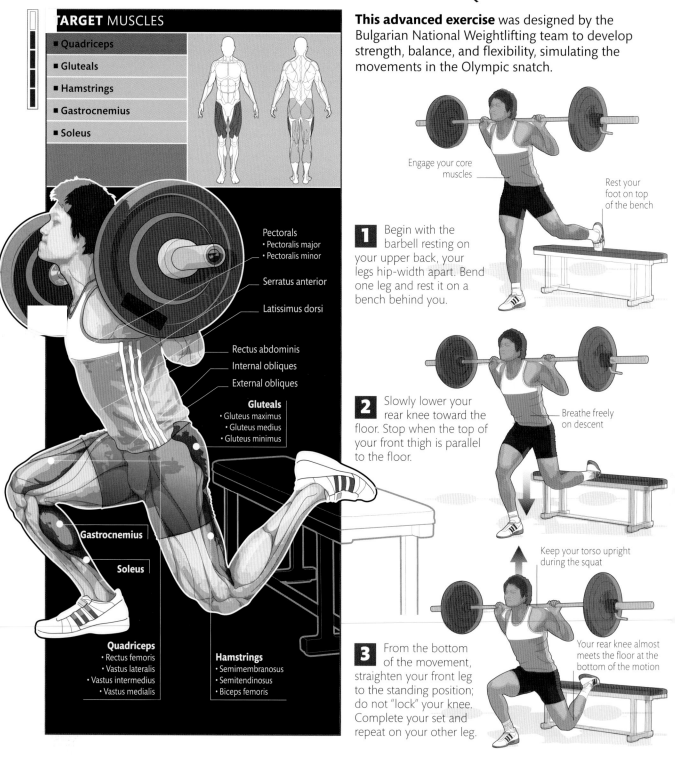

TARGET MUSCLES

- Quadriceps
- Gluteals
- Hamstrings
- Gastrocnemius
- Soleus

This advanced exercise was designed by the Bulgarian National Weightlifting team to develop strength, balance, and flexibility, simulating the movements in the Olympic snatch.

Pectorals
• Pectoralis major
• Pectoralis minor

Serratus anterior

Latissimus dorsi

Rectus abdominis

Internal obliques

External obliques

Gluteals
• Gluteus maximus
• Gluteus medius
• Gluteus minimus

Gastrocnemius

Soleus

Quadriceps
• Rectus femoris
• Vastus lateralis
• Vastus intermedius
• Vastus medialis

Hamstrings
• Semimembranosus
• Semitendinosus
• Biceps femoris

Engage your core muscles

Rest your foot on top of the bench

1 Begin with the barbell resting on your upper back, your legs hip-width apart. Bend one leg and rest it on a bench behind you.

Breathe freely on descent

2 Slowly lower your rear knee toward the floor. Stop when the top of your front thigh is parallel to the floor.

Keep your torso upright during the squat

Your rear knee almost meets the floor at the bottom of the motion

3 From the bottom of the movement, straighten your front leg to the standing position; do not "lock" your knee. Complete your set and repeat on your other leg.

BULGARIAN DUMBBELL SPLIT SQUAT

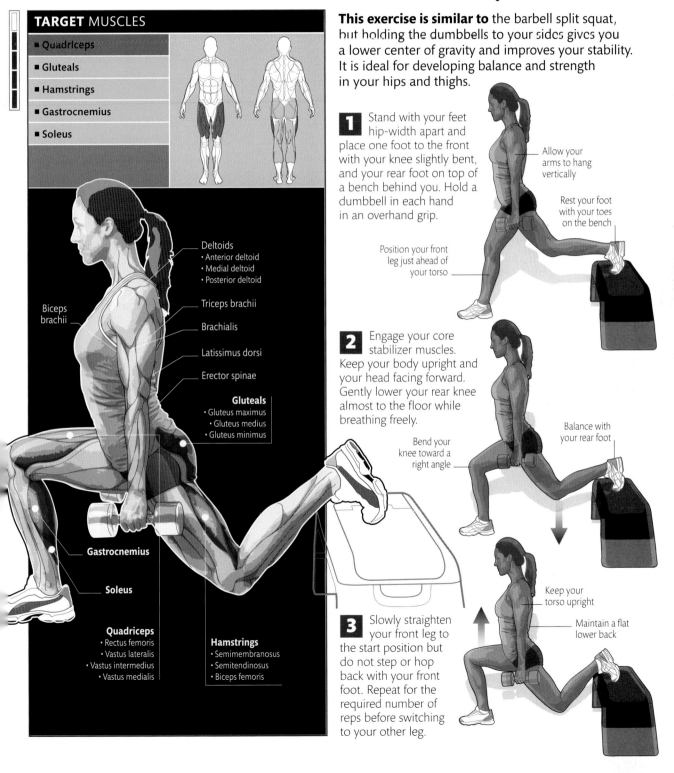

TARGET MUSCLES

- Quadriceps
- Gluteals
- Hamstrings
- Gastrocnemius
- Soleus

This exercise is similar to the barbell split squat, but holding the dumbbells to your sides gives you a lower center of gravity and improves your stability. It is ideal for developing balance and strength in your hips and thighs.

1 Stand with your feet hip-width apart and place one foot to the front with your knee slightly bent, and your rear foot on top of a bench behind you. Hold a dumbbell in each hand in an overhand grip.

Allow your arms to hang vertically

Rest your foot with your toes on the bench

Position your front leg just ahead of your torso

2 Engage your core stabilizer muscles. Keep your body upright and your head facing forward. Gently lower your rear knee almost to the floor while breathing freely.

Bend your knee toward a right angle

Balance with your rear foot

3 Slowly straighten your front leg to the start position but do not step or hop back with your front foot. Repeat for the required number of reps before switching to your other leg.

Keep your torso upright

Maintain a flat lower back

Deltoids
• Anterior deltoid
• Medial deltoid
• Posterior deltoid

Biceps brachii

Triceps brachii

Brachialis

Latissimus dorsi

Erector spinae

Gluteals
• Gluteus maximus
• Gluteus medius
• Gluteus minimus

Gastrocnemius

Soleus

Quadriceps
• Rectus femoris
• Vastus lateralis
• Vastus intermedius
• Vastus medialis

Hamstrings
• Semimembranosus
• Semitendinosus
• Biceps femoris

BARBELL LUNGE

TARGET MUSCLES

- Quadriceps
- Gluteals
- Hamstrings

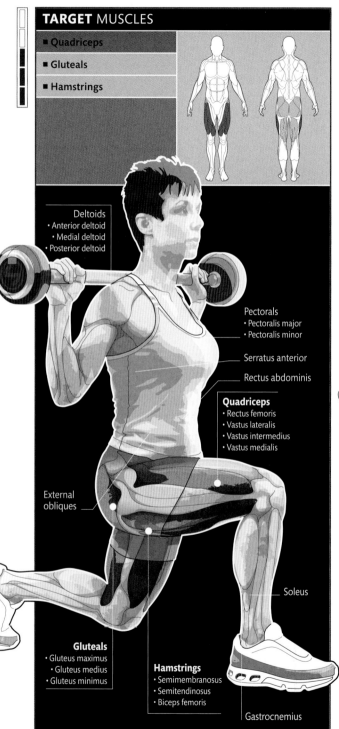

Deltoids
• Anterior deltoid
• Medial deltoid
• Posterior deltoid

Pectorals
• Pectoralis major
• Pectoralis minor

Serratus anterior

Rectus abdominis

Quadriceps
• Rectus femoris
• Vastus lateralis
• Vastus intermedius
• Vastus medialis

External obliques

Soleus

Gluteals
• Gluteus maximus
• Gluteus medius
• Gluteus minimus

Hamstrings
• Semimembranosus
• Semitendinosus
• Biceps femoris

Gastrocnemius

This underused exercise develops and tones the muscles of your legs and glutes. It is a dynamic movement that is useful in training for racket sports, since it improves your ability to reach those difficult shots.

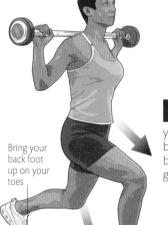

Bring your back foot up on your toes

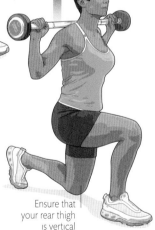

Look straight ahead

Keep your knees slightly bent

1 Stand with your feet hip-width apart and your knees soft. Rest the barbell across your upper back, holding it with a wide grip, knuckles facing back.

2 Engage your core muscles and take one long step forward. At the same time, lower your rear knee toward the floor, breathing freely.

Ensure that your rear thigh is vertical

3 Let your rear knee almost touch the floor, then straighten your front leg and step back to the start position. Complete your set and repeat for your other leg.

WARNING!

Do not attempt this exercise with a weight that makes you feel you are being "forced" downward or that makes you unstable—you should feel in control of the barbell at all times. Ensure that you keep your torso upright throughout.

OVERHEAD BARBELL LUNGE

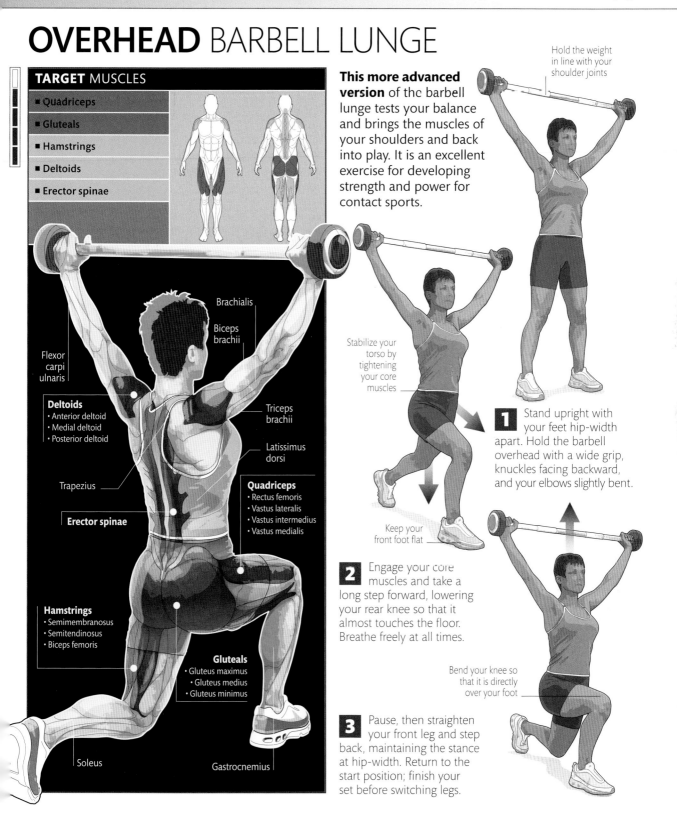

TARGET MUSCLES

- Quadriceps
- Gluteals
- Hamstrings
- Deltoids
- Erector spinae

This more advanced version of the barbell lunge tests your balance and brings the muscles of your shoulders and back into play. It is an excellent exercise for developing strength and power for contact sports.

Hold the weight in line with your shoulder joints

Flexor carpi ulnaris

Brachialis

Biceps brachii

Deltoids
- Anterior deltoid
- Medial deltoid
- Posterior deltoid

Triceps brachii

Latissimus dorsi

Trapezius

Quadriceps
- Rectus femoris
- Vastus lateralis
- Vastus intermedius
- Vastus medialis

Erector spinae

Hamstrings
- Semimembranosus
- Semitendinosus
- Biceps femoris

Gluteals
- Gluteus maximus
- Gluteus medius
- Gluteus minimus

Soleus

Gastrocnemius

Stabilize your torso by tightening your core muscles

Keep your front foot flat

1 Stand upright with your feet hip-width apart. Hold the barbell overhead with a wide grip, knuckles facing backward, and your elbows slightly bent.

2 Engage your core muscles and take a long step forward, lowering your rear knee so that it almost touches the floor. Breathe freely at all times.

Bend your knee so that it is directly over your foot

3 Pause, then straighten your front leg and step back, maintaining the stance at hip-width. Return to the start position; finish your set before switching legs.

FORWARD LUNGE

TARGET MUSCLES

- Quadriceps
- Gluteals
- Hamstrings

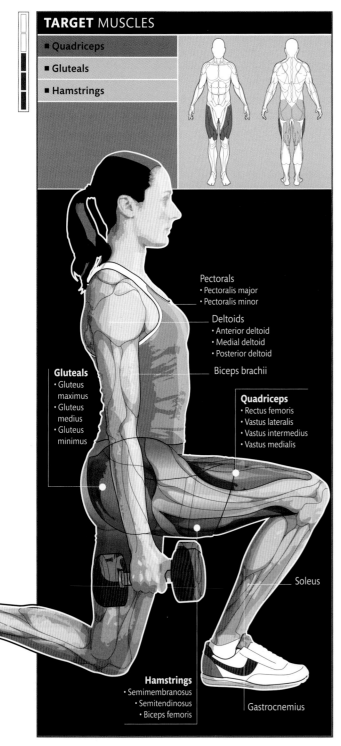

Pectorals
• Pectoralis major
• Pectoralis minor

Deltoids
• Anterior deltoid
• Medial deltoid
• Posterior deltoid

Biceps brachii

Gluteals
• Gluteus maximus
• Gluteus medius
• Gluteus minimus

Quadriceps
• Rectus femoris
• Vastus lateralis
• Vastus intermedius
• Vastus medialis

Soleus

Hamstrings
• Semimembranosus
• Semitendinosus
• Biceps femoris

Gastrocnemius

This full body exercise is effective in developing strength in your leg and hip muscles. Holding the dumbbells by your sides rather than over your shoulders makes it easier for you to hold your body upright. Be sure to practice the movement before using weights.

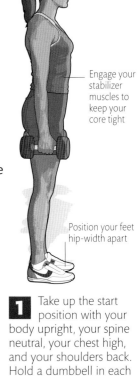

Engage your stabilizer muscles to keep your core tight

Position your feet hip-width apart

1 Take up the start position with your body upright, your spine neutral, your chest high, and your shoulders back. Hold a dumbbell in each hand, with your arms by your sides.

Pull your shoulders back

Keep your back leg straight

2 Take a step forward, holding your upper body upright. Descend under tight control by bending at your hips, knees, and ankles. Don't lean forward at any point.

3 Descend until both knees reach an angle of 90 degrees. Your back knee should be directly under your hip and just off the floor. Hold before you return to the start.

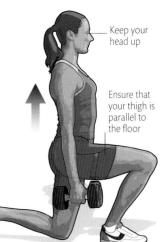

Keep your head up

Ensure that your thigh is parallel to the floor

LATERAL LUNGE

TARGET MUSCLES

- Quadriceps
- Hamstrings
- Gastrocnemius

This more advanced lunge appeals to sports performers who need to develop their agility and the ability to change direction while running. It demands good hip and ankle flexibility.

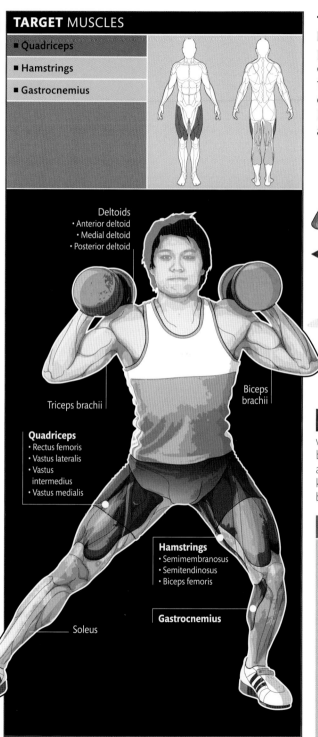

Deltoids
- Anterior deltoid
- Medial deltoid
- Posterior deltoid

Triceps brachii

Biceps brachii

Quadriceps
- Rectus femoris
- Vastus lateralis
- Vastus intermedius
- Vastus medialis

Hamstrings
- Semimembranosus
- Semitendinosus
- Biceps femoris

Gastrocnemius

Soleus

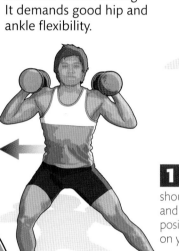

1 Start with your body upright, your legs shoulder-width apart, and your spine in a neutral position. Hold the dumbbells on your shoulders.

2 Take a lunge step out directly to the side while retaining an upright body position. Don't allow your lunging knee to go far beyond your toes.

VARIATION

If you lack the hip mobility needed to lunge with the dumbbells positioned above your shoulders, try this alternative, in which you hold the dumbbells below your body with your arms straight.

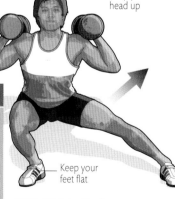

Keep your head up

Keep your feet flat

3 Sit into the lunge position until the thigh of your "standing" leg is parallel to the floor. Push off your lunging foot and return to the start position. Complete the set on one side, then switch legs.

BARBELL STEP-UP

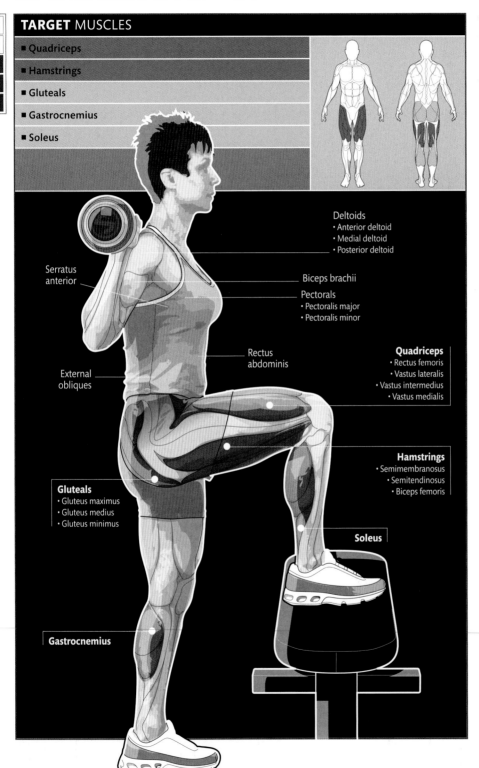

TARGET MUSCLES

- Quadriceps
- Hamstrings
- Gluteals
- Gastrocnemius
- Soleus

Serratus anterior

External obliques

Deltoids
- Anterior deltoid
- Medial deltoid
- Posterior deltoid

Biceps brachii

Pectorals
- Pectoralis major
- Pectoralis minor

Rectus abdominis

Quadriceps
- Rectus femoris
- Vastus lateralis
- Vastus intermedius
- Vastus medialis

Hamstrings
- Semimembranosus
- Semitendinosus
- Biceps femoris

Gluteals
- Gluteus maximus
- Gluteus medius
- Gluteus minimus

Soleus

Gastrocnemius

This excellent exercise targets the main muscles of your leg—the quads, hamstrings, and glutes. The muscles of your calves assist while your core muscles stop your body from leaning forward or twisting. The exercise helps develop, and also puts demands on, your heart and lungs. Beginners should start with body weight until they are familiar with the movement.

VARIATION

Try this exercise holding dumbbells at your sides. They are easier to "load" and hold in place than a barbell, and can be safely jettisoned if you start to feel yourself losing balance. You can also make this exercise easier by using just your own body weight to work against gravity.

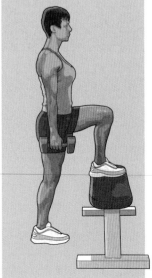

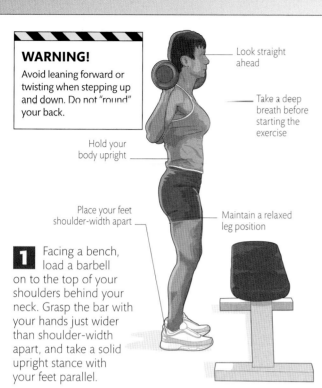

Look straight ahead

Take a deep breath before starting the exercise

Hold your body upright

Place your feet shoulder-width apart

Maintain a relaxed leg position

1 Facing a bench, load a barbell on to the top of your shoulders behind your neck. Grasp the bar with your hands just wider than shoulder-width apart, and take a solid upright stance with your feet parallel.

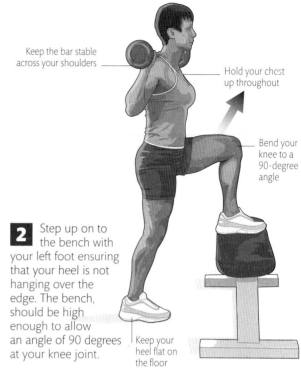

Keep the bar stable across your shoulders

Hold your chest up throughout

Bend your knee to a 90-degree angle

2 Step up on to the bench with your left foot ensuring that your heel is not hanging over the edge. The bench, should be high enough to allow an angle of 90 degrees at your knee joint.

Keep your heel flat on the floor

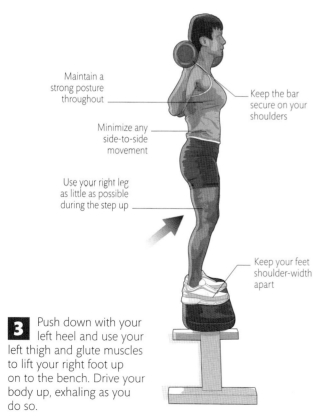

Maintain a strong posture throughout

Keep the bar secure on your shoulders

Minimize any side-to-side movement

Use your right leg as little as possible during the step up

Keep your feet shoulder-width apart

3 Push down with your left heel and use your left thigh and glute muscles to lift your right foot up on to the bench. Drive your body up, exhaling as you do so.

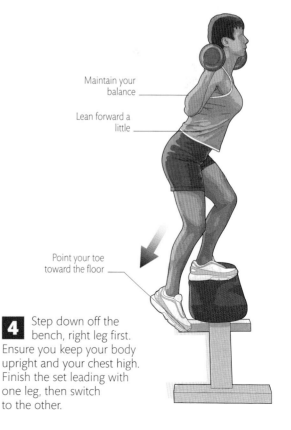

Maintain your balance

Lean forward a little

Point your toe toward the floor

4 Step down off the bench, right leg first. Ensure you keep your body upright and your chest high. Finish the set leading with one leg, then switch to the other.

45-DEGREE LEG PRESS

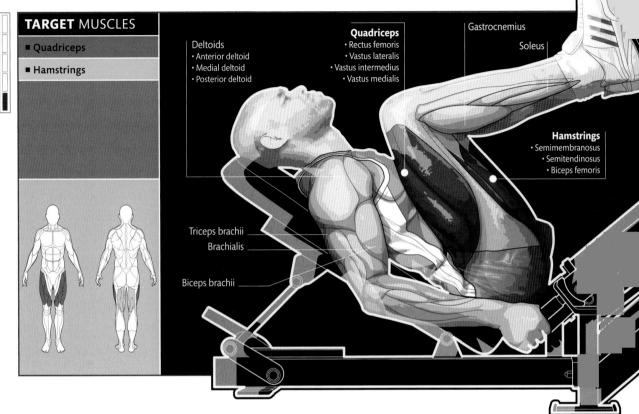

TARGET MUSCLES

- Quadriceps
- Hamstrings

Deltoids
- Anterior deltoid
- Medial deltoid
- Posterior deltoid

Quadriceps
- Rectus femoris
- Vastus lateralis
- Vastus intermedius
- Vastus medialis

Gastrocnemius

Soleus

Hamstrings
- Semimembranosus
- Semitendinosus
- Biceps femoris

Triceps brachii

Brachialis

Biceps brachii

This simple movement is a good confidence builder for beginners who are preparing for more functional leg exercises, such as the squat. It places little stress on the lower back and is suitable for those who have not yet developed high core strength. It also allows relatively heavy weights to be used early on, providing welcome motivation for the novice. As when using all exercise machines, ensure that the leg press is set to match your height and limb length.

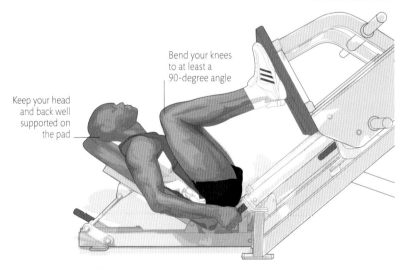

Bend your knees to at least a 90-degree angle

Keep your head and back well supported on the pad

1 Select your desired weight on the stack and sit on the machine. Place your feet hip-width apart on the platform and take the weight on your legs. Release the safety lock on the machine and hold the handle supports.

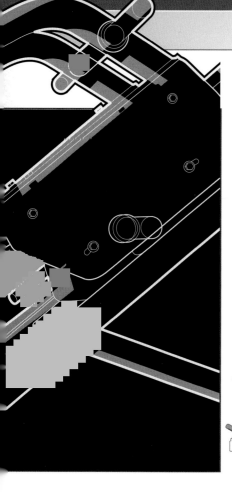

WARNING!

Keep your lower back pressed firmly against the pads throughout the exercise; avoid raising your head from the support and cease lowering the weight if you feel your lower back begin to lift off the backrest. Do not lock out your knees at the top of the movement and be sure to raise and lower the weight slowly from the stack, without "clacking" at the bottom of the motion.

VARIATION

You can perform the leg press one leg at a time, which helps you to address any strength imbalances between them. Imbalances can reduce sports performance and make you more prone to injury. You can also change your foot position in the two-leg version to modify the focus of the exercise: spreading your feet wider and pointing your toes out will work your inner thighs more, while placing your feet higher on the platform will emphasize your glutes.

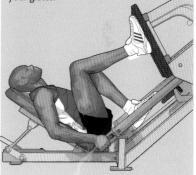

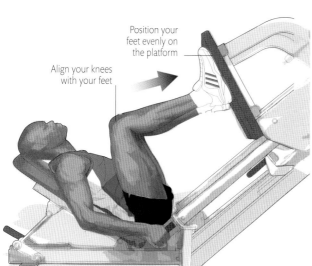

Position your feet evenly on the platform

Align your knees with your feet

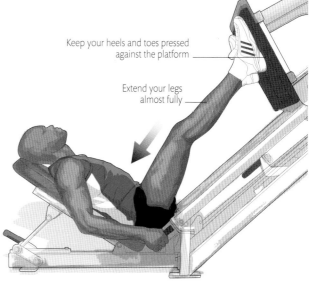

Keep your heels and toes pressed against the platform

Extend your legs almost fully

2 Extend your legs to push the platform away from you. Push slowly and continuously, keeping your heels and your toes on the platform; do not allow your knees to splay outward as you push.

3 Continue pushing until your legs are almost fully extended. Pause for a moment at the top of the movement and then return to the start position slowly and under control.

MACHINE LEG CURL

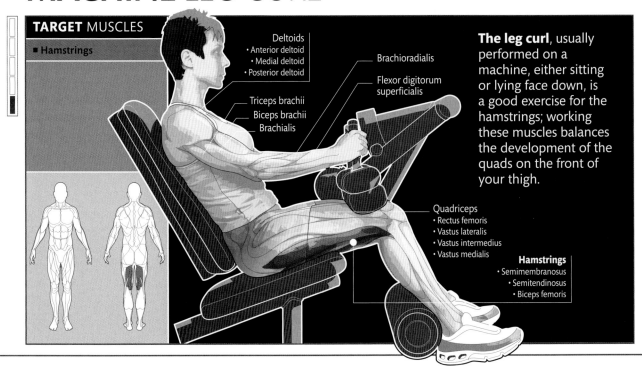

TARGET MUSCLES

■ Hamstrings

Deltoids
• Anterior deltoid
• Medial deltoid
• Posterior deltoid

Brachioradialis

Flexor digitorum superficialis

Triceps brachii
Biceps brachii
Brachialis

Quadriceps
• Rectus femoris
• Vastus lateralis
• Vastus intermedius
• Vastus medialis

Hamstrings
• Semimembranosus
• Semitendinosus
• Biceps femoris

The leg curl, usually performed on a machine, either sitting or lying face down, is a good exercise for the hamstrings; working these muscles balances the development of the quads on the front of your thigh.

MACHINE LEG EXTENSION

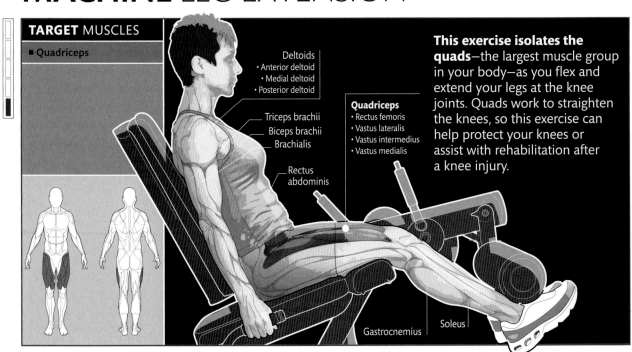

TARGET MUSCLES

■ Quadriceps

Deltoids
• Anterior deltoid
• Medial deltoid
• Posterior deltoid

Quadriceps
• Rectus femoris
• Vastus lateralis
• Vastus intermedius
• Vastus medialis

Triceps brachii
Biceps brachii
Brachialis

Rectus abdominis

Gastrocnemius

Soleus

This exercise isolates the quads—the largest muscle group in your body—as you flex and extend your legs at the knee joints. Quads work to straighten the knees, so this exercise can help protect your knees or assist with rehabilitation after a knee injury.

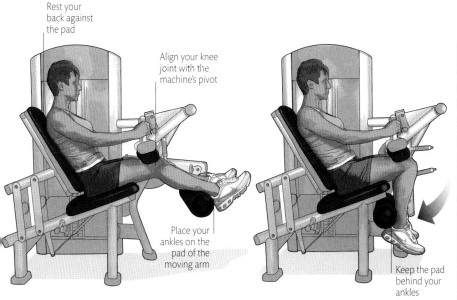

Rest your back against the pad

Align your knee joint with the machine's pivot

Place your ankles on the pad of the moving arm

Keep the pad behind your ankles

VARIATION

You can perform a similar exercise using a cable pulley machine. This is more challenging because you have to stabilize your whole body—the machine does not support you in a fixed position. Attach an ankle strap to your ankle and ensure that the knee of your moving leg points down so that your hamstring pulls your heel toward your glutes. Move slowly, taking slightly longer to lower your leg than to raise it.

1 Select a weight from the stack and sit on the machine. Adjust the moving arm so that it is under your ankles and doesn't slide up your calves. Position the lap pad above your knees.

2 Bring the moving arm back in a smooth motion to contract your hamstrings fully, then return it under control to the start position. Keep your back stable against the seat.

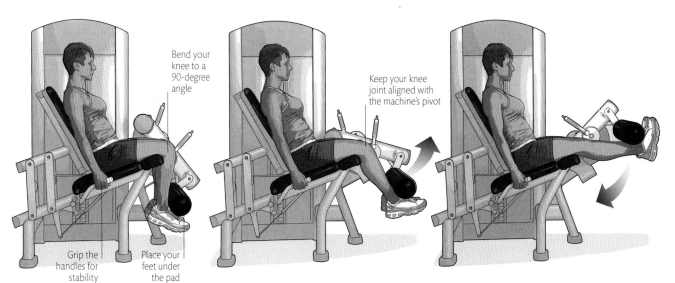

Bend your knee to a 90-degree angle

Keep your knee joint aligned with the machine's pivot

Grip the handles for stability

Place your feet under the pad

1 Select a weight from the stack and sit on the machine with your back against the pad. Adjust the moving arm to suit the length of your lower leg.

2 Using a controlled movement— and no jerking—bring your lower leg up while pressing your back and buttocks against the pads.

3 Continue the movement until your legs are parallel to the floor. Exhale and relax, allowing your legs to return to the start position.

HIP ABDUCTOR

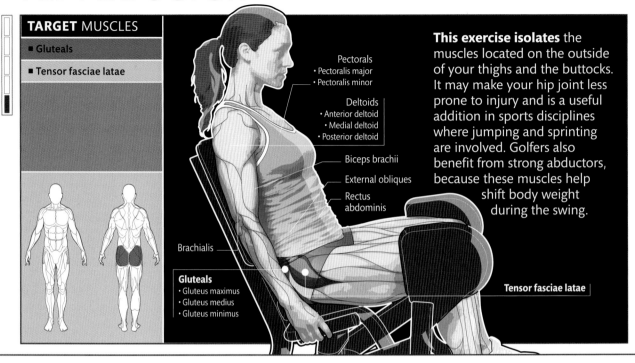

TARGET MUSCLES

- Gluteals
- Tensor fasciae latae

Pectorals
· Pectoralis major
· Pectoralis minor

Deltoids
· Anterior deltoid
· Medial deltoid
· Posterior deltoid

Biceps brachii

External obliques

Rectus
abdominis

Brachialis

Gluteals
· Gluteus maximus
· Gluteus medius
· Gluteus minimus

Tensor fasciae latae

This exercise isolates the muscles located on the outside of your thighs and the buttocks. It may make your hip joint less prone to injury and is a useful addition in sports disciplines where jumping and sprinting are involved. Golfers also benefit from strong abductors, because these muscles help shift body weight during the swing.

HIP ADDUCTOR

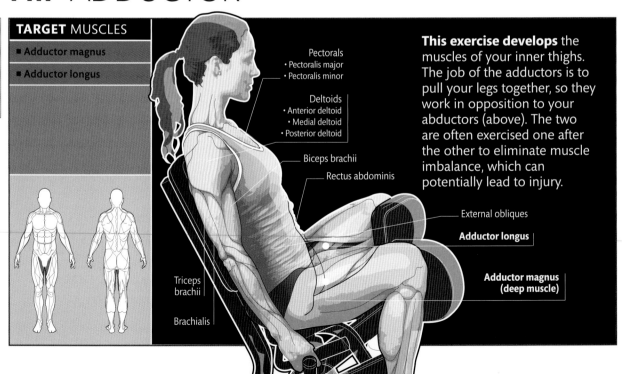

TARGET MUSCLES

- Adductor magnus
- Adductor longus

Pectorals
· Pectoralis major
· Pectoralis minor

Deltoids
· Anterior deltoid
· Medial deltoid
· Posterior deltoid

Biceps brachii

Rectus abdominis

External obliques

Adductor longus

**Adductor magnus
(deep muscle)**

Triceps
brachii

Brachialis

This exercise develops the muscles of your inner thighs. The job of the adductors is to pull your legs together, so they work in opposition to your abductors (above). The two are often exercised one after the other to eliminate muscle imbalance, which can potentially lead to injury.

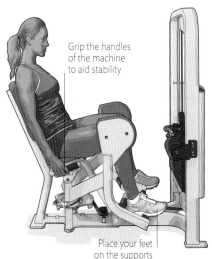

Grip the handles of the machine to aid stability

Place your feet on the supports

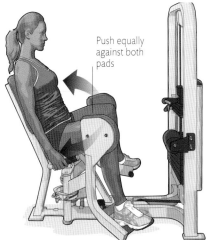

Push equally against both pads

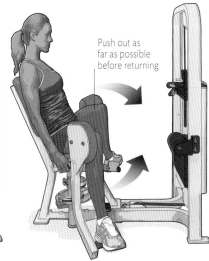

Push out as far as possible before returning

1 Set the desired resistance on the weight stack. Sit on the machine and adjust the height of the seat so that the sides of your knees rest comfortably against the pads.

2 Press your upper body back into the seat and tense your core muscles for stability. Push out steadily against the pads to achieve a full range of movement while breathing freely.

3 Slowly resist the inward force of the pads as you move slowly back to the start position. Try to equalize the force borne on each of your legs.

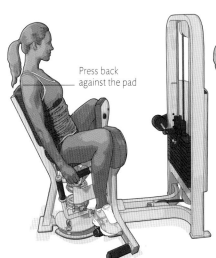

Press back against the pad

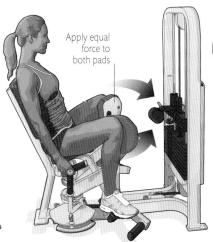

Apply equal force to both pads

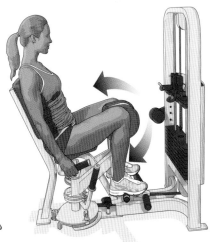

1 Select the desired resistance on the weight stack. Sit on the machine and adjust the height of the seat so that your knees rest comfortably against the pads.

2 Grip the side handles to stabilize your upper body and steadily push your legs against the pads to bring them together while breathing freely. Do not bash the pads together.

3 In a slow, controlled manner, allow the pads to return to the starting position. Keep your core muscles tensed throughout the movement.

CALF RAISE

TARGET MUSCLES

- Gastrocnemius
- Soleus

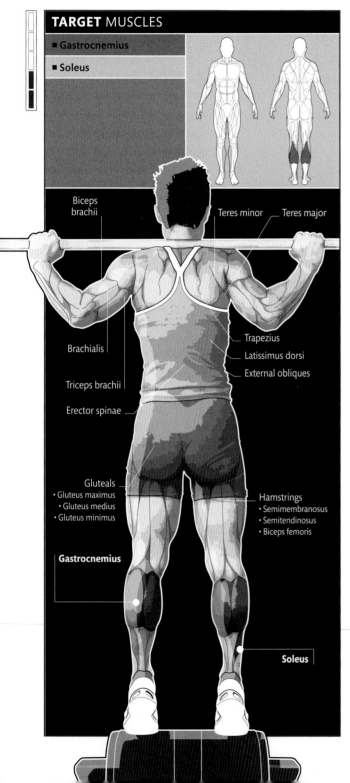

Biceps brachii

Teres minor

Teres major

Brachialis

Trapezius

Latissimus dorsi

Triceps brachii

External obliques

Erector spinae

Gluteals
- Gluteus maximus
- Gluteus medius
- Gluteus minimus

Hamstrings
- Semimembranosus
- Semitendinosus
- Biceps femoris

Gastrocnemius

Soleus

This exercise develops the muscles of your lower leg. The movement tests your balance, especially when performed with heavier free weights, so work on a Smith machine to stabilize your body.

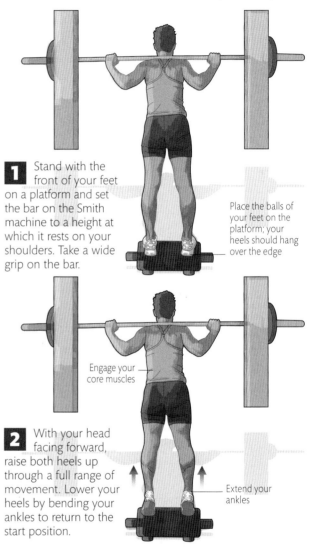

1 Stand with the front of your feet on a platform and set the bar on the Smith machine to a height at which it rests on your shoulders. Take a wide grip on the bar.

Place the balls of your feet on the platform; your heels should hang over the edge

Engage your core muscles

2 With your head facing forward, raise both heels up through a full range of movement. Lower your heels by bending your ankles to return to the start position.

Extend your ankles

VARIATION

This exercise can be performed on a special calf raise machine on which you lift weighted pads rather than a barbell. Set the desired resistance and stand tall under the pads, gripping the handles provided and keeping your elbows bent. Contract your calf muscles and fully extend your ankles. Hold the top position before lowering your body under full control.

STRAIGHT-LEG DEADLIFT

TARGET MUSCLES

- Hamstrings
- Gluteals
- Erector spinae
- Quadriceps

This underestimated exercise strengthens your lower back and develops your legs and glutes. Many football linebackers include this in their workout regimens.

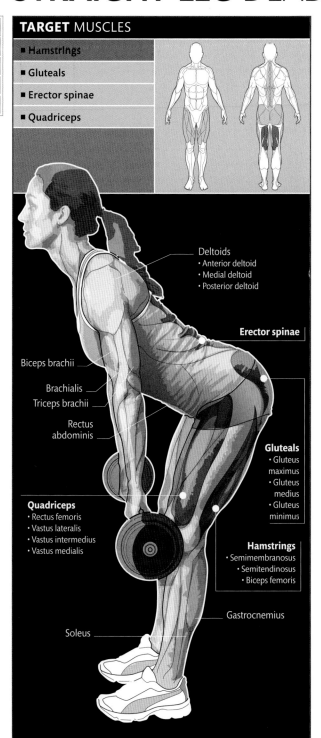

Deltoids
• Anterior deltoid
• Medial deltoid
• Posterior deltoid

Erector spinae

Biceps brachii

Brachialis
Triceps brachii

Rectus abdominis

Quadriceps
• Rectus femoris
• Vastus lateralis
• Vastus intermedius
• Vastus medialis

Gluteals
• Gluteus maximus
• Gluteus medius
• Gluteus minimus

Hamstrings
• Semimembranosus
• Semitendinosus
• Biceps femoris

Gastrocnemius

Soleus

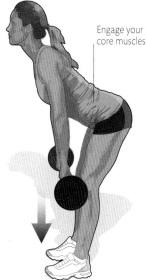

Engage your core muscles

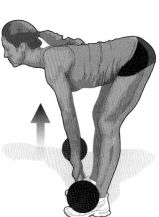

Keep your back straight throughout

1 Stand upright with your feet hip-width apart and the barbell resting across your upper thighs. Hold the bar with an overhand grip.

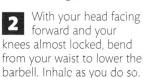

2 With your head facing forward and your knees almost locked, bend from your waist to lower the barbell. Inhale as you do so.

VARIATION

If you have good hip mobility, try standing on an elevated platform. This will allow the barbell to travel beyond the level of your feet and make your muscles work harder. However, do not be tempted to extend your muscles beyond what feels comfortable, and try to keep your motion fluid, without "bouncing" the barbell.

3 Maintaining control over your core stability, slowly pivot at your hips to raise your upper body to the start position. Breathe out as you do so.

BARBELL DEADLIFT

TARGET MUSCLES

- Gluteals
- Trapezius
- Erector spinae
- Rectus abdominis
- Hamstrings
- Quadriceps

Sometimes called the "king of exercises" because of its effectiveness in building leg and back strength, the deadlift is also one of the three lifts performed in competitive powerlifting.

1 Squat down so that your feet are under the bar, and the bar rests against your shins. Grip the bar using an alternate hook grip to prevent it from rotating; your hands should be wider than shoulder-width apart.

Keep your back flat and tight throughout

Grip the bar with an alternate hook—one hand over, one under the bar

3 Continue the lift as if pushing the floor away from you with your feet, until you stand up straight with your knees locked.

Brace your shoulders back

Grip tightly so that the bar does not rotate in your hands

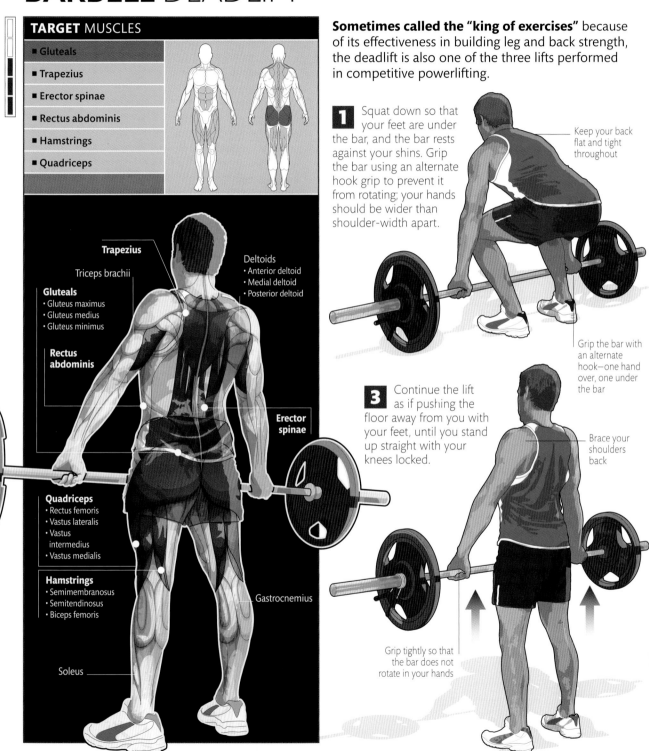

Trapezius

Triceps brachii

Gluteals
- Gluteus maximus
- Gluteus medius
- Gluteus minimus

Rectus abdominis

Deltoids
- Anterior deltoid
- Medial deltoid
- Posterior deltoid

Erector spinae

Quadriceps
- Rectus femoris
- Vastus lateralis
- Vastus intermedius
- Vastus medialis

Hamstrings
- Semimembranosus
- Semitendinosus
- Biceps femoris

Gastrocnemius

Soleus

2 Begin lifting the bar with a long, strong leg push, extending your knees and hips. Your knees should be bent as you lift the bar past them.

Pull your shoulder blades together

Push your hips in toward the bar

Keep the bar close to your body throughout the lift

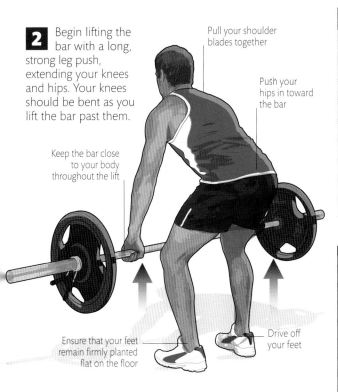

Ensure that your feet remain firmly planted flat on the floor

Drive off your feet

VARIATION

Using dumbbells for the deadlift recruits more muscles to control and stabilize movement. It is a good way of developing strength and technique for heavier barbell lifts. Start with light weights to determine your range of motion. As with the barbell lift, keep your back flat and the weights close to your body; do not pause at the bottom of the movement or allow the weights to "bounce" as you lower them.

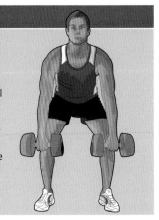

WARNING!

Correct lifting technique is essential in this movement. Never lift with your spine flexed forward: not only will the exercise be ineffective, but you also risk spinal injury. Always raise and lower your shoulders and hips together. Keep the bar close to your body and do not drop it at the end of the movement; always lower it under control.

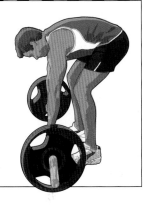

4 Unlock your knees. Maintaining a tight, flat back and keeping your head up, start to lower the bar under control. Your knees should be bent as you lower the bar past them.

Move your hips back and down

Lower the bar under control

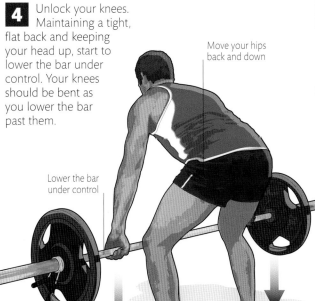

5 Slowly move your hips and shoulders together when lowering the bar back down to the start position. Do not drop the bar.

Pull your shoulders back

Bend at your knees

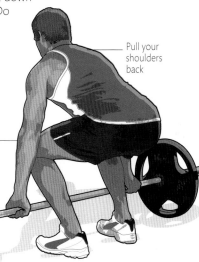

ROMANIAN DEADLIFT

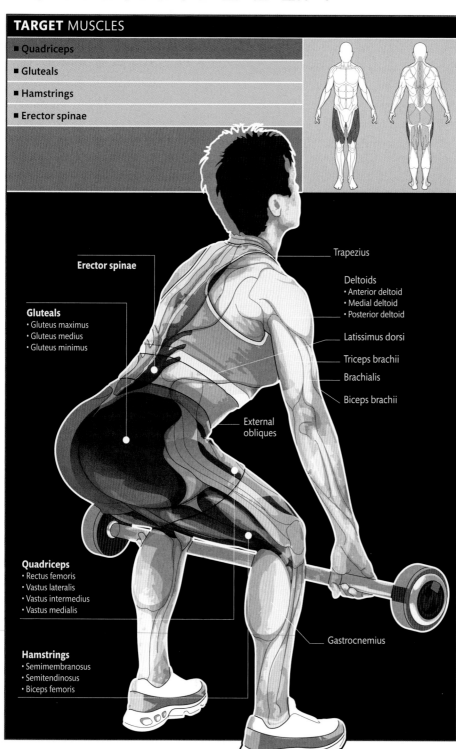

TARGET MUSCLES

- Quadriceps
- Gluteals
- Hamstrings
- Erector spinae

Erector spinae

Gluteals
- Gluteus maximus
- Gluteus medius
- Gluteus minimus

Quadriceps
- Rectus femoris
- Vastus lateralis
- Vastus intermedius
- Vastus medialis

Hamstrings
- Semimembranosus
- Semitendinosus
- Biceps femoris

Trapezius

Deltoids
- Anterior deltoid
- Medial deltoid
- Posterior deltoid

Latissimus dorsi

Triceps brachii

Brachialis

Biceps brachii

External obliques

Gastrocnemius

This movement does a good job of balancing work on your quads with development of your hamstrings and glutes— the muscles that extend your hips. The Romanian deadlift makes an excellent, though difficult, addition to your general training program, especially if you wish to improve your power and leg speed.

VARIATION

If using heavy weights, you should work off a rack adjusted to suit your height. When using heavy weights, reverse the grip on one hand (one over, one under grip) to stop the bar from rolling. You can also use wrist straps, which provide protection and enhance your grip.

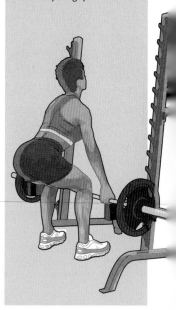

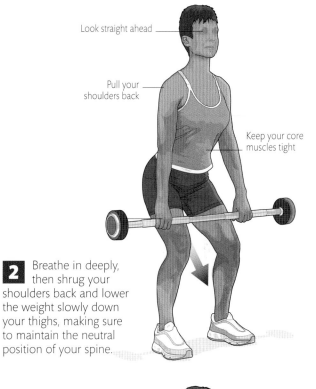

Keep your shoulders back and your spine neutral

Hold your chest up

Allow your arms to hang straight down

Take an overhand grip on the bar with your hands just wider than shoulder-width apart

Look straight ahead

Pull your shoulders back

Keep your core muscles tight

1 Stand straight with the barbell resting across your upper thighs. Your knees should be unlocked and slightly bent and your feet around shoulder-width apart.

2 Breathe in deeply, then shrug your shoulders back and lower the weight slowly down your thighs, making sure to maintain the neutral position of your spine.

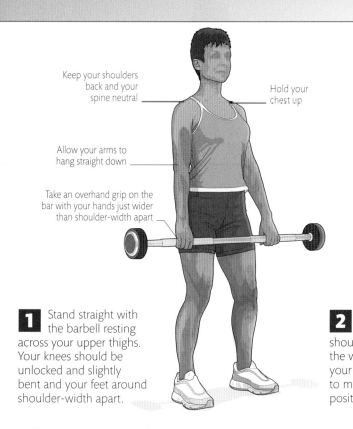
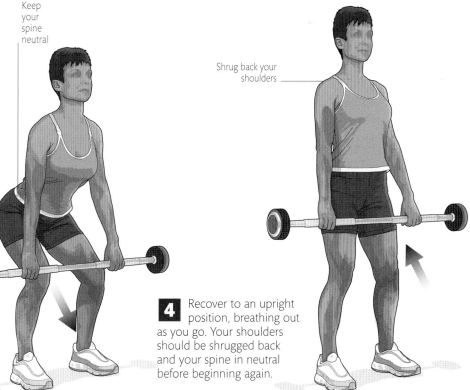

WARNING!

Safe and effective performance of this exercise depends on you keeping your back neutral. Do not bend over or be tempted to take the weight down below your knees. Be aware that this is an advanced move, first developed to help weightlifters train for the first part of the clean or snatch. When beginning, perfect the move with an unloaded bar and do not attempt too many repetitions.

Keep your spine neutral

Shrug back your shoulders

3 Lower the bar toward your knees, keeping it very close to your body. Your shoulders should come forward, ahead of the bar, as your hips ease back.

4 Recover to an upright position, breathing out as you go. Your shoulders should be shrugged back and your spine in neutral before beginning again.

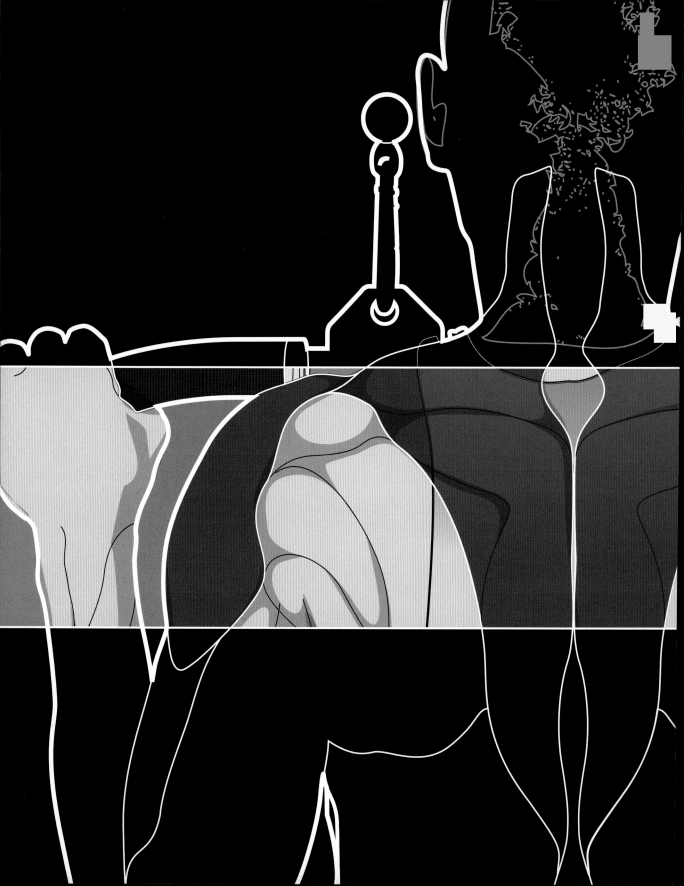

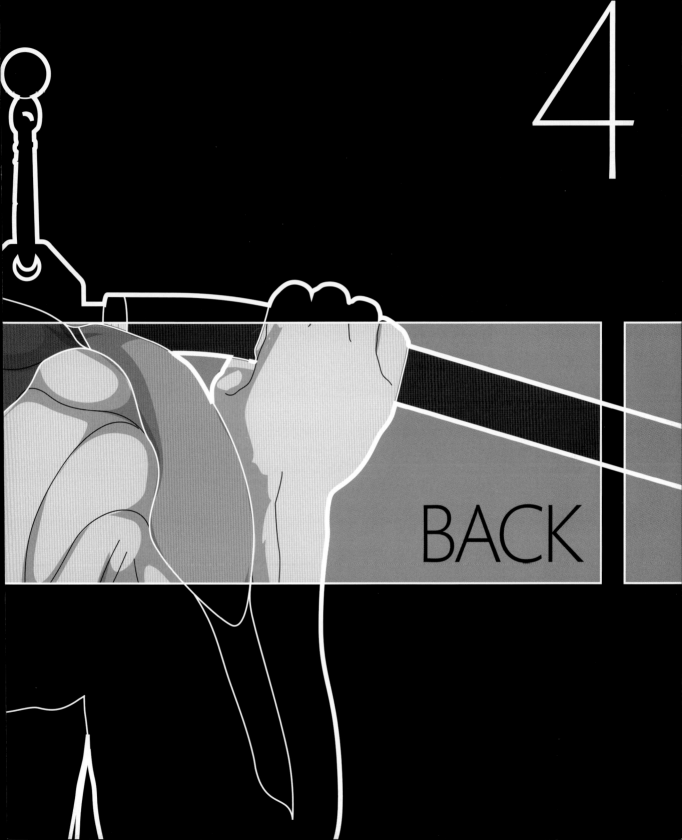

4

BACK

ASSISTED CHIN-UP

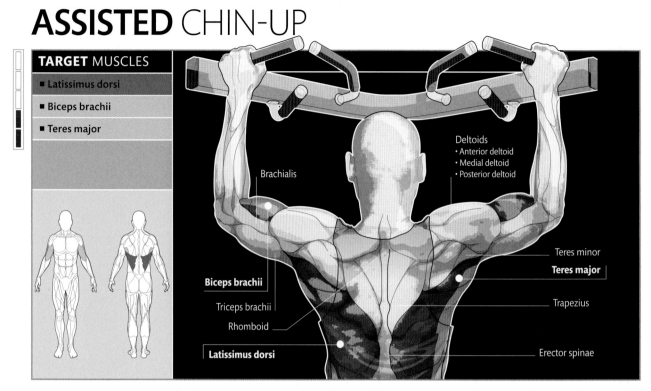

TARGET MUSCLES

- Latissimus dorsi
- Biceps brachii
- Teres major

Brachialis

Deltoids
• Anterior deltoid
• Medial deltoid
• Posterior deltoid

Teres minor

Teres major

Biceps brachii

Triceps brachii

Trapezius

Rhomboid

Latissimus dorsi

Erector spinae

This is a great way to work your big back muscles and practise the movement of the regular chin-up (see page 94) if you lack the strength to lift your whole body weight. Remember that adding weight to the stack makes the exercise easier.

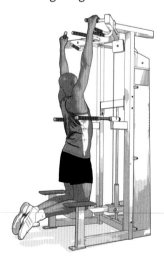

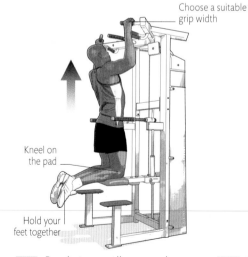

Kneel on the pad

Choose a suitable grip width

Hold your feet together

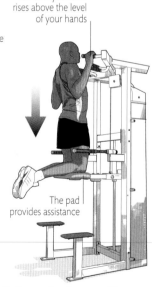

Pull until your chin rises above the level of your hands

The pad provides assistance

1 Select the weight from the stack; and stand on the foot rests. Choose your grip (see page 94) and place one knee then the other on the pad and ensure your arms are straight.

2 Bend at your elbows and shoulders and use your lats to pull your body up. Keep your body straight; breathe out going up and in going down.

3 Pull your body up until your chin is above the line of the hand grips. Pause, then lower your body by reversing the movement until your arms are fully straight.

LAT PULL-DOWN

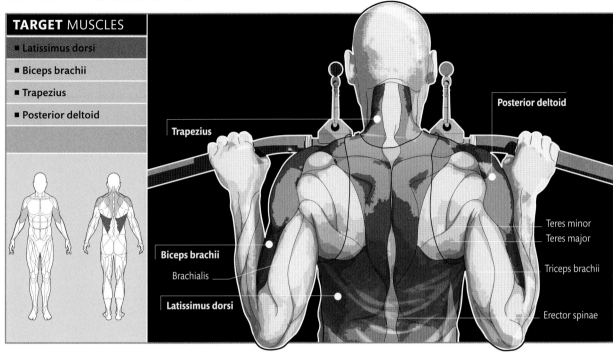

TARGET MUSCLES

- Latissimus dorsi
- Biceps brachii
- Trapezius
- Posterior deltoid

Trapezius

Posterior deltoid

Biceps brachii

Brachialis

Latissimus dorsi

Teres minor

Teres major

Triceps brachii

Erector spinae

This is another good exercise for your back if you lack the upper body strength to lift your own bodyweight in the regular chin-up. You can increase the resistance to build strength gradually.

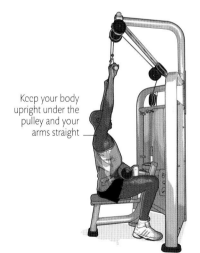

Keep your body upright under the pulley and your arms straight

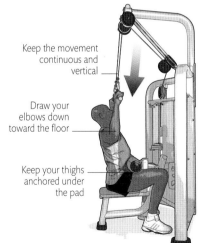

Keep the movement continuous and vertical

Draw your elbows down toward the floor

Keep your thighs anchored under the pad

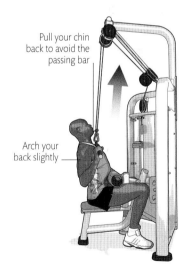

Pull your chin back to avoid the passing bar

Arch your back slightly

1 Select the desired resistance on the stack. Grip the bar a little wider than shoulder-width then sit down and place your upper thighs under the pad.

2 Easing your body back slightly, pull the bar down to the top of your chest, making sure your elbows are drawn in to your upper body as far as possible.

3 Once the bar touches the upper part of your chest, allow it to return under slowly and under full control until your arms are completely extended.

CHIN-UP

TARGET MUSCLES

- Latissimus dorsi
- Teres major
- Trapezius
- Biceps brachii

One of the most effective strength builders for the back, this challenging exercise is ideal in training for sports that involve gripping and grappling. When starting out, begin with the assisted version (see page 92) to build strength and promote muscular development.

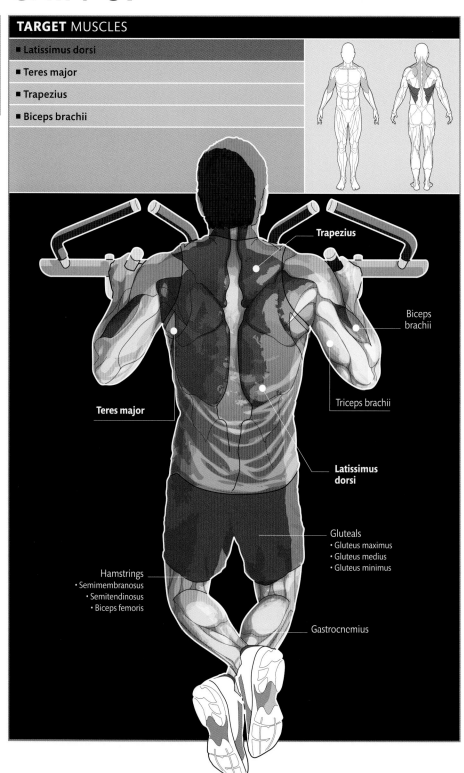

Trapezius

Biceps brachii

Triceps brachii

Teres major

Latissimus dorsi

Gluteals
· Gluteus maximus
· Gluteus medius
· Gluteus minimus

Hamstrings
· Semimembranosus
· Semitendinosus
· Biceps femoris

Gastrocnemius

VARIATION

Try varying your grip and hand spacing. An overhand grip uses your biceps less so is tougher than an underhand grip. A narrow grip hits the smaller muscles in your shoulders, while a wide grip is more challenging on your lats but stresses your elbows.

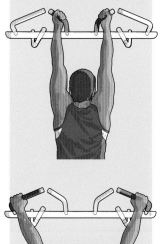

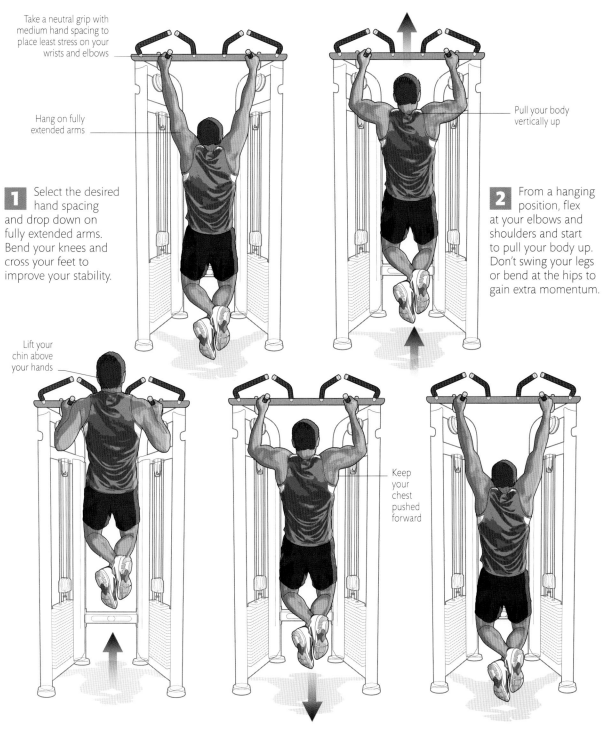

Take a neutral grip with medium hand spacing to place least stress on your wrists and elbows

Hang on fully extended arms

1 Select the desired hand spacing and drop down on fully extended arms. Bend your knees and cross your feet to improve your stability.

Pull your body vertically up

2 From a hanging position, flex at your elbows and shoulders and start to pull your body up. Don't swing your legs or bend at the hips to gain extra momentum.

Lift your chin above your hands

Keep your chest pushed forward

3 Continue pulling your body up vertically until your chin passes the level of your hands. Keep your shoulders back.

4 Pause at the top of the movement, then begin to lower your body slowly and under control. Look ahead, not down to the floor.

5 Return to the start position with your legs in line with your torso and your arms fully extended—don't cheat by stopping short on your descent.

SEATED PULLEY ROW

TARGET MUSCLES

- Latissimus dorsi
- Teres major
- Trapezius

This is a key muscle builder and strength developer for your back. However, good technique is important if you are to achieve optimum results safely.

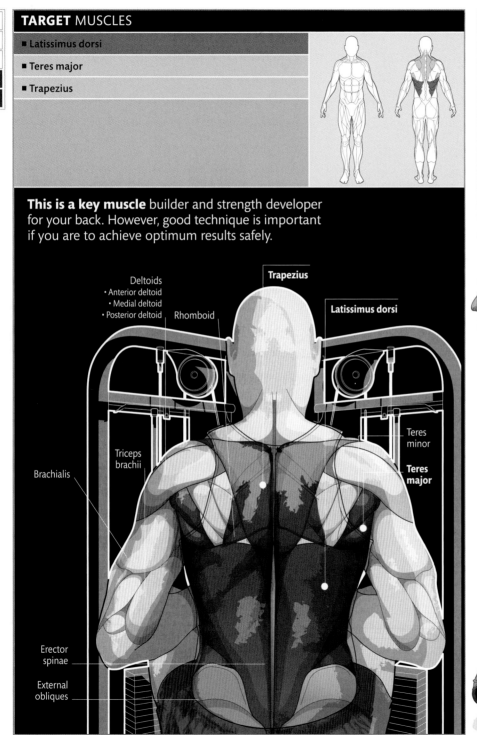

Deltoids
· Anterior deltoid
· Medial deltoid
· Posterior deltoid

Rhomboid

Trapezius

Latissimus dorsi

Teres minor

Teres major

Triceps brachii

Brachialis

Erector spinae

External obliques

VARIATION

The one-arm seated pulley row allows you to work your arms separately. This helps to balance your lat development because your weaker side cannot be supported by your stronger side. Select a lower weight than you would use for the two-handed exercise and hold your "spare" arm ahead of you or rest it on your thigh. Be careful to maintain good form throughout; and when you have completed your set with one arm, work the other side equally.

WARNING!

To keep from damaging your back, make sure that you keep your legs bent at the knee, and do not bend your back. Don't allow the weight to pull you in, and avoid leaning back on the pull to get extra leverage. The path of the handles (or bar) should be straight back and horizontal, and your movement should be slow and continuous, not jerky.

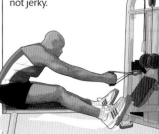

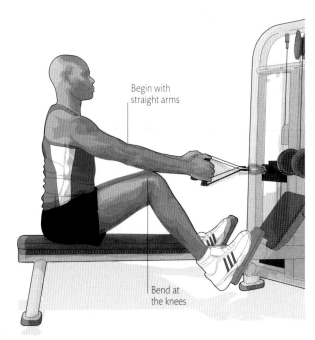

Begin with
straight arms

Bend at
the knees

1 Select the desired resistance from the stack.
Push with your legs until your arms are fully
extended and your back is in a neutral position.
Bend your knees to an angle of around 90 degrees.

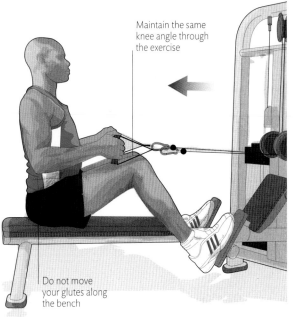

Maintain the same
knee angle through
the exercise

Do not move
your glutes along
the bench

2 Draw your elbows back, maintaining a
neutral spine position and an upright body.
Keep your feet braced flat against the foot rests of
the rowing machine.

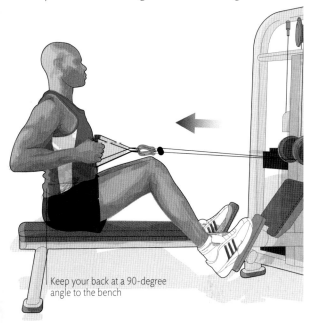

Keep your back at a 90-degree
angle to the bench

3 Pull the handles (or bar) back into your
body at the level of your upper abdomen.
Draw your elbows back as far as possible.
Breathe out as you pull.

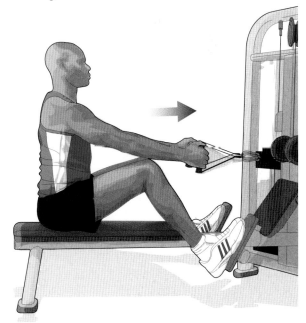

4 In the return phase of the exercise, allow
your arms to straighten in a controlled
manner, breathing in as you do so. Don't let
the weight pull you in toward the stack.

STANDING PULLEY ROW

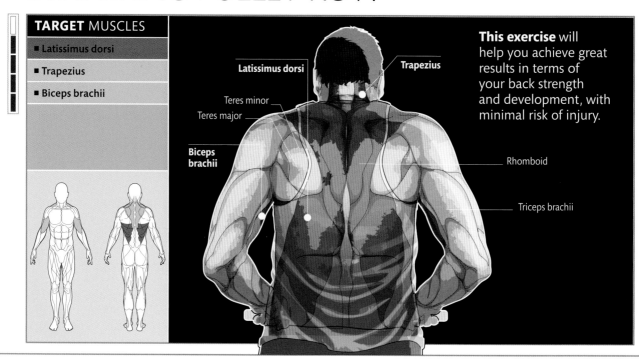

TARGET MUSCLES

- Latissimus dorsi
- Trapezius
- Biceps brachii

Latissimus dorsi

Trapezius

Teres minor

Teres major

Biceps brachii

Rhomboid

Triceps brachii

This exercise will help you achieve great results in terms of your back strength and development, with minimal risk of injury.

ONE-ARM ROW

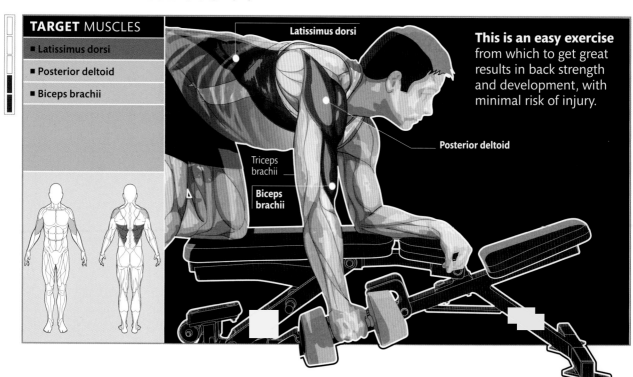

TARGET MUSCLES

- Latissimus dorsi
- Posterior deltoid
- Biceps brachii

Latissimus dorsi

Posterior deltoid

Triceps brachii

Biceps brachii

This is an easy exercise from which to get great results in back strength and development, with minimal risk of injury.

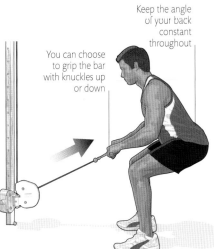
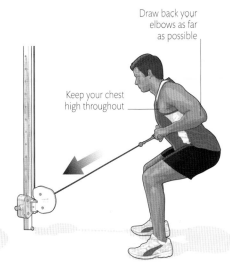
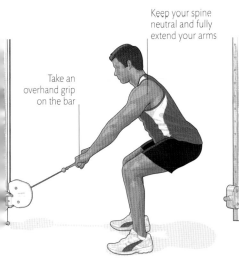
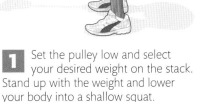

Keep your spine neutral and fully extend your arms

Take an overhand grip on the bar

Keep the angle of your back constant throughout

You can choose to grip the bar with knuckles up or down

Draw back your elbows as far as possible

Keep your chest high throughout

1 Set the pulley low and select your desired weight on the stack. Stand up with the weight and lower your body into a shallow squat.

2 Maintain the shallow squat position, ensuring that your back stays flat. Pull the bar toward you, aiming for your upper abdomen.

3 Pull the bar all the way into your body. Pause, then return to the start position with straight arms, slowly and under full control.

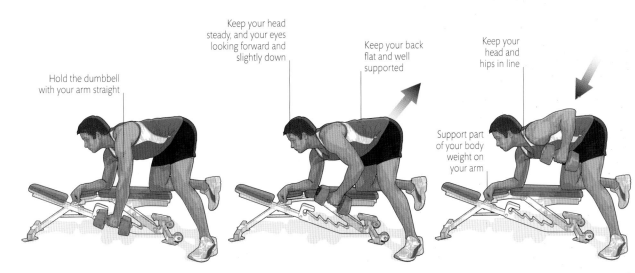

Keep your head steady, and your eyes looking forward and slightly down

Keep your back flat and well supported

Keep your head and hips in line

Hold the dumbbell with your arm straight

Support part of your body weight on your arm

1 Rest one knee on a bench. Holding your back flat, brace your body with your free arm. Hold the dumbbell with one hand.

2 Hold your back flat and your shoulders level. Raise the dumbbell toward your body with your elbow pointing up.

3 Pull your elbow as high as possible before returning, under control, to the start position. Complete your set, then repeat with your other arm.

BENT-OVER ROW

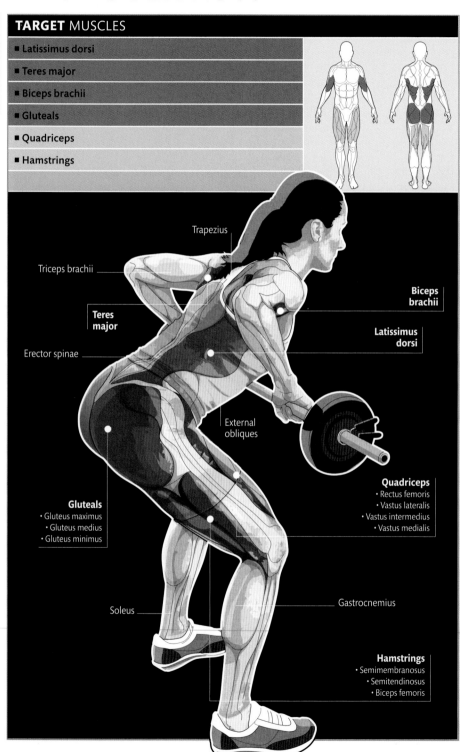

TARGET MUSCLES

- Latissimus dorsi
- Teres major
- Biceps brachii
- Gluteals
- Quadriceps
- Hamstrings

This is one of the most important exercises for the large muscles of your back—the latissimus dorsi—and will give you the classic "V" shape. It is a multijoint exercise that builds good posture, helps prevent back injuries, and also provides a thorough lower-body and core workout.

Trapezius

Triceps brachii

Teres major

Erector spinae

Biceps brachii

Latissimus dorsi

External obliques

Gluteals
· Gluteus maximus
· Gluteus medius
· Gluteus minimus

Quadriceps
· Rectus femoris
· Vastus lateralis
· Vastus intermedius
· Vastus medialis

Soleus

Gastrocnemius

Hamstrings
· Semimembranosus
· Semitendinosus
· Biceps femoris

WARNING!

Keep your back straight; if you allow it to become rounded and lose its flat, neutral position, the forces acting on the base of your spine increase dramatically and the risk of injury is high. Do not allow your shoulders to collapse forward either during or after the lift, when you return the bar to the floor.

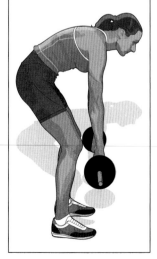

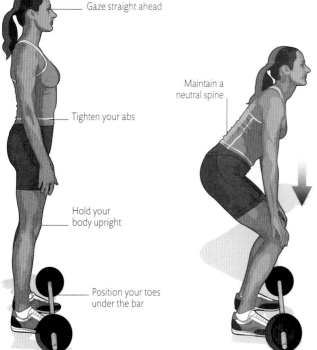

Gaze straight ahead

Tighten your abs

Hold your body upright

Position your toes under the bar

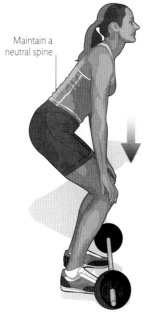

Maintain a neutral spine

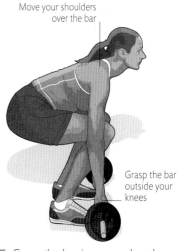

Move your shoulders over the bar

Grasp the bar outside your knees

1 Stand upright with your head level, your core muscles engaged, and your toes under the bar. Shrug your shoulders back and slightly down, hollowing your back.

2 Bending your knees over the bar, lower your body, keeping your spine neutral. Keep your feet shoulder-width apart and your gaze straight ahead.

3 Grasp the bar in an overhand grip, with your arms outside your knees. Keep your back flat, your heels pressed down on the floor, and your head forward.

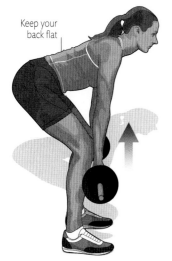

Keep your back flat

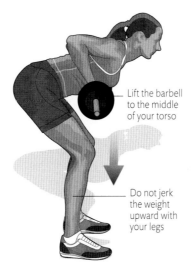

Lift the barbell to the middle of your torso

Do not jerk the weight upward with your legs

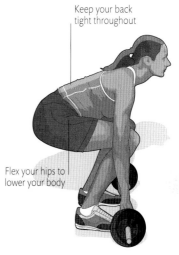

Keep your back tight throughout

Flex your hips to lower your body

4 Partially straighten your legs, keeping the angle of your back constant until the bar is just below your knees. Your body should feel stable and braced at your hips.

5 Bring the barbell up, flexing your arms and raising your elbows, until it touches your body. Pause, then let your elbows extend back to the start position (Step 3), and repeat.

6 At the end of your set, lower the barbell to the ground by bending your knees, keeping your back at a constant angle. Don't swing the weight at any point in the exercise.

BARBELL PULL-OVER

TARGET MUSCLES

- Pectorals
- Latissimus dorsi
- Triceps

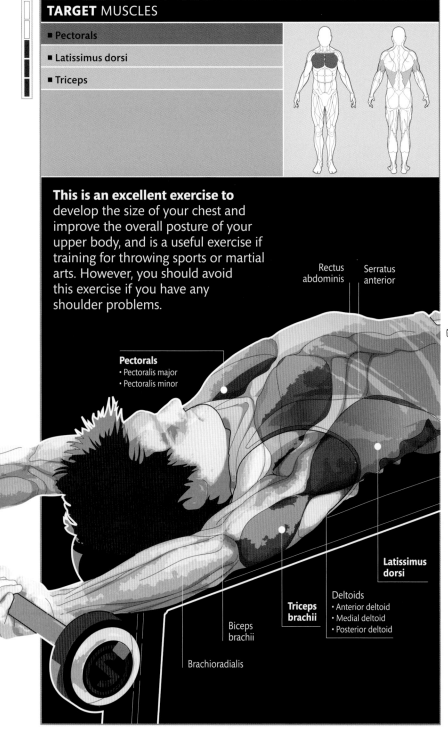

This is an excellent exercise to develop the size of your chest and improve the overall posture of your upper body, and is a useful exercise if training for throwing sports or martial arts. However, you should avoid this exercise if you have any shoulder problems.

Rectus abdominis

Serratus anterior

Pectorals
• Pectoralis major
• Pectoralis minor

Latissimus dorsi

Deltoids
• Anterior deltoid
• Medial deltoid
• Posterior deltoid

Triceps brachii

Biceps brachii

Brachioradialis

VARIATION

You can perform this exercise with a narrow grip on the barbell, using an EZ bar, or with a single dumbbell. In all of these variations you can bend your arms slightly on the downward movement past the head. This allows a greater range of movement and puts more emphasis on the triceps. In each case, ensure that your feet stay planted on the floor.

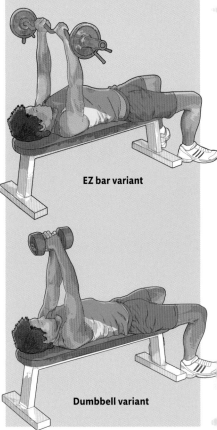

EZ bar variant

Dumbbell variant

WARNING!

Using an excessive weight in this exercise can cause your lower back to arch, which could damage your intervertebral discs. Always use a weight that is light enough to enable you to maintain good form throughout the full range of movement.

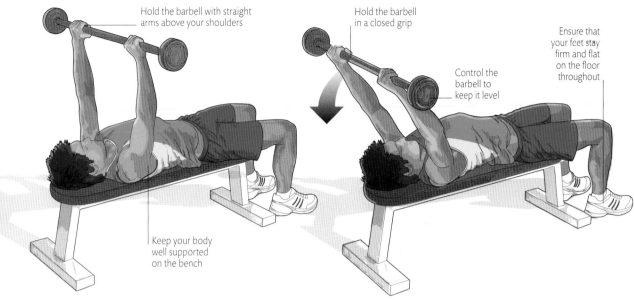

Hold the barbell with straight arms above your shoulders

Hold the barbell in a closed grip

Ensure that your feet stay firm and flat on the floor throughout

Control the barbell to keep it level

Keep your body well supported on the bench

1 Lie on a bench with your head close to one end, and your shoulders, glutes, and head in contact with the pad. Place your feet flat on the floor for stability. Hold the barbell slightly wider than shoulder-width and in line with the upper part of your chest.

2 Lower the barbell overhead to a horizontal position or as far as your shoulder mobility will allow. You should feel a gentle stretch in your chest. Try to keep your arms straight, but you can bend slightly at your elbows if this is more comfortable. Breathe in as you lower the weight.

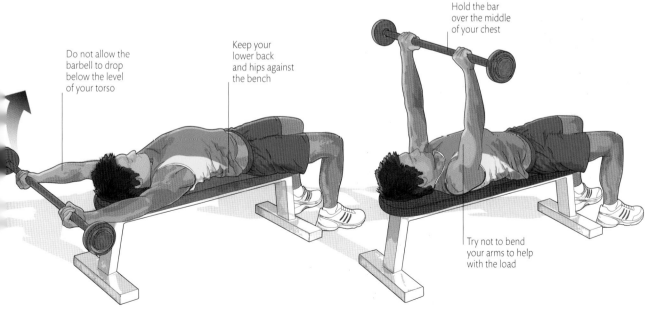

Do not allow the barbell to drop below the level of your torso

Keep your lower back and hips against the bench

Hold the bar over the middle of your chest

Try not to bend your arms to help with the load

3 Pause momentarily at the extreme of the movement then, keeping your arms straight, raise the barbell to the upright position. Breathe out as you do so.

4 Back at the start position, take a little time to check your body alignment and foot placement before starting on the next repetition.

GOOD MORNING BARBELL

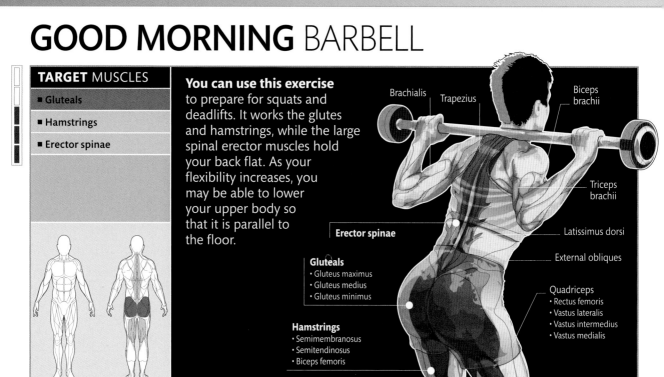

TARGET MUSCLES

- Gluteals
- Hamstrings
- Erector spinae

You can use this exercise to prepare for squats and deadlifts. It works the glutes and hamstrings, while the large spinal erector muscles hold your back flat. As your flexibility increases, you may be able to lower your upper body so that it is parallel to the floor.

Brachialis

Trapezius

Biceps brachii

Triceps brachii

Erector spinae

Latissimus dorsi

External obliques

Gluteals
- Gluteus maximus
- Gluteus medius
- Gluteus minimus

Quadriceps
- Rectus femoris
- Vastus lateralis
- Vastus intermedius
- Vastus medialis

Hamstrings
- Semimembranosus
- Semitendinosus
- Biceps femoris

BACK EXTENSION

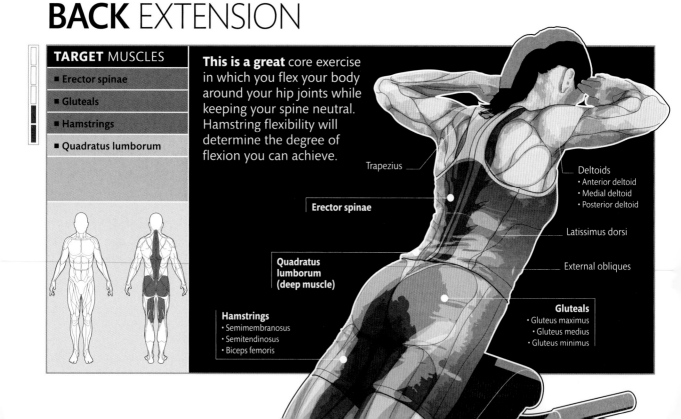

TARGET MUSCLES

- Erector spinae
- Gluteals
- Hamstrings
- Quadratus lumborum

This is a great core exercise in which you flex your body around your hip joints while keeping your spine neutral. Hamstring flexibility will determine the degree of flexion you can achieve.

Trapezius

Deltoids
- Anterior deltoid
- Medial deltoid
- Posterior deltoid

Erector spinae

Latissimus dorsi

External obliques

Quadratus lumborum (deep muscle)

Gluteals
- Gluteus maximus
- Gluteus medius
- Gluteus minimus

Hamstrings
- Semimembranosus
- Semitendinosus
- Biceps femoris

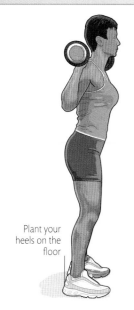
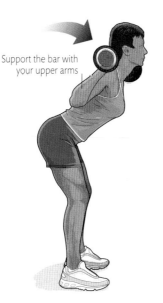
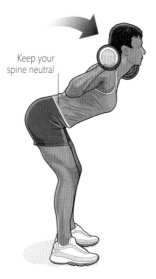
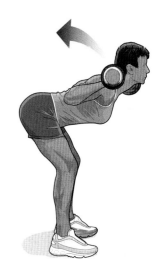

Plant your heels on the floor

Support the bar with your upper arms

Keep your spine neutral

1 Holding your body upright, position the barbell behind your neck and resting on your upper back. Keep your knees slightly bent and your spine neutral.

2 Bending slightly at your knees and hips, start to lean forward under control. Keep your chin up—it will stop you from rounding your back.

3 Lean forward by pivoting at your hip. Continue lowering your chest, keeping your back neutral and allowing your knees to bend slightly.

4 Flex as far as possible: with practice your back may be parallel to the floor. Return to the start position, breathing out as you go.

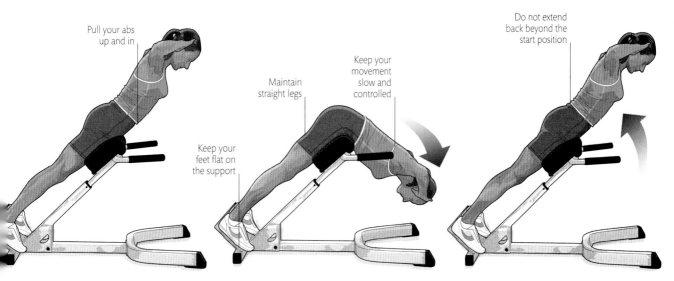

Pull your abs up and in

Maintain straight legs

Keep your movement slow and controlled

Keep your feet flat on the support

Do not extend back beyond the start position

1 Position your thighs on the pads of the Roman chair so that your hips are free to flex. Your feet should be flat on the foot supports, your spine neutral, and your elbows pointing out.

2 Flex at your hips and drop your upper body toward the floor. Keep your back flat. Stop bending when the flexibility of your hamstrings restricts further movement.

3 Return to the start position, contracting your hamstrings, glutes, and spinal erectors. Do not extend beyond the start position as you may injure your back.

PRONE ROW

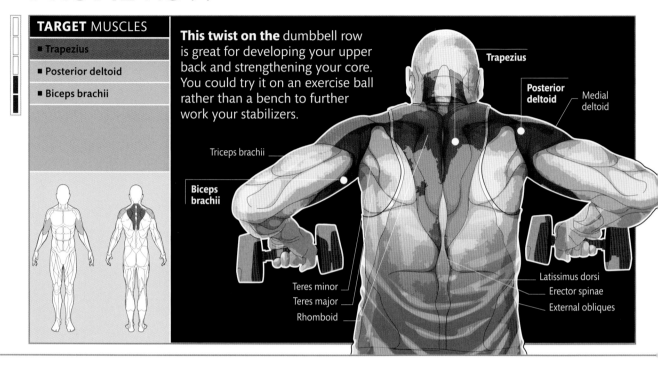

TARGET MUSCLES

- Trapezius
- Posterior deltoid
- Biceps brachii

This twist on the dumbbell row is great for developing your upper back and strengthening your core. You could try it on an exercise ball rather than a bench to further work your stabilizers.

Trapezius

Posterior deltoid

Medial deltoid

Triceps brachii

Biceps brachii

Teres minor

Teres major

Rhomboid

Latissimus dorsi

Erector spinae

External obliques

STRAIGHT-ARM PULL-DOWN

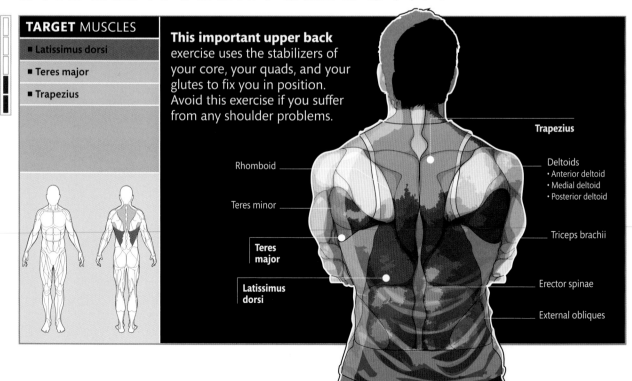

TARGET MUSCLES

- Latissimus dorsi
- Teres major
- Trapezius

This important upper back exercise uses the stabilizers of your core, your quads, and your glutes to fix you in position. Avoid this exercise if you suffer from any shoulder problems.

Rhomboid

Teres minor

Teres major

Latissimus dorsi

Trapezius

Deltoids
- Anterior deltoid
- Medial deltoid
- Posterior deltoid

Triceps brachii

Erector spinae

External obliques

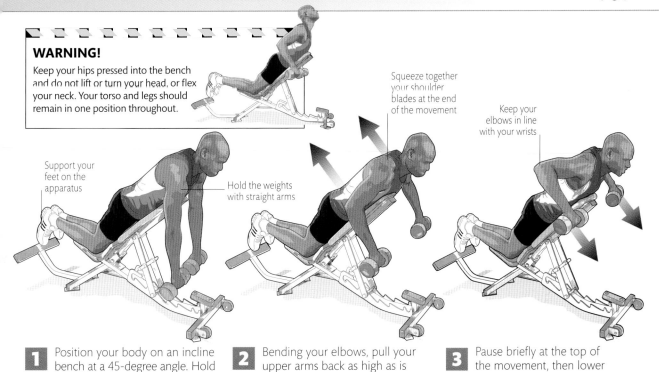

WARNING!

Keep your hips pressed into the bench and do not lift or turn your head, or flex your neck. Your torso and legs should remain in one position throughout.

Support your feet on the apparatus

Hold the weights with straight arms

Squeeze together your shoulder blades at the end of the movement

Keep your elbows in line with your wrists

1 Position your body on an incline bench at a 45-degree angle. Hold the dumbbells in an overhand grip and lie chest-down against the pad.

2 Bending your elbows, pull your upper arms back as high as is comfortable, while keeping them at right angles to your torso.

3 Pause briefly at the top of the movement, then lower the weights slowly and under control to the start position.

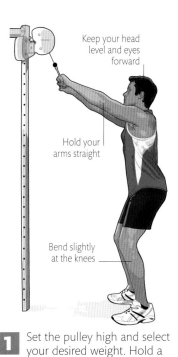

Keep your head level and eyes forward

Hold your arms straight

Bend slightly at the knees

Maintain straight arms throughout the movement

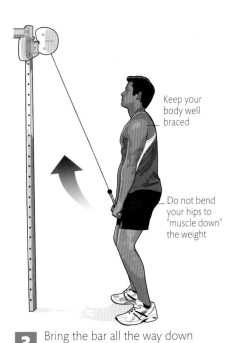

Keep your body well braced

Do not bend your hips to "muscle down" the weight

1 Set the pulley high and select your desired weight. Hold a straight bar in an overhand grip. Brace your legs and glutes.

2 Bring the bar down slowly in a controlled movement. Do not lean forward or allow your weight to shift forward into the movement.

3 Bring the bar all the way down to your upper thighs in an arc. Pause, then return slowly to the start postion, following the same arc.

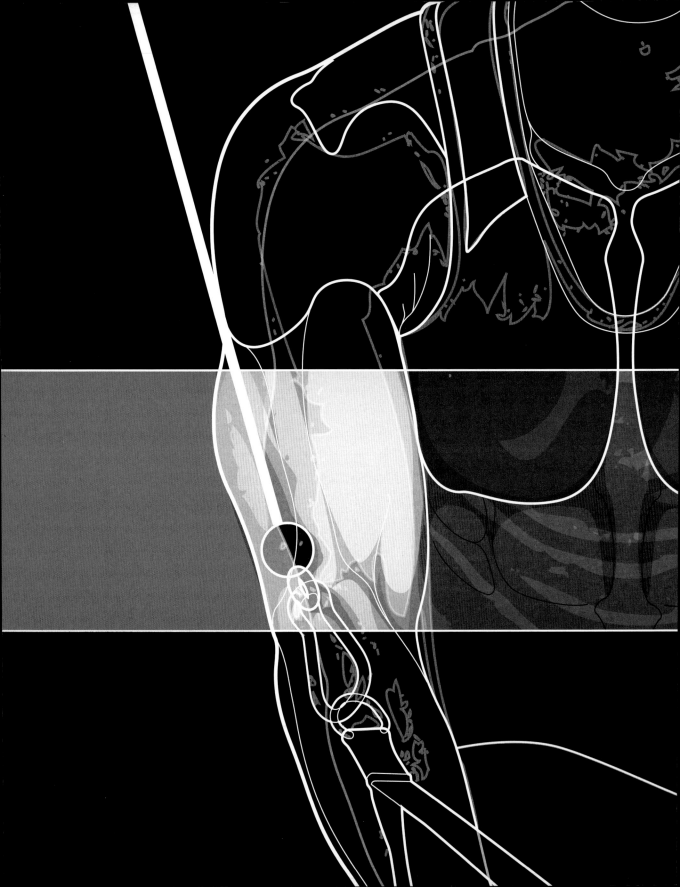

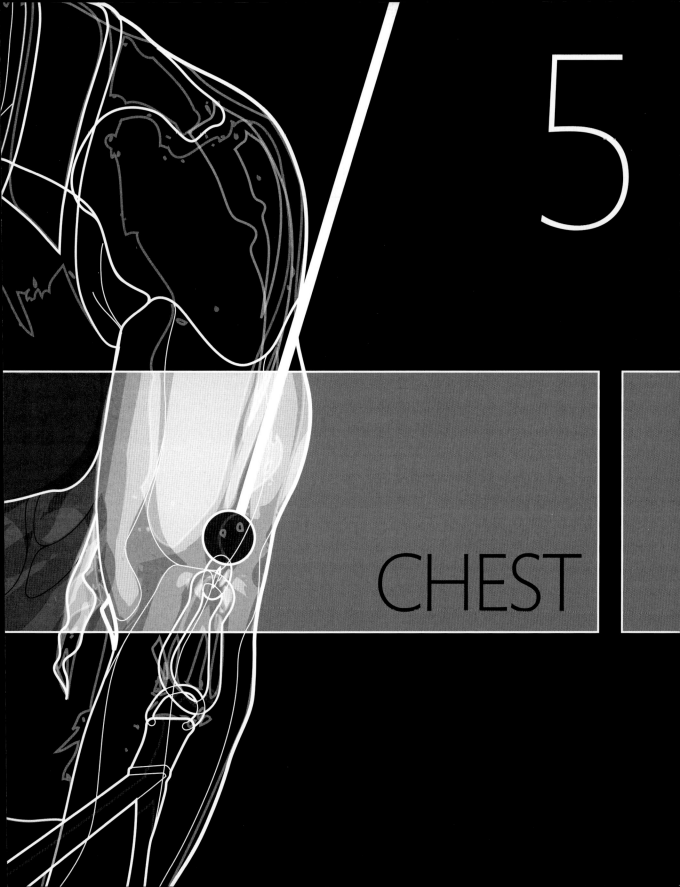

5

CHEST

BARBELL BENCH PRESS

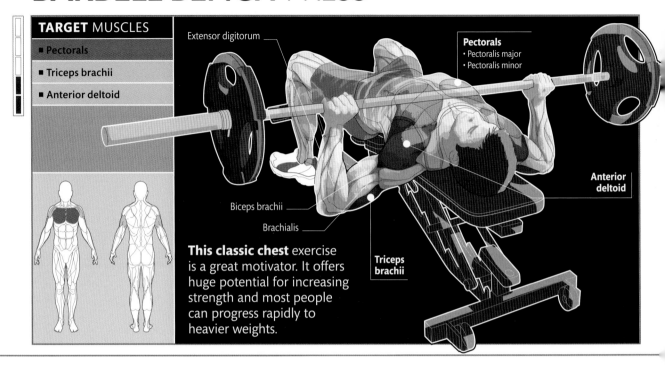

TARGET MUSCLES

- Pectorals
- Triceps brachii
- Anterior deltoid

Extensor digitorum

Pectorals
- Pectoralis major
- Pectoralis minor

Anterior deltoid

Biceps brachii

Brachialis

Triceps brachii

This classic chest exercise is a great motivator. It offers huge potential for increasing strength and most people can progress rapidly to heavier weights.

DUMBBELL BENCH PRESS

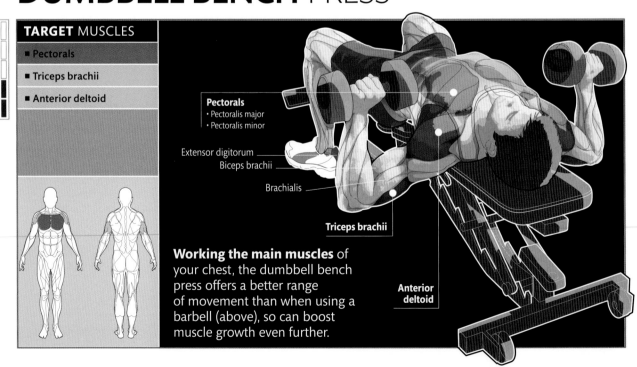

TARGET MUSCLES

- Pectorals
- Triceps brachii
- Anterior deltoid

Pectorals
- Pectoralis major
- Pectoralis minor

Extensor digitorum
Biceps brachii

Brachialis

Triceps brachii

Anterior deltoid

Working the main muscles of your chest, the dumbbell bench press offers a better range of movement than when using a barbell (above), so can boost muscle growth even further.

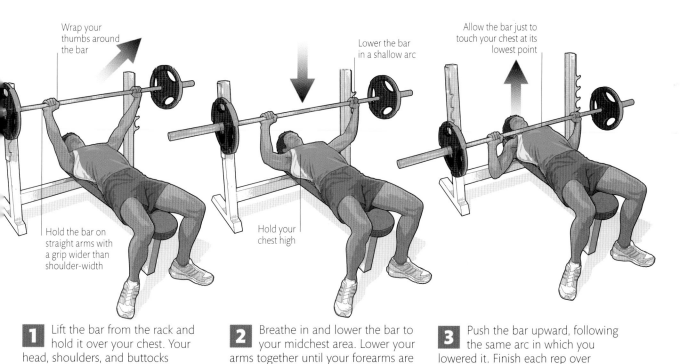

Wrap your thumbs around the bar

Hold the bar on straight arms with a grip wider than shoulder-width

Lower the bar in a shallow arc

Hold your chest high

Allow the bar just to touch your chest at its lowest point

1 Lift the bar from the rack and hold it over your chest. Your head, shoulders, and buttocks should be solidly on the bench.

2 Breathe in and lower the bar to your midchest area. Lower your arms together until your forearms are vertical at the low point.

3 Push the bar upward, following the same arc in which you lowered it. Finish each rep over your chest with straight arms.

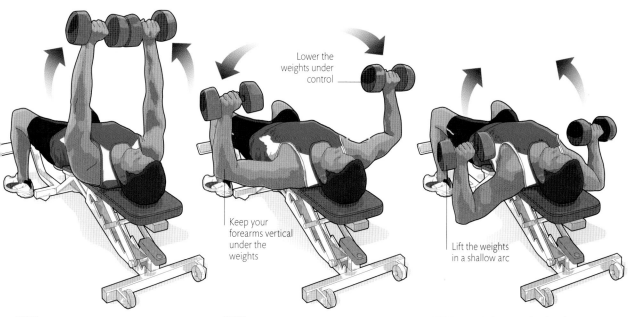

Lower the weights under control

Keep your forearms vertical under the weights

Lift the weights in a shallow arc

1 Raise the dumbbells over your chest. Stabilize your body by keeping your shoulders, head, and hips pressed against the bench.

2 Lower the weights together slowly and under control, keeping them aligned across the middle of your chest.

3 Press the weights back up in a shallow arc until they are together above your chest once again.

INCLINE BARBELL BENCH PRESS

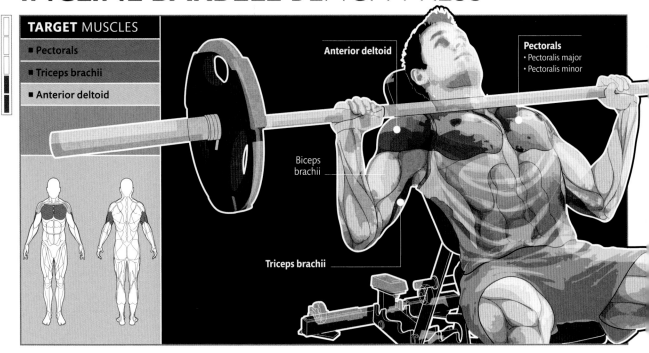

TARGET MUSCLES

- Pectorals
- Triceps brachii
- Anterior deltoid

Anterior deltoid

Pectorals
- Pectoralis major
- Pectoralis minor

Biceps brachii

Triceps brachii

This is one of the basic movements
for developing your chest. You will be able to lift
less at an incline than flat because the smaller
muscles of your shoulders come into play.

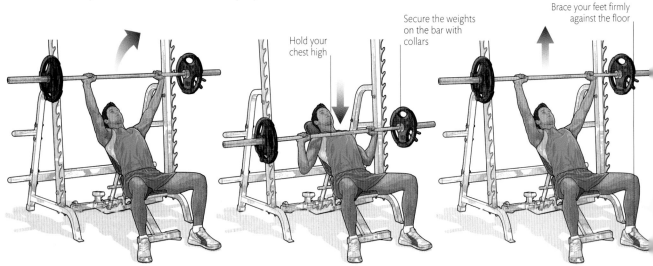

Hold your chest high

Secure the weights on the bar with collars

Brace your feet firmly against the floor

1 Grip the bar securely with your hands more than shoulder-width apart. Place your feet flat on the floor and lift the bar from the rack.

2 Lower the bar to the top of your chest so that your forearms are nearly vertical under the bar. Press your shoulders against the bench.

3 Keeping your head pressed against the bench and your spine neutral, straighten your arms evenly until the bar reaches the start position.

INCLINE DUMBBELL BENCH PRESS

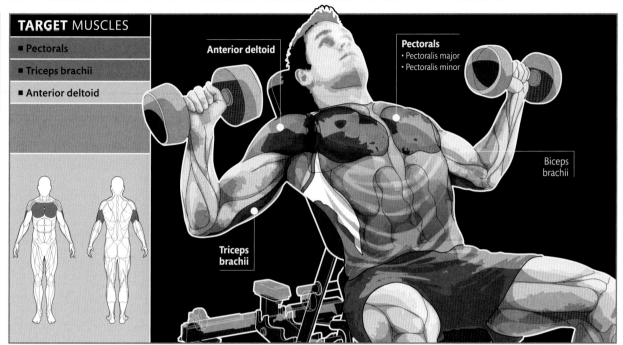

TARGET MUSCLES

- Pectorals
- Triceps brachii
- Anterior deltoid

Anterior deltoid

Pectorals
- Pectoralis major
- Pectoralis minor

Biceps brachii

Triceps brachii

Similar to the incline barbell press, this exercise allows a greater range of motion and so is of even greater value in functional terms for sports training purposes.

WARNING!

Make sure that you raise and lower the weights evenly. Avoid jerking or twisting your body to "muscle" them upward. Keep your body well balanced by holding the weights directly over your shoulders at the start.

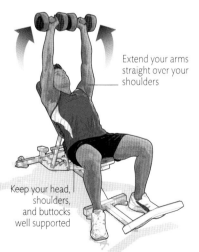

Extend your arms straight over your shoulders

Keep your head, shoulders, and buttocks well supported

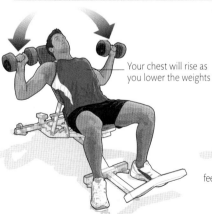

Your chest will rise as you lower the weights

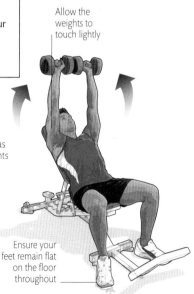

Allow the weights to touch lightly

Ensure your feet remain flat on the floor throughout

1 Lift the dumbbells over your shoulder joints on straight arms. The dumbbells should touch at the top of the movement.

2 Lower the dumbbells slowly and evenly to the point at which your upper arms are near vertical and the weights are level with your shoulders.

3 Push the weights upward in a shallow arc back to the start position. Fully extend your arms and let the dumbbells touch lightly.

INCLINE FLY

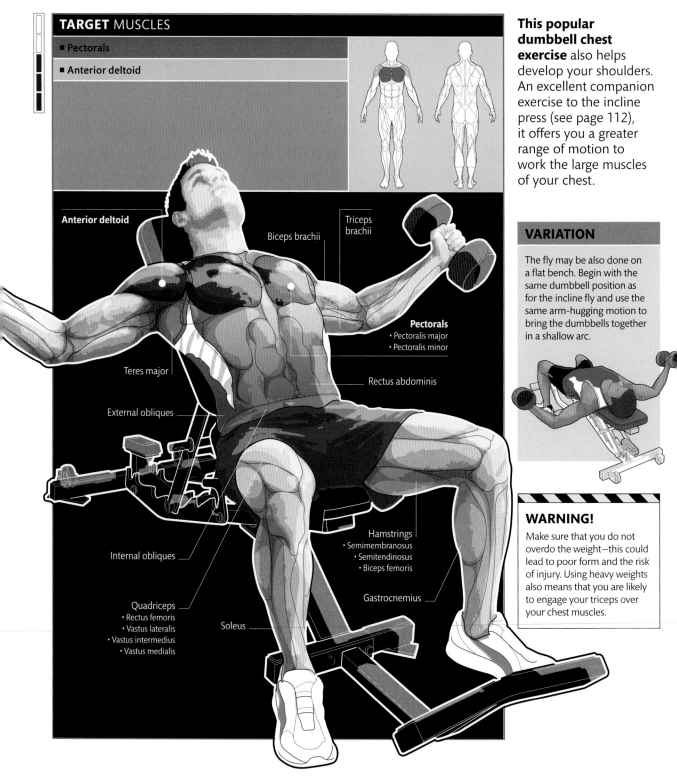

TARGET MUSCLES

- ■ Pectorals
- ■ Anterior deltoid

This popular dumbbell chest exercise also helps develop your shoulders. An excellent companion exercise to the incline press (see page 112), it offers you a greater range of motion to work the large muscles of your chest.

Anterior deltoid

Triceps brachii

Biceps brachii

Pectorals
- Pectoralis major
- Pectoralis minor

Teres major

Rectus abdominis

External obliques

Internal obliques

Hamstrings
- Semimembranosus
- Semitendinosus
- Biceps femoris

Gastrocnemius

Quadriceps
- Rectus femoris
- Vastus lateralis
- Vastus intermedius
- Vastus medialis

Soleus

VARIATION

The fly may be also done on a flat bench. Begin with the same dumbbell position as for the incline fly and use the same arm-hugging motion to bring the dumbbells together in a shallow arc.

WARNING!

Make sure that you do not overdo the weight—this could lead to poor form and the risk of injury. Using heavy weights also means that you are likely to engage your triceps over your chest muscles.

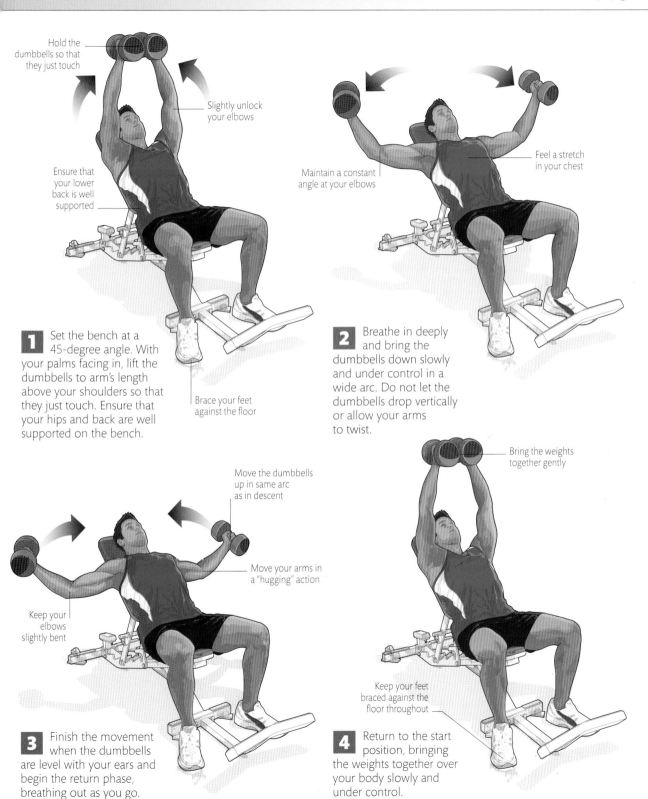

Hold the dumbbells so that they just touch

Slightly unlock your elbows

Ensure that your lower back is well supported

1 Set the bench at a 45-degree angle. With your palms facing in, lift the dumbbells to arm's length above your shoulders so that they just touch. Ensure that your hips and back are well supported on the bench.

Brace your feet against the floor

Maintain a constant angle at your elbows

Feel a stretch in your chest

2 Breathe in deeply and bring the dumbbells down slowly and under control in a wide arc. Do not let the dumbbells drop vertically or allow your arms to twist.

Move the dumbbells up in same arc as in descent

Move your arms in a "hugging" action

Keep your elbows slightly bent

3 Finish the movement when the dumbbells are level with your ears and begin the return phase, breathing out as you go.

Bring the weights together gently

Keep your feet braced against the floor throughout

4 Return to the start position, bringing the weights together over your body slowly and under control.

CABLE CROSS-OVER

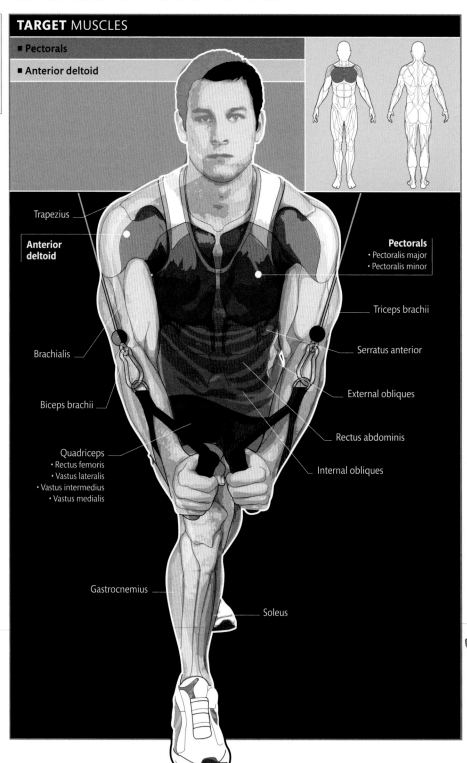

TARGET MUSCLES

- Pectorals
- Anterior deltoid

Trapezius

Anterior deltoid

Brachialis

Biceps brachii

Quadriceps
- Rectus femoris
- Vastus lateralis
- Vastus intermedius
- Vastus medialis

Gastrocnemius

Soleus

Pectorals
- Pectoralis major
- Pectoralis minor

Triceps brachii

Serratus anterior

External obliques

Rectus abdominis

Internal obliques

In this chest and shoulder exercise, your body is not supported by a bench, so the stabilizing muscles of your core and legs have to work to keep you in position. Using the cable machine also works your muscles over a large range of motion.

VARIATION

You can perform the cable cross-over exercise at varying heights by setting the pulley to a low position or to waist height. These different start positions allow you to work your chest muscles from slightly different angles.

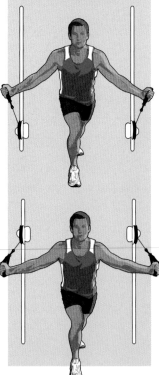

1 Set the pulley to its highest position and select your desired weight on the stack. Leaning slightly forward and with your legs braced, bring the pulley handles down across your body. Breathe in and let your arms travel back in a wide arc so that they are just behind the line of your torso. This is the start position.

WARNING!

Choose a weight that is not so heavy as to pull your body back from its braced position. Do not use the momentum of your body to complete the movement because you will almost certainly lose balance and risk injury.

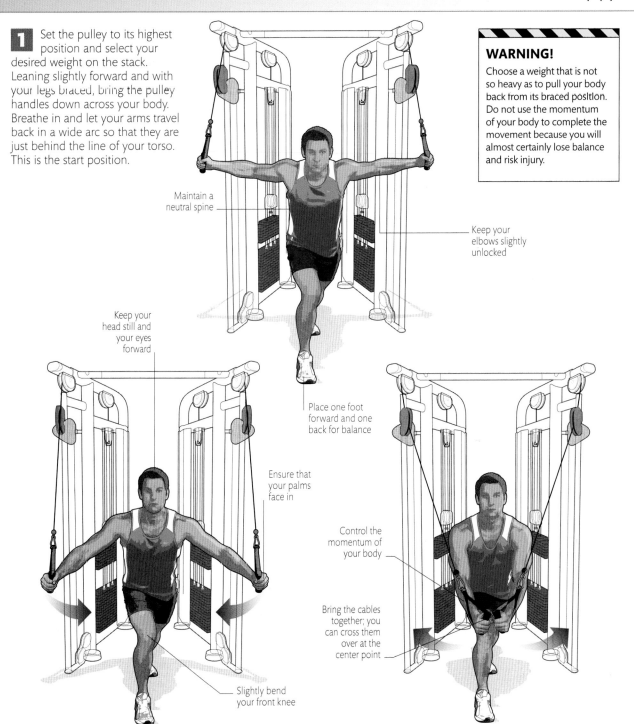

Maintain a neutral spine

Keep your elbows slightly unlocked

Keep your head still and your eyes forward

Place one foot forward and one back for balance

Ensure that your palms face in

Control the momentum of your body

Bring the cables together; you can cross them over at the center point

Slightly bend your front knee

2 Bring your arms down and across your body in a wide arc—like a hugging motion. Keep your head up and maintain a slight bend in your arms as you pull the handles forward and down at a slight angle. Breathe out on the effort.

3 Bring your hands to the front of your body before starting the return phase, reversing the arc of movement in Step 2. Make sure that your arms move at the same speed and that your elbows stay in the same slightly bent position throughout the movement.

MACHINE BENCH PRESS

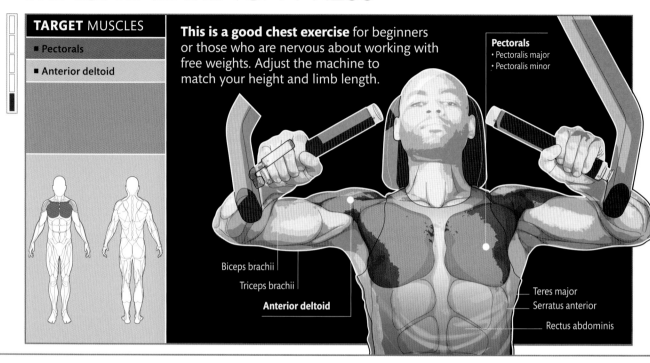

TARGET MUSCLES

- Pectorals
- Anterior deltoid

This is a good chest exercise for beginners or those who are nervous about working with free weights. Adjust the machine to match your height and limb length.

Pectorals
- Pectoralis major
- Pectoralis minor

Biceps brachii

Triceps brachii

Anterior deltoid

Teres major

Serratus anterior

Rectus abdominis

MACHINE FLY

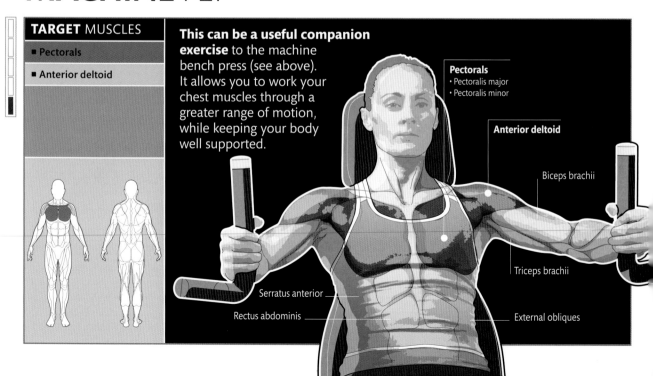

TARGET MUSCLES

- Pectorals
- Anterior deltoid

This can be a useful companion exercise to the machine bench press (see above). It allows you to work your chest muscles through a greater range of motion, while keeping your body well supported.

Pectorals
- Pectoralis major
- Pectoralis minor

Anterior deltoid

Biceps brachii

Triceps brachii

Serratus anterior

Rectus abdominis

External obliques

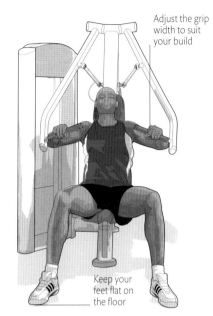

Adjust the grip width to suit your build

Keep your feet flat on the floor

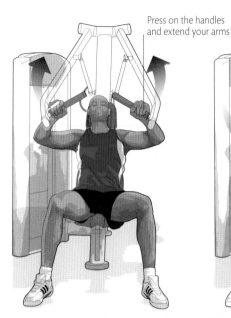

Press on the handles and extend your arms

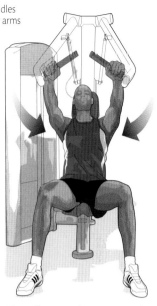

1 Set your desired weight on the stack. Take an overhand grip on the handles, which should be at midchest level.

2 Breathe in deeply, then breathe out as you press the handles in a slow and controlled movement; keep your body tight against the pads.

3 Fully extend your arms then return the handles to the start position, breathing in. Don't let the weight rest on the stack before starting another rep.

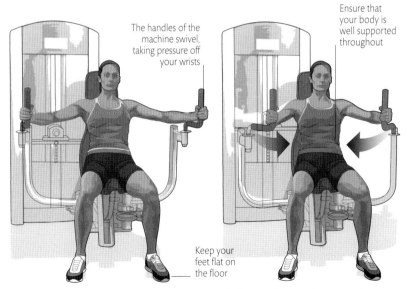

The handles of the machine swivel, taking pressure off your wrists

Ensure that your body is well supported throughout

Keep your feet flat on the floor

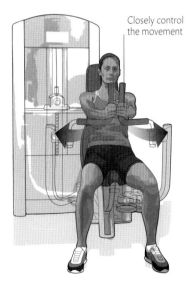

Closely control the movement

1 Set your desired weight on the stack. Allow your arms to spread in a wide arc so that the handles are just behind the line of your torso.

2 Breathe out, bringing the handles together in a wide arc, with your elbows slightly bent, in a hugging motion.

3 When the movement is complete and your knuckles touch, contract your chest muscles and begin the return phase, back to the start position.

PUSH-UP

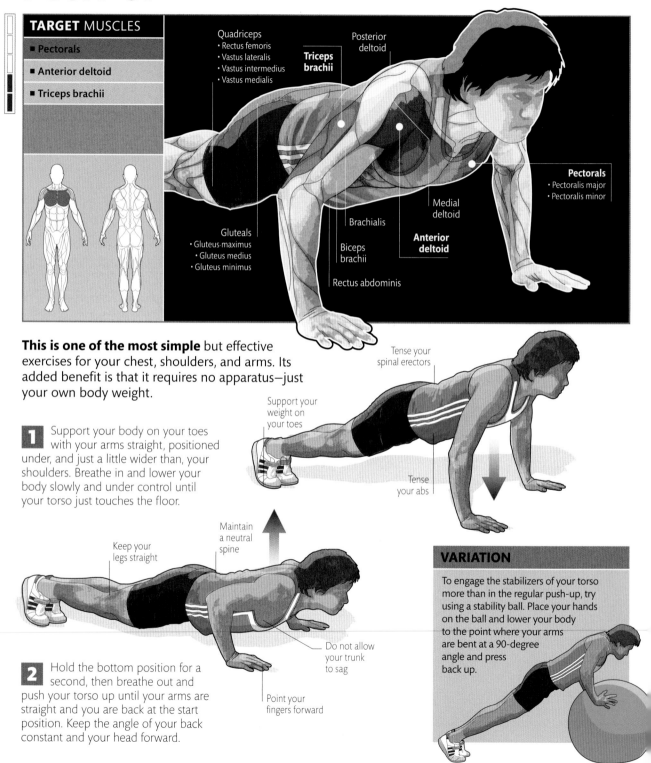

TARGET MUSCLES

- **Pectorals**
- **Anterior deltoid**
- **Triceps brachii**

Quadriceps
- Rectus femoris
- Vastus lateralis
- Vastus intermedius
- Vastus medialis

Triceps brachii

Posterior deltoid

Pectorals
- Pectoralis major
- Pectoralis minor

Medial deltoid

Brachialis

Anterior deltoid

Gluteals
- Gluteus maximus
- Gluteus medius
- Gluteus minimus

Biceps brachii

Rectus abdominis

This is one of the most simple but effective exercises for your chest, shoulders, and arms. Its added benefit is that it requires no apparatus—just your own body weight.

Tense your spinal erectors

Support your weight on your toes

Tense your abs

1 Support your body on your toes with your arms straight, positioned under, and just a little wider than, your shoulders. Breathe in and lower your body slowly and under control until your torso just touches the floor.

Keep your legs straight

Maintain a neutral spine

Do not allow your trunk to sag

Point your fingers forward

2 Hold the bottom position for a second, then breathe out and push your torso up until your arms are straight and you are back at the start position. Keep the angle of your back constant and your head forward.

VARIATION

To engage the stabilizers of your torso more than in the regular push-up, try using a stability ball. Place your hands on the ball and lower your body to the point where your arms are bent at a 90-degree angle and press back up.

FRAME-SUPPORTED PUSH-UP

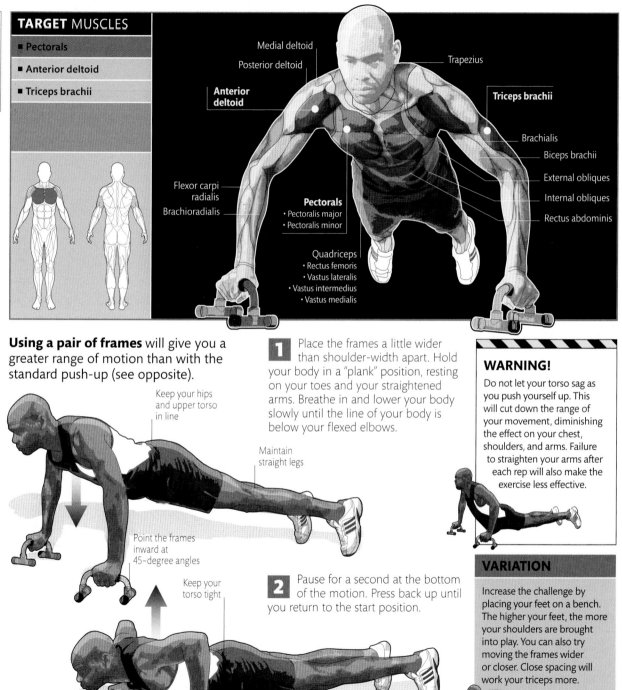

TARGET MUSCLES

- Pectorals
- Anterior deltoid
- Triceps brachii

Medial deltoid
Posterior deltoid
Trapezius
Anterior deltoid
Triceps brachii
Brachialis
Biceps brachii
External obliques
Internal obliques
Rectus abdominis
Flexor carpi radialis
Brachioradialis
Pectorals
• Pectoralis major
• Pectoralis minor
Quadriceps
• Rectus femoris
• Vastus lateralis
• Vastus intermedius
• Vastus medialis

Using a pair of frames will give you a greater range of motion than with the standard push-up (see opposite).

Keep your hips and upper torso in line

Maintain straight legs

Point the frames inward at 45-degree angles

Keep your torso tight

Support your weight on your toes

1 Place the frames a little wider than shoulder-width apart. Hold your body in a "plank" position, resting on your toes and your straightened arms. Breathe in and lower your body slowly until the line of your body is below your flexed elbows.

2 Pause for a second at the bottom of the motion. Press back up until you return to the start position.

WARNING!

Do not let your torso sag as you push yourself up. This will cut down the range of your movement, diminishing the effect on your chest, shoulders, and arms. Failure to straighten your arms after each rep will also make the exercise less effective.

VARIATION

Increase the challenge by placing your feet on a bench. The higher your feet, the more your shoulders are brought into play. You can also try moving the frames wider or closer. Close spacing will work your triceps more.

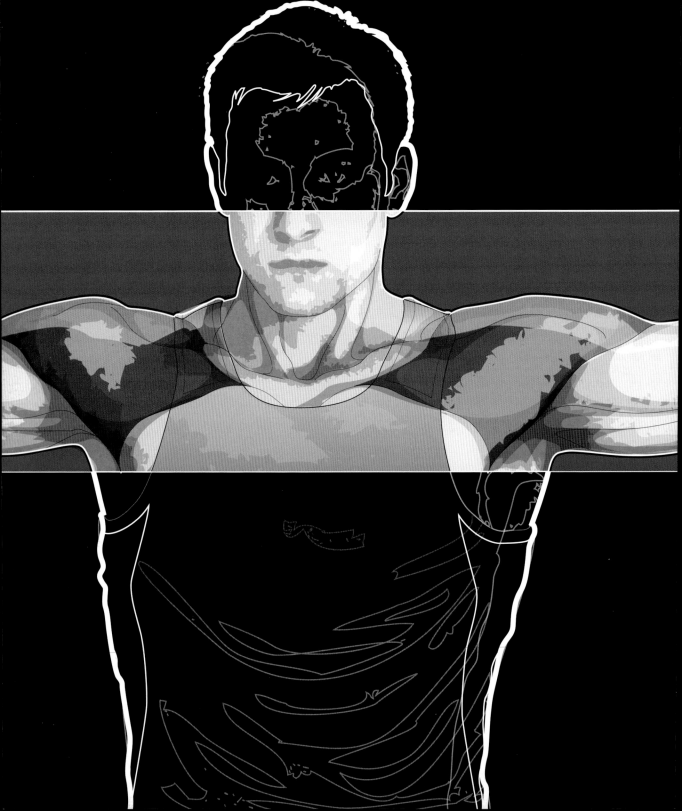

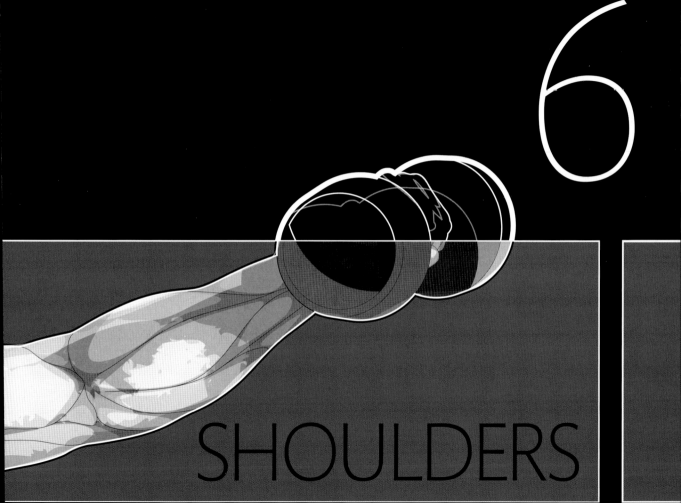

6

SHOULDERS

MILITARY BARBELL PRESS

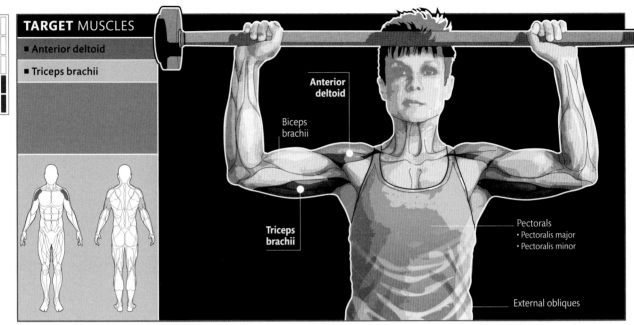

TARGET MUSCLES

- Anterior deltoid
- Triceps brachii

Anterior deltoid

Biceps brachii

Triceps brachii

Pectorals
- Pectoralis major
- Pectoralis minor

External obliques

The military or barbell press is simple but very effective, and is one of the basic exercises around which all shoulder routines are constructed.

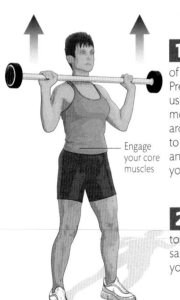

Engage your core muscles

Keep your feet flat on the floor, a little more than shoulder-width apart

Keep the bar over your center of gravity

1 Hold the bar across the front of your shoulders. Press the bar upward using your shoulders, moving it in a shallow arc around your face to a position above and slightly behind your head.

2 Gripping tightly, lower the bar back to the start position in the same shallow arc past your head.

WARNING!

Ensure your back is in a neutral position. Bending your back not only engages your chest, aiding the shoulders, and thus reducing the effectiveness of the exercise, but it also places great stress on your lower spine. Keep your wrists rigid and directly under the bar at all times—turning them back can lead to a risk of wrist injury. Finally, make sure to move your head back a fraction as you lift the bar in order to keep from hitting your chin.

VARIATION

You can perform the military press seated on a bench. The seated position means that you are not able to "help" the bar up by using your legs and so tends to isolate the effects of the exercise. Keep your back in an upright position and plant your feet securely on the floor.

DUMBBELL SHOULDER PRESS

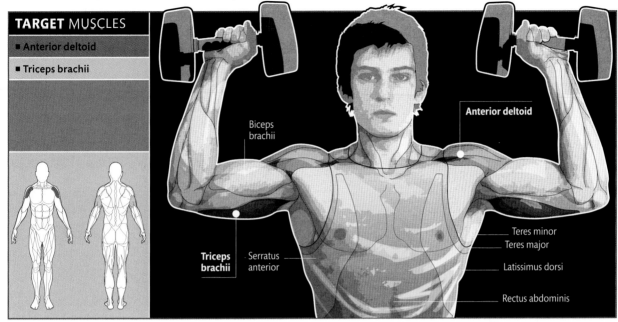

TARGET MUSCLES

- Anterior deltoid
- Triceps brachii

Biceps brachii

Anterior deltoid

Triceps brachii

Serratus anterior

Teres minor

Teres major

Latissimus dorsi

Rectus abdominis

You can perform this variant of the shoulder press seated (as shown), standing, or with alternate presses. The main advantage that it offers over the military press is that you do not need to move the bar around your face on the way up and down.

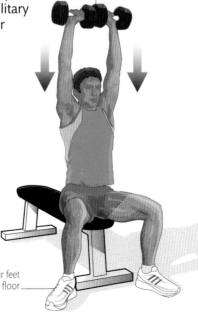

Allow the dumbbells to touch lightly behind your head

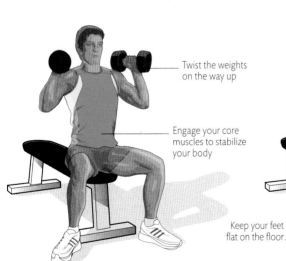

Twist the weights on the way up

Engage your core muscles to stabilize your body

Keep your feet flat on the floor

1 Sit on the end of a bench holding the dumbbells at shoulder height. Press the weights upward to arm's length with your shoulders, breathing out.

2 Briefly hold the weights at arm's length without locking out your elbows, then slowly lower the dumbbells to the start position.

VARIATION

If you lack the confidence to use free weights, try the overhead press on a machine. This is a less effective exercise than the seated or standing press, especially if you are training for sports, because your back is supported by the equipment and so you do not engage your stabilizers. As with all machine exercises, you should only use a machine that adjusts to your height and limb length.

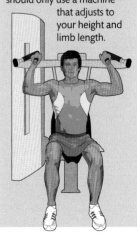

UPRIGHT ROW

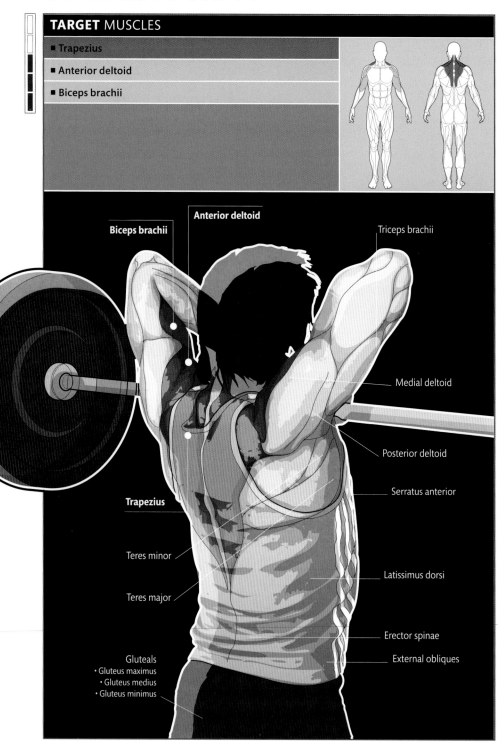

TARGET MUSCLES

- Trapezius
- Anterior deltoid
- Biceps brachii

Biceps brachii

Anterior deltoid

Triceps brachii

Medial deltoid

Posterior deltoid

Serratus anterior

Trapezius

Teres minor

Teres major

Latissimus dorsi

Erector spinae

External obliques

Gluteals
• Gluteus maximus
• Gluteus medius
• Gluteus minimus

This exercise is great for developing strength around your shoulder and upper back, and helps improve your posture. It should be avoided, however, if you suffer from shoulder pain or stiffness.

VARIATION

Using dumbbells for the upright row works each arm independently, and prevents your elbows from rising much farther than parallel to the floor, arguably making this a safer exercise because you are less likely to damage your rotator cuffs.

VARIATION

Using a low cable pulley for the upright row offers you a steadier and more stable resistance through the movement than is possible when working with a barbell. Make sure that you stand close to the pulley and keep the bar tight to your body. Use a close grip to preferentially work your upper back; or a wider grip to engage your shoulders in the exercise.

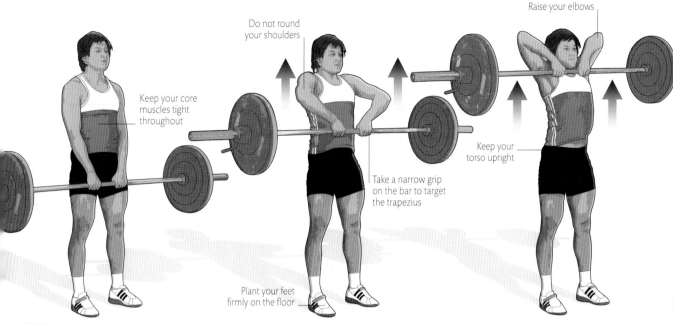

Keep your core muscles tight throughout

Do not round your shoulders

Take a narrow grip on the bar to target the trapezius

Plant your feet firmly on the floor

Raise your elbows

Keep your torso upright

1 Place your feet hip-width apart and take a narrow overhand grip on the bar, with your palms facing toward your body. Lift the bar so that it rests across your thighs.

2 Pull the bar up toward your chin in a smooth motion. Lift it close to your body, keeping your elbows high and over the bar. Keep your back tight and upright.

3 Continue pulling the bar up until it reaches your chin, keeping your hands below the level of your elbows. Pause briefly at the top of the movement.

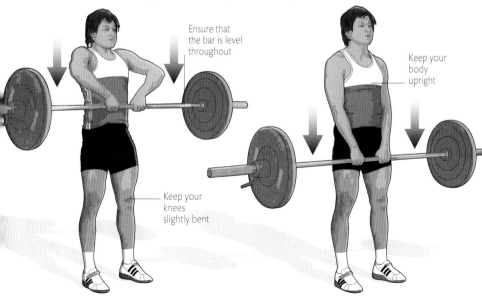

Ensure that the bar is level throughout

Keep your body upright

Keep your knees slightly bent

4 Lower the bar to the start position under close control. Use a smooth motion, keeping your elbows over the bar and your back tight.

5 Return to the start position with your arms fully extended. Exhale slowly as you do so. Return the bar to the floor at the end of your set.

WARNING!

The upright row demands good technique if you are to avoid back and shoulder injury, and it should not be done if you have a history of shoulder pain. Work within your limits and never arch your back or jerk the weight; if you are at all nervous about injury, do not lift the bar above midchest height—this avoids the extreme internal rotation of the shoulder at the top of the movement. Stop the exercise immediately if you experience any pain.

DUMBBELL SHOULDER SHRUG

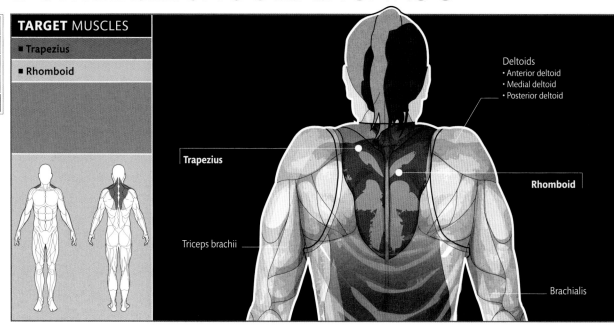

TARGET MUSCLES

- **Trapezius**
- **Rhomboid**

Deltoids
- Anterior deltoid
- Medial deltoid
- Posterior deltoid

Trapezius

Rhomboid

Triceps brachii

Brachialis

This highly specific exercise uses limited motion to work your trapezius, which lies at the back of your neck. A strong trapezius will help protect your neck and spine—making it useful for all contact sports.

VARIATION

You can perform the shrug with a barbell held in an overhand grip across the front of your thighs. The movement pathway is vertical, as with the dumbbell variant. Do not jerk the weight or arch your back—this motion will be much less effective at working your trapezius muscle.

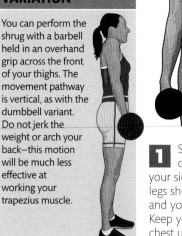

Allow your arms to hang straight by your sides

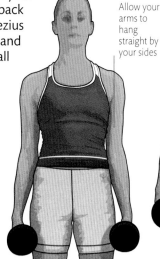

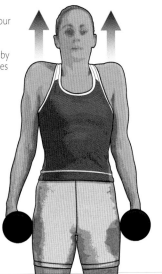

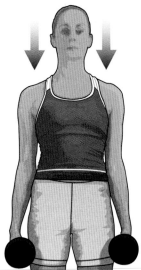

1 Stand upright with the dumbbells hanging by your sides. Stand with your legs shoulder-width apart and your knees slightly bent. Keep your abs tight and your chest up.

2 Holding the dumbbells in an overhand grip, with your thumbs wrapped around each bar, shrug the weights upward by drawing your shoulders vertically up toward your ears.

3 Hold the weights up for 1–2 seconds at the highest point before lowering them to the start position under control, following the same line of movement in which they were raised.

SHOULDER SHRUG FROM HANG

TARGET MUSCLES

- Trapezius
- Rhomboid
- Gastrocnemius

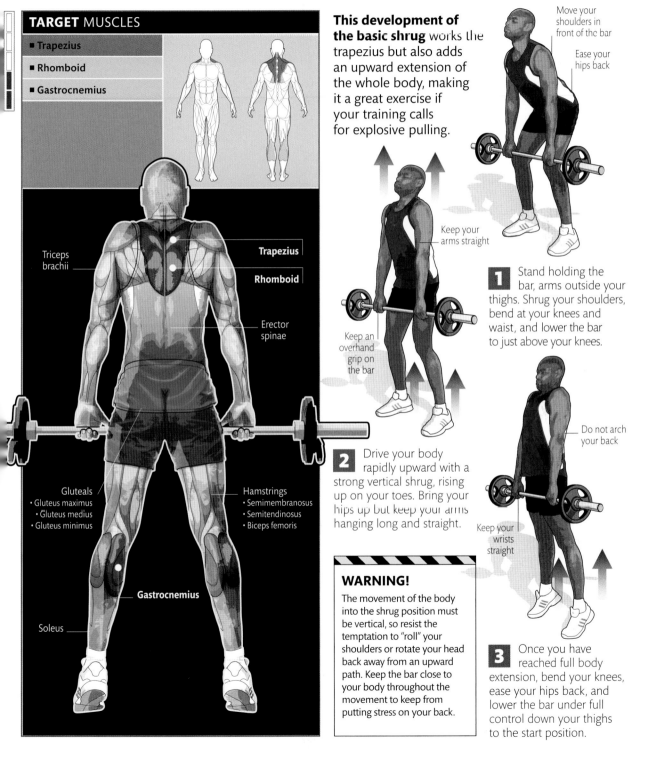

Triceps brachii

Trapezius

Rhomboid

Erector spinae

Gluteals
- Gluteus maximus
- Gluteus medius
- Gluteus minimus

Hamstrings
- Semimembranosus
- Semitendinosus
- Biceps femoris

Gastrocnemius

Soleus

This development of the basic shrug works the trapezius but also adds an upward extension of the whole body, making it a great exercise if your training calls for explosive pulling.

Move your shoulders in front of the bar

Ease your hips back

Keep your arms straight

Keep an overhand grip on the bar

1 Stand holding the bar, arms outside your thighs. Shrug your shoulders, bend at your knees and waist, and lower the bar to just above your knees.

2 Drive your body rapidly upward with a strong vertical shrug, rising up on your toes. Bring your hips up but keep your arms hanging long and straight.

Do not arch your back

Keep your wrists straight

WARNING!

The movement of the body into the shrug position must be vertical, so resist the temptation to "roll" your shoulders or rotate your head back away from an upward path. Keep the bar close to your body throughout the movement to keep from putting stress on your back.

3 Once you have reached full body extension, bend your knees, ease your hips back, and lower the bar under full control down your thighs to the start position.

FRONT DUMBBELL RAISE

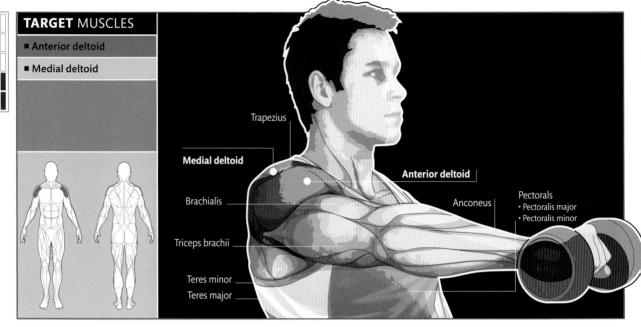

TARGET MUSCLES

- Anterior deltoid
- Medial deltoid

Trapezius

Medial deltoid

Anterior deltoid

Brachialis

Anconeus

Pectorals
- Pectoralis major
- Pectoralis minor

Triceps brachii

Teres minor

Teres major

This exercise develops and defines the smaller muscles of your shoulders, which help you perform other exercises correctly. You can lift both arms at once or alternate left and right.

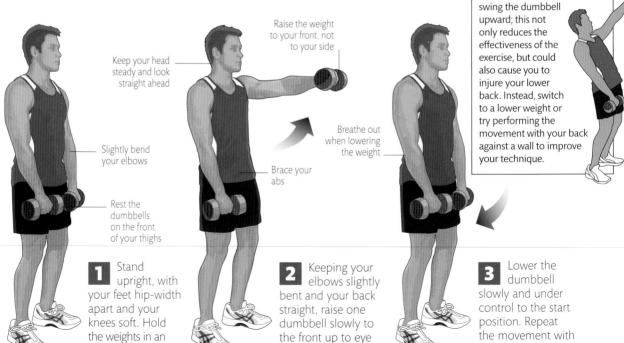

Keep your head steady and look straight ahead

Slightly bend your elbows

Rest the dumbbells on the front of your thighs

Raise the weight to your front, not to your side

Breathe out when lowering the weight

Brace your abs

1 Stand upright, with your feet hip-width apart and your knees soft. Hold the weights in an overhand grip.

2 Keeping your elbows slightly bent and your back straight, raise one dumbbell slowly to the front up to eye level while breathing in.

3 Lower the dumbbell slowly and under control to the start position. Repeat the movement with your other arm.

WARNING!

Try not to lean back and swing the dumbbell upward; this not only reduces the effectiveness of the exercise, but could also cause you to injure your lower back. Instead, switch to a lower weight or try performing the movement with your back against a wall to improve your technique.

LATERAL DUMBBELL RAISE

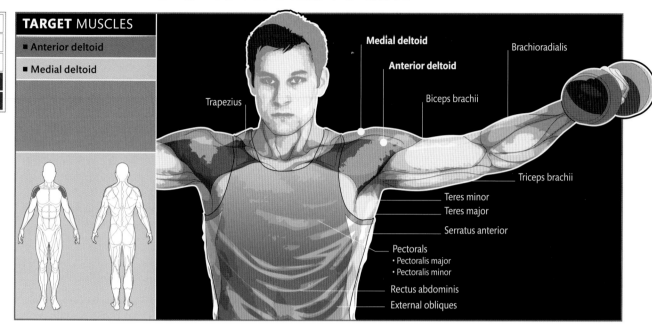

TARGET MUSCLES
- Anterior deltoid
- Medial deltoid

Medial deltoid

Anterior deltoid

Brachioradialis

Trapezius

Biceps brachii

Triceps brachii

Teres minor
Teres major

Serratus anterior

Pectorals
• Pectoralis major
• Pectoralis minor

Rectus abdominis

External obliques

This is a good exercise to develop the width of your upper back and is a valuable aid in most racket and field sports where power—the combination of strength and speed—can give you a competitive edge.

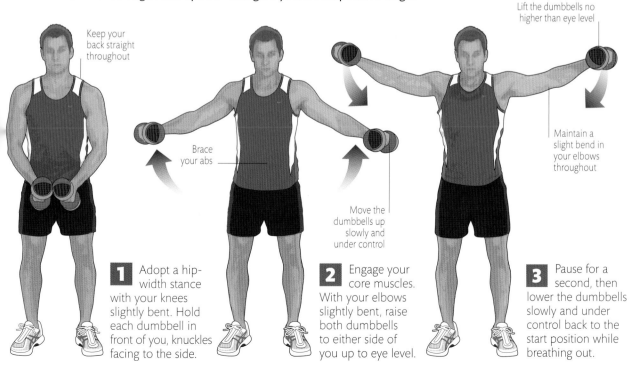

Keep your back straight throughout

Brace your abs

Move the dumbbells up slowly and under control

Lift the dumbbells no higher than eye level

Maintain a slight bend in your elbows throughout

1 Adopt a hip-width stance with your knees slightly bent. Hold each dumbbell in front of you, knuckles facing to the side.

2 Engage your core muscles. With your elbows slightly bent, raise both dumbbells to either side of you up to eye level.

3 Pause for a second, then lower the dumbbells slowly and under control back to the start position while breathing out.

REAR LATERAL RAISE

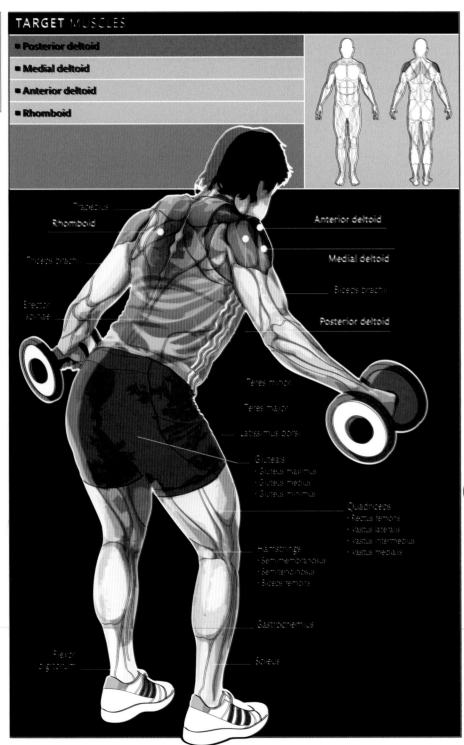

TARGET MUSCLES

- Posterior deltoid
- Medial deltoid
- Anterior deltoid
- Rhomboid

Trapezius
Rhomboid
Triceps brachii
Erector spinae

Anterior deltoid
Medial deltoid
Biceps brachii
Posterior deltoid

Teres minor
Teres major
Latissimus dorsi
Gluteals
· Gluteus maximus
· Gluteus medius
· Gluteus minimus

Hamstrings
· Semimembranosus
· Semitendinosus
· Biceps femoris

Quadriceps
· Rectus femoris
· Vastus lateralis
· Vastus intermedius
· Vastus medialis

Gastrocnemius

Flexor digitorum

Soleus

This is a great raw strength exercise that develops your shoulders and the muscles in the middle section of your back—principally, your rhomboids. You can perform the exercise standing, seated, or lying, but in all cases ensure that you maintain good body position to avoid engaging the larger muscles of your back.

VARIATION

Performing this exercise lying prone on a bench puts more emphasis on your medial deltoids and rhomboids. This variant is best performed with your legs fixed, making it a more advanced isolation exercise. You may also perform the exercise sitting at the end of a bench; here, keep your torso bent over to work your posterior deltoids, or more upright to emphasize your medial deltoids.

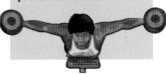

WARNING!

Rounding your back during this exercise may cause injury to your back or spine. Keep the movement of the weights slow and well balanced on both sides, trying not to move your knees, head, or spine; your elbows should be slightly bent and fixed at this angle throughout. Do not allow your shoulders to rise.

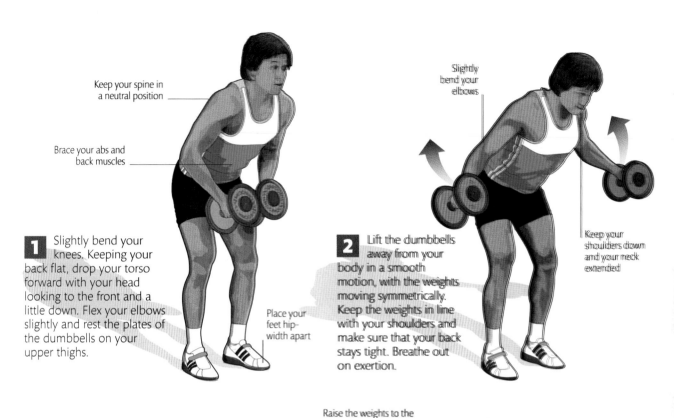

Keep your spine in a neutral position

Brace your abs and back muscles

1 Slightly bend your knees. Keeping your back flat, drop your torso forward with your head looking to the front and a little down. Flex your elbows slightly and rest the plates of the dumbbells on your upper thighs.

Place your feet hip-width apart

Slightly bend your elbows

2 Lift the dumbbells away from your body in a smooth motion, with the weights moving symmetrically. Keep the weights in line with your shoulders and make sure that your back stays tight. Breathe out on exertion.

Keep your shoulders down and your neck extended

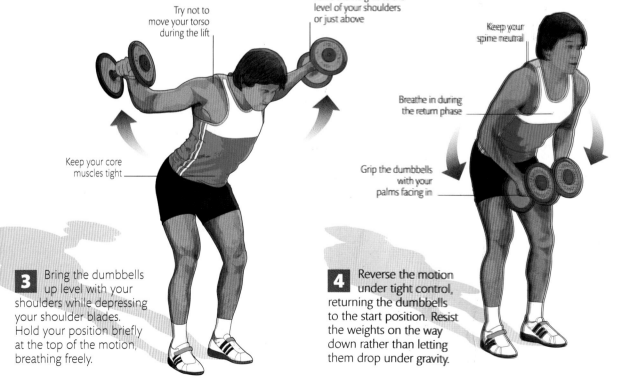

Try not to move your torso during the lift

Raise the weights to the level of your shoulders or just above

Keep your core muscles tight

3 Bring the dumbbells up level with your shoulders while depressing your shoulder blades. Hold your position briefly at the top of the motion, breathing freely.

Keep your spine neutral

Breathe in during the return phase

Grip the dumbbells with your palms facing in

4 Reverse the motion under tight control, returning the dumbbells to the start position. Resist the weights on the way down rather than letting them drop under gravity.

SCARECROW ROTATION

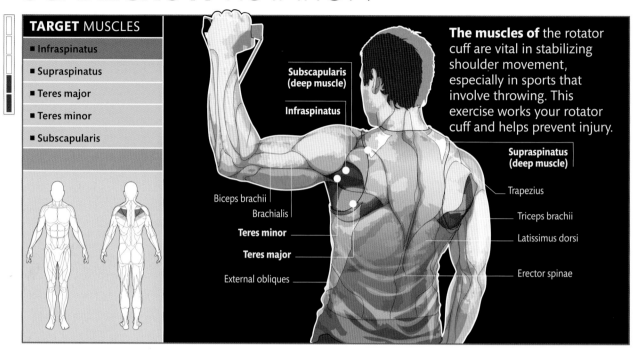

TARGET MUSCLES

- Infraspinatus
- Supraspinatus
- Teres major
- Teres minor
- Subscapularis

Subscapularis (deep muscle)

Infraspinatus

Biceps brachii

Brachialis

Teres minor

Teres major

External obliques

The muscles of the rotator cuff are vital in stabilizing shoulder movement, especially in sports that involve throwing. This exercise works your rotator cuff and helps prevent injury.

Supraspinatus (deep muscle)

Trapezius

Triceps brachii

Latissimus dorsi

Erector spinae

EXTERNAL DUMBBELL ROTATION

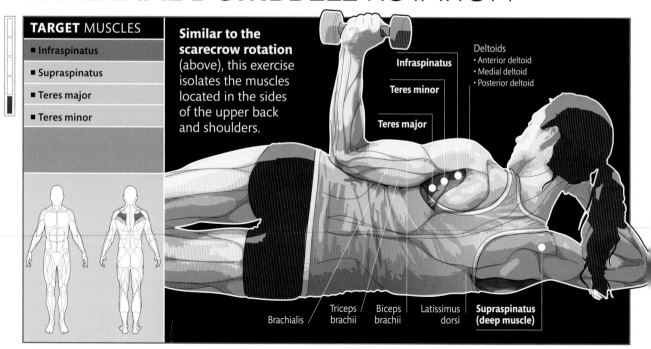

TARGET MUSCLES

- Infraspinatus
- Supraspinatus
- Teres major
- Teres minor

Similar to the scarecrow rotation (above), this exercise isolates the muscles located in the sides of the upper back and shoulders.

Infraspinatus

Teres minor

Teres major

Deltoids
- Anterior deltoid
- Medial deltoid
- Posterior deltoid

Brachialis

Triceps brachii

Biceps brachii

Latissimus dorsi

Supraspinatus (deep muscle)

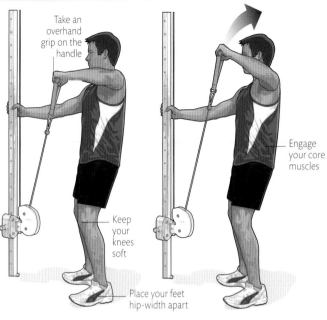

Take an overhand grip on the handle

Keep your knees soft

Place your feet hip-width apart

Engage your core muscles

Move your forearm to a vertical position

1 Stand facing a low pulley and grip the handle in one hand. Raise your elbow to the side in line with your shoulder.

2 Keeping your upper arm motionless, slowly pivot your forearm upward to a vertical position, breathing freely as you go.

3 Lower your forearm to the start position, breathing freely. Complete the set and repeat with your other arm.

VARIATION

You can increase the range of movement for this exercise by working with dumbbells on a bench. Support your body on an incline bench at an angle of 45 degrees and pivot your forearms, as described in the main exercise. Try to fit the scarecrow rotation into your regimen; it is often omitted because the muscles targeted are deep, so developing them does not directly enhance your appearance. However, damage to the rotator cuff is a very common injury and one that takes a lot of rehabilitation.

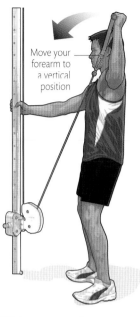

1 Lie on an exercise mat on one side, leaning neither forward nor backward. With your upper arm to your side and your forearm to the front of your body, take an overhand grip on a dumbbell; form a right angle at your elbow.

2 Keeping your upper arm as still as possible and your elbow fixed against your side, gently raise your forearm through a comfortable range of movement in a smooth, controlled action.

3 Maintaining your elbow at a right angle and pressed against your side, lower the dumbbell slowly to the start position and complete the set. Repeat with your other arm.

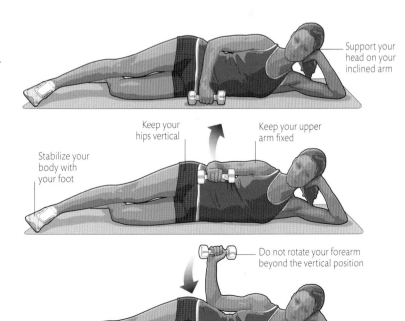

Support your head on your inclined arm

Keep your hips vertical

Keep your upper arm fixed

Stabilize your body with your foot

Do not rotate your forearm beyond the vertical position

INTERNAL ROTATION

TARGET MUSCLES

- Pectorals
- Supraspinatus
- Infraspinatus
- Subscapularis
- Teres major
- Teres minor

The purpose of this exercise is to develop your rotator cuff muscles and your pecs. A simple pulley exercise, it is mainly used in bodybuilding or in rehabilitation for a rotator cuff injury.

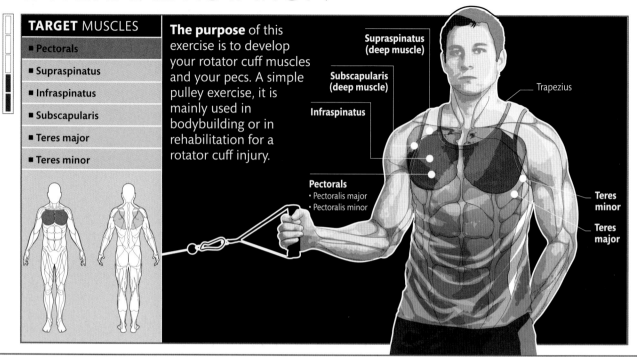

Supraspinatus (deep muscle)

Subscapularis (deep muscle)

Infraspinatus

Pectorals
• Pectoralis major
• Pectoralis minor

Trapezius

Teres minor

Teres major

EXTERNAL ROTATION

TARGET MUSCLES

- Infraspinatus
- Supraspinatus
- Subscapularis
- Teres major
- Teres minor

This exercise develops the muscles at the rear of your shoulder. It is often used in the rehabilitation of the shoulder after injury but also makes good preparation for throwing and racket sports.

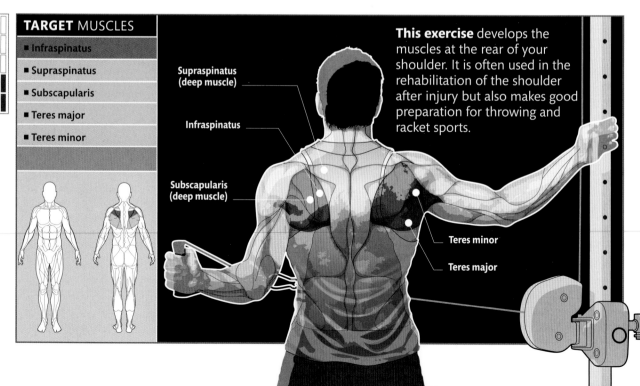

Supraspinatus (deep muscle)

Infraspinatus

Subscapularis (deep muscle)

Teres minor

Teres major

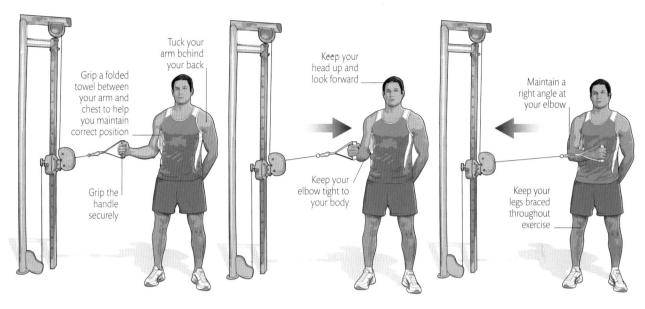

Grip a folded towel between your arm and chest to help you maintain correct position

Tuck your arm behind your back

Grip the handle securely

Keep your head up and look forward

Keep your elbow tight to your body

Maintain a right angle at your elbow

Keep your legs braced throughout exercise

1 Stand sideways to a pulley set at about waist height. Bend your elbow to 90 degrees and turn your arm out away from your body.

2 Keep your shoulders, hips, and feet in line. Pull the handle slowly and under control toward the middle of your body.

3 Bring your lower arm across as far as comfortable. Return slowly to the start position. Finish the set and then repeat for your other arm.

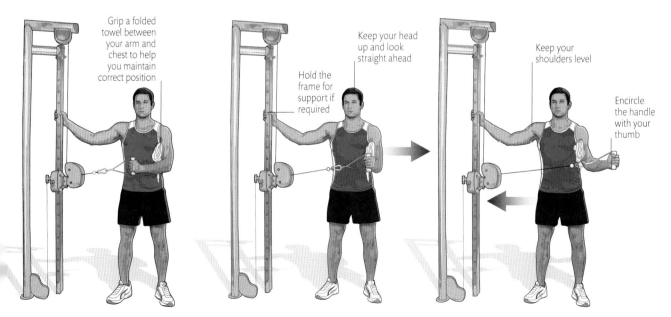

Grip a folded towel between your arm and chest to help you maintain correct position

Keep your head up and look straight ahead

Hold the frame for support if required

Keep your shoulders level

Encircle the handle with your thumb

1 Stand sideways to a pulley set at about waist height. Reach across your body and grip the handle, with your knuckles facing toward the pulley.

2 Keep your shoulders, hips, and feet in line. With your elbow bent and tight to your body, move your lower arm across and away from your body.

3 When you reach your full range of movement return to the start position under control. Finish the set and repeat for your other arm.

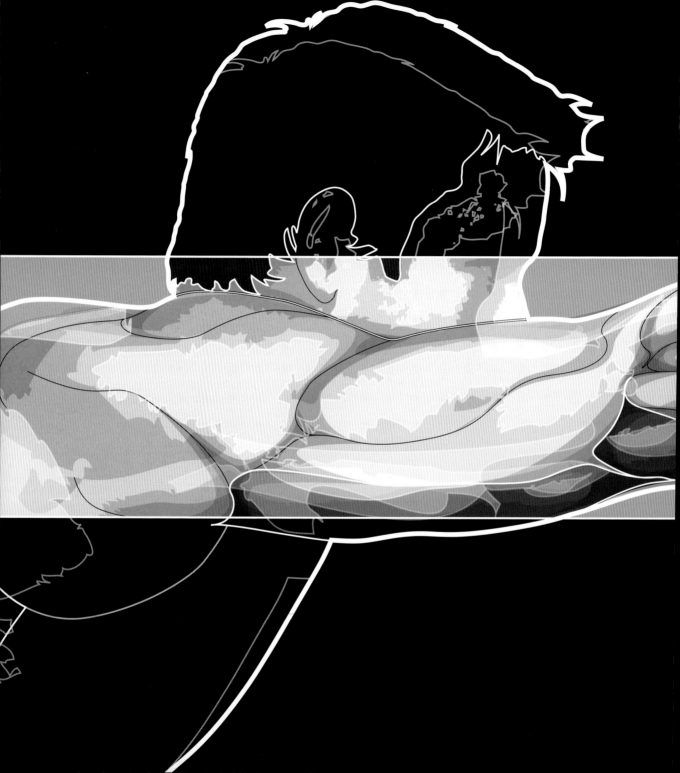

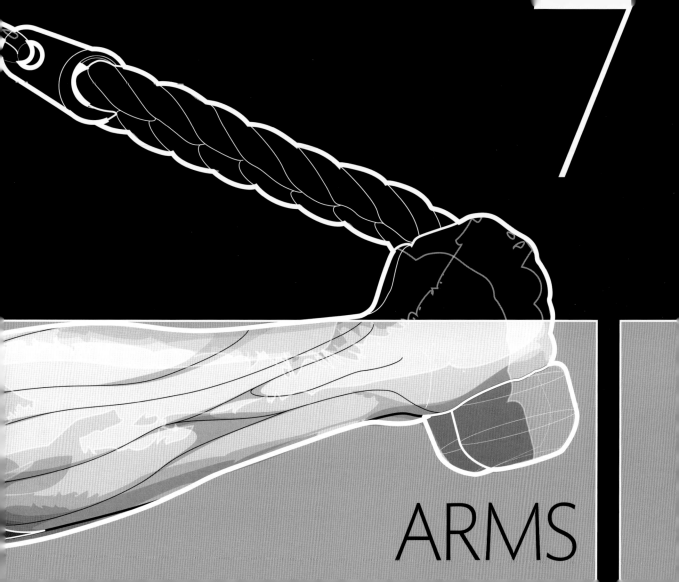

7

ARMS

BENCH DIP

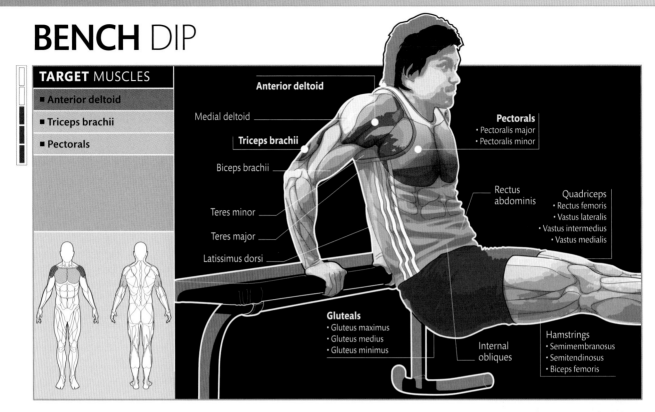

TARGET MUSCLES

- Anterior deltoid
- Triceps brachii
- Pectorals

Anterior deltoid

Medial deltoid

Triceps brachii

Biceps brachii

Teres minor

Teres major

Latissimus dorsi

Pectorals
• Pectoralis major
• Pectoralis minor

Rectus abdominis

Quadriceps
• Rectus femoris
• Vastus lateralis
• Vastus intermedius
• Vastus medialis

Gluteals
• Gluteus maximus
• Gluteus medius
• Gluteus minimus

Internal obliques

Hamstrings
• Semimembranosus
• Semitendinosus
• Biceps femoris

Bench dips are a good general upper body exercise and ideal training for the bench press. You can perform this exercise using just one bench to support your arms, though a second, lower bench beneath your feet makes the movement easier.

WARNING!

Make sure that the benches or other supports you use are strong and stable enough to carry your weight and that they are of sufficient height to allow you a full range of motion.

Do not force your shoulder joints beyond their normal range of movement and avoid rounding your back or allowing it to move away too far from the edge of the bench.

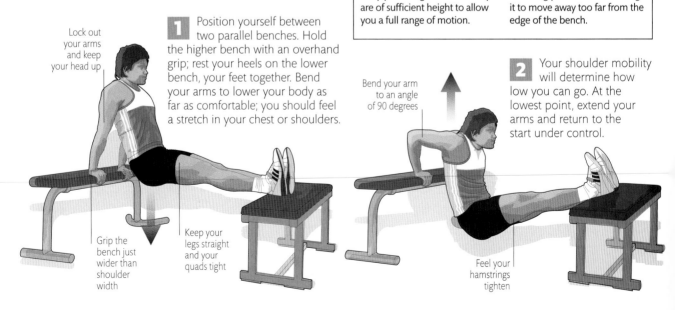

1 Position yourself between two parallel benches. Hold the higher bench with an overhand grip; rest your heels on the lower bench, your feet together. Bend your arms to lower your body as far as comfortable; you should feel a stretch in your chest or shoulders.

Lock out your arms and keep your head up

Grip the bench just wider than shoulder width

Keep your legs straight and your quads tight

Bend your arm to an angle of 90 degrees

2 Your shoulder mobility will determine how low you can go. At the lowest point, extend your arms and return to the start under control.

Feel your hamstrings tighten

BAR DIP

TARGET MUSCLES

- Triceps
- Anterior deltoid
- Pectorals

Bar dips help to build upper body strength and are ideal in training for throwing events. Good technique takes practice; if you are just starting out, let the knee pad on an assisted dip machine take part of your weight as you build strength.

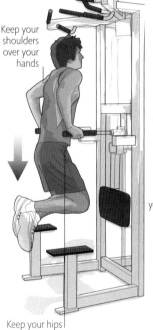

1 Grip the parallel bars with your palms facing each other. Hold your weight on locked arms and cross your feet to help keep you stable.

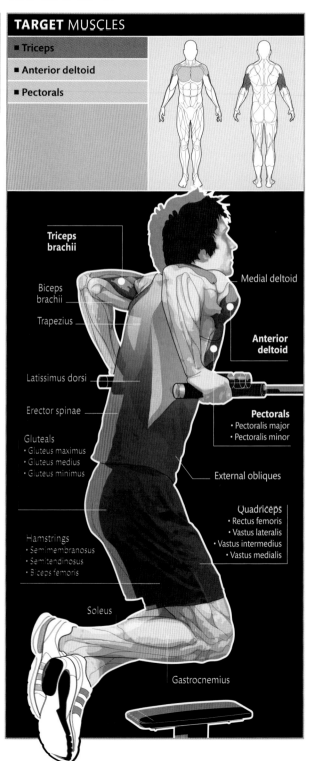

Triceps brachii

Biceps brachii

Trapezius

Medial deltoid

Anterior deltoid

Latissimus dorsi

Erector spinae

Pectorals
• Pectoralis major
• Pectoralis minor

Gluteals
• Gluteus maximus
• Gluteus medius
• Gluteus minimus

External obliques

Quadriceps
• Rectus femoris
• Vastus lateralis
• Vastus intermedius
• Vastus medialis

Hamstrings
• Semimembranosus
• Semitendinosus
• Biceps femoris

Soleus

Gastrocnemius

Keep your shoulders over your hands

2 Take a deep breath. Keeping your body straight, unlock your elbows and start to lower your body between the bars, trying to maintain an upright posture.

Do not let your elbows splay out beyond your wrists

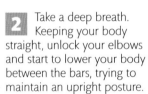

Keep your hips beneath your shoulders

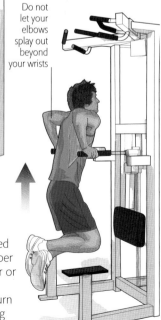

3 Once you have lowered yourself until your upper arms are parallel to the floor or you cannot go any farther, immediately push up to return to the start position, exhaling as you go.

DUMBBELL TRICEPS EXTENSION

TARGET MUSCLES

- Triceps brachii
- Anconeus

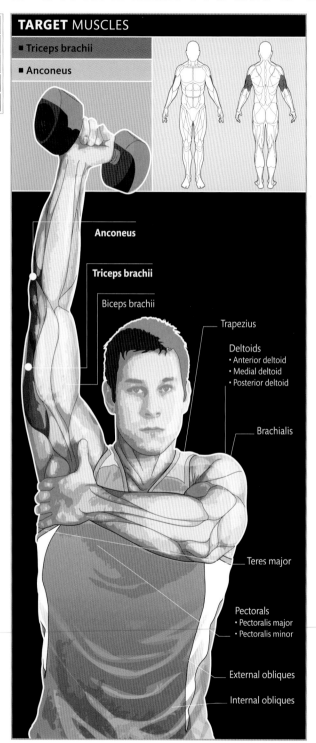

Anconeus

Triceps brachii

Biceps brachii

Trapezius

Deltoids
- Anterior deltoid
- Medial deltoid
- Posterior deltoid

Brachialis

Teres major

Pectorals
- Pectoralis major
- Pectoralis minor

External obliques

Internal obliques

This exercise targets your triceps, which constitute most of the mass of your upper arm. Performed standing rather than seated or lying, this movement also engages your core muscles, providing the added benefit of building trunk strength.

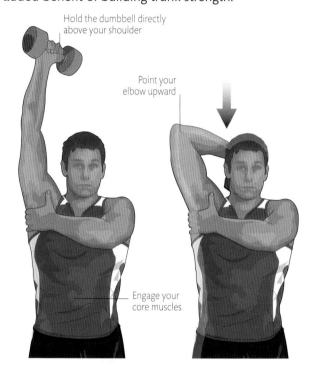

Hold the dumbbell directly above your shoulder

Point your elbow upward

Engage your core muscles

1 Stand with your feet hip-width apart and your knees relaxed. Hold a dumbbell in one hand and raise it overhead to arm's length. Use your free arm to brace across your body.

2 Lower the dumbbell behind your head, keeping your back straight. Pause briefly at the bottom of the motion, then slowly raise the dumbbell to the start position.

VARIATION

If you are a beginner, keeping your body balanced while performing the exercise standing up can be tricky. To improve your stability, try holding on to a solid support with your free hand or perform the exercise sitting on a bench, preferably one with a back support.

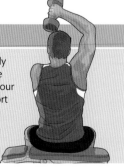

BARBELL TRICEPS EXTENSION

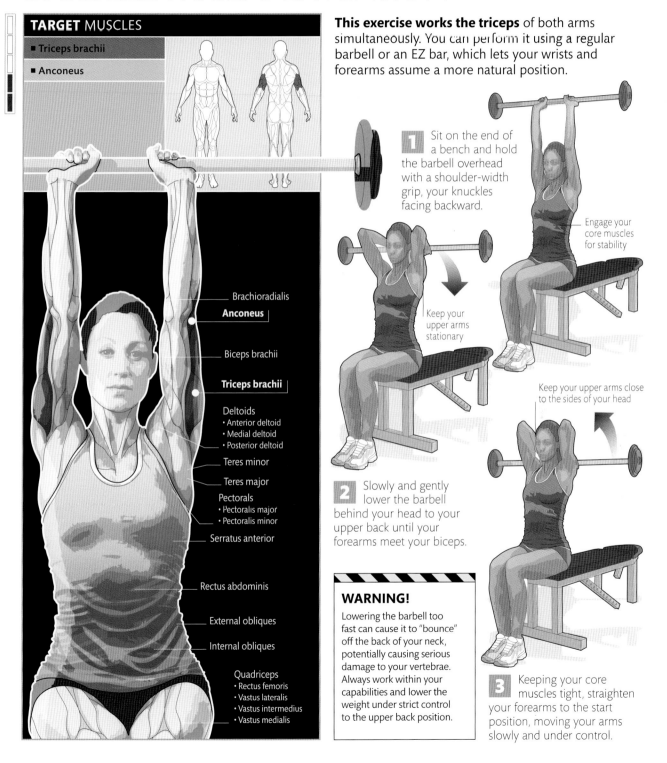

TARGET MUSCLES

- Triceps brachii
- Anconeus

This exercise works the triceps of both arms simultaneously. You can perform it using a regular barbell or an EZ bar, which lets your wrists and forearms assume a more natural position.

Brachioradialis

Anconeus

Biceps brachii

Triceps brachii

Deltoids
- Anterior deltoid
- Medial deltoid
- Posterior deltoid

Teres minor

Teres major

Pectorals
- Pectoralis major
- Pectoralis minor

Serratus anterior

Rectus abdominis

External obliques

Internal obliques

Quadriceps
- Rectus femoris
- Vastus lateralis
- Vastus intermedius
- Vastus medialis

1 Sit on the end of a bench and hold the barbell overhead with a shoulder-width grip, your knuckles facing backward.

Engage your core muscles for stability

Keep your upper arms stationary

Keep your upper arms close to the sides of your head

2 Slowly and gently lower the barbell behind your head to your upper back until your forearms meet your biceps.

WARNING!

Lowering the barbell too fast can cause it to "bounce" off the back of your neck, potentially causing serious damage to your vertebrae. Always work within your capabilities and lower the weight under strict control to the upper back position.

3 Keeping your core muscles tight, straighten your forearms to the start position, moving your arms slowly and under control.

PRONE TRICEPS EXTENSION

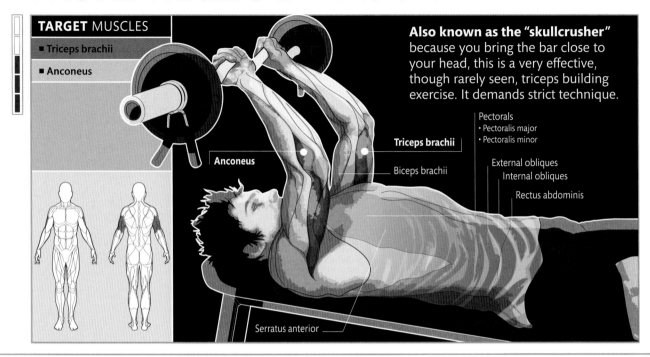

TARGET MUSCLES

- Triceps brachii
- Anconeus

Also known as the "skullcrusher" because you bring the bar close to your head, this is a very effective, though rarely seen, triceps building exercise. It demands strict technique.

Anconeus

Triceps brachii

Biceps brachii

Pectorals
• Pectoralis major
• Pectoralis minor

External obliques
Internal obliques

Rectus abdominis

Serratus anterior

TRICEPS KICKBACK

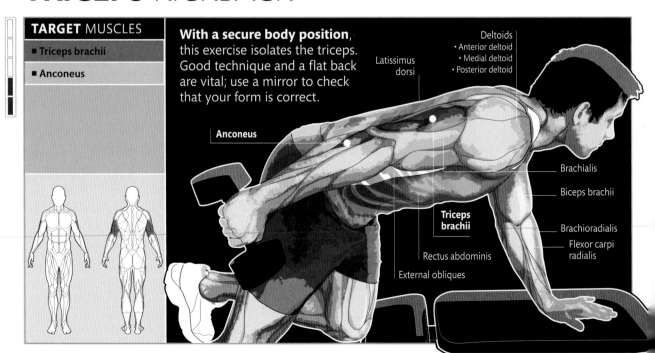

TARGET MUSCLES

- Triceps brachii
- Anconeus

With a secure body position, this exercise isolates the triceps. Good technique and a flat back are vital; use a mirror to check that your form is correct.

Anconeus

Latissimus dorsi

Deltoids
• Anterior deltoid
• Medial deltoid
• Posterior deltoid

Triceps brachii

Rectus abdominis

External obliques

Brachialis

Biceps brachii

Brachioradialis

Flexor carpi radialis

Position your hands so that your knuckles point backward

Pivot only at the elbow

Keep your core muscles engaged

Do not allow your elbows to splay out

WARNING!

This exercise is not called the skullcrusher for nothing! Keep your movement under close control and slow the descent of the bar as it nears your head. Be sure to lower the bar toward your forehead, not to the level of your nose; this helps to ease the strain on your wrists.

1 Lie on a bench with your feet flat on the floor and take a shoulder-width grip on the EZ bar with your arms straight above your chest.

2 Fix your shoulders and core. Bend at your elbows only—not your shoulders—to lower the barbell slowly to just above your forehead.

3 Pause at the bottom of the movement, then slowly straighten your forearms under control back to the start position.

Kneel on the bench to stabilize your body

Keep your upper arm in line with your back

Keep your upper body almost parallel to the floor

Hold the weight with an overhand grip

WARNING!

Raise and lower the dumbbell slowly; swinging the weight can cause twisting of your trunk making your lower back unstable and prone to injury.

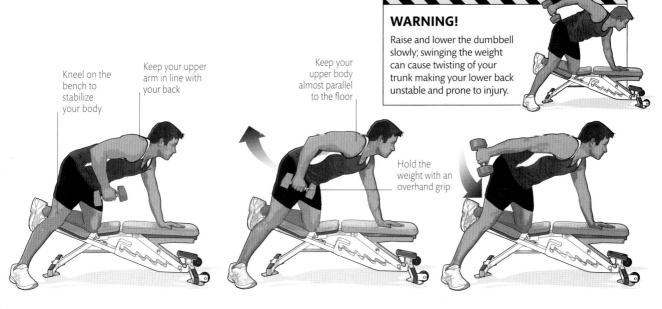

1 Support your left knee and left hand on a bench; bend from the hips, while gripping a dumbbell in your right hand.

2 Brace your body. Pivot at your elbow to straighten your arm, lifting the weight slowly and under close control to a horizontal position.

3 Pause briefly at the top of the motion; slowly bring the dumbbell back to the start position. Complete the set, then repeat with your other arm.

CLOSE-GRIP BENCH PRESS

TARGET MUSCLES

- Triceps
- Deltoids
- Pectorals

This exercise is similar at first glance to the regular bench press, but bringing your hands closer together on the bar places far more emphasis on the triceps and anterior deltoids than on the chest. The close-grip bench press helps build big triceps and is a good assistance exercise for competition power lifting.

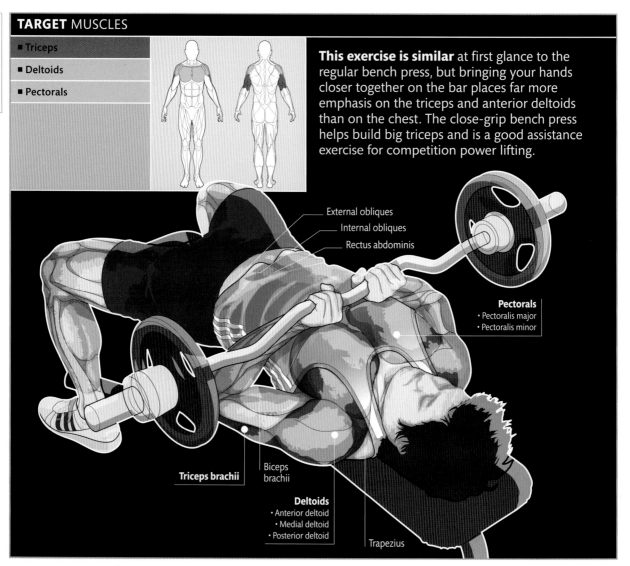

- External obliques
- Internal obliques
- Rectus abdominis

Pectorals
- Pectoralis major
- Pectoralis minor

Triceps brachii

Biceps brachii

Deltoids
- Anterior deltoid
- Medial deltoid
- Posterior deltoid

Trapezius

VARIATION

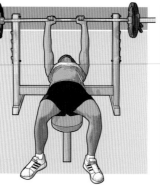

You can use an Olympic bar or a straight training bar for this exercise. Grip the bar a little narrower than shoulder-width, but don't place your hands too close together, because the exercise will become less effective for your triceps and will likely place excessive stress on your wrists.

VARIATION

The close-grip push-up is a related exercise that targets the the triceps with a resistance of approximately two-thirds of your body weight. By adjusting the position of your hands and the direction of your elbows, you can isolate very specific areas of your triceps and deltoids. The exercise is also very safe and does not require the use of any equipment.

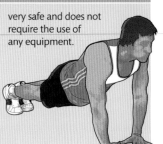

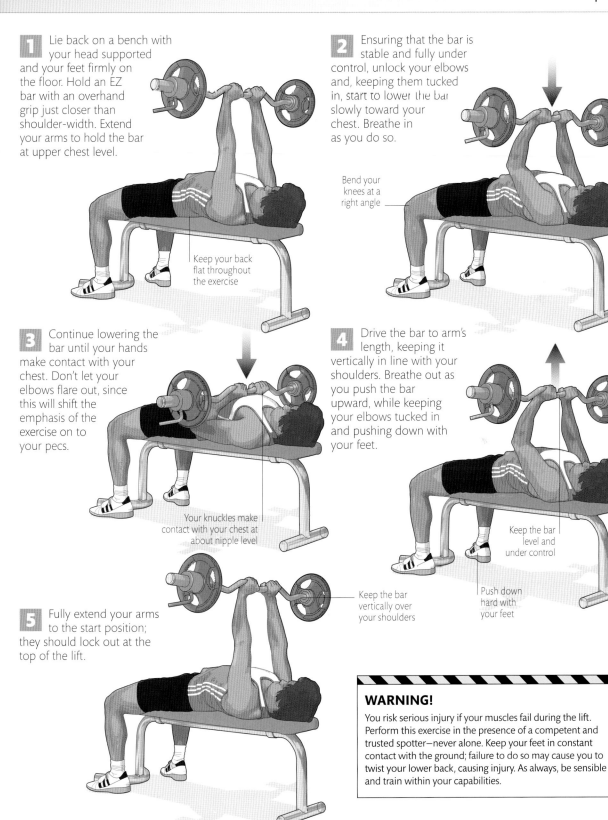

1 Lie back on a bench with your head supported and your feet firmly on the floor. Hold an EZ bar with an overhand grip just closer than shoulder-width. Extend your arms to hold the bar at upper chest level.

Keep your back flat throughout the exercise

2 Ensuring that the bar is stable and fully under control, unlock your elbows and, keeping them tucked in, start to lower the bar slowly toward your chest. Breathe in as you do so.

Bend your knees at a right angle

3 Continue lowering the bar until your hands make contact with your chest. Don't let your elbows flare out, since this will shift the emphasis of the exercise on to your pecs.

Your knuckles make contact with your chest at about nipple level

4 Drive the bar to arm's length, keeping it vertically in line with your shoulders. Breathe out as you push the bar upward, while keeping your elbows tucked in and pushing down with your feet.

Keep the bar level and under control

Keep the bar vertically over your shoulders

Push down hard with your feet

5 Fully extend your arms to the start position; they should lock out at the top of the lift.

WARNING!

You risk serious injury if your muscles fail during the lift. Perform this exercise in the presence of a competent and trusted spotter—never alone. Keep your feet in constant contact with the ground; failure to do so may cause you to twist your lower back, causing injury. As always, be sensible and train within your capabilities.

TRICEPS PUSH-DOWN

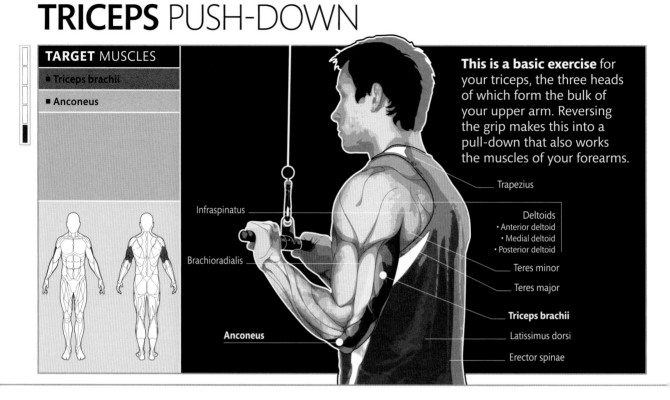

TARGET MUSCLES
- Triceps brachii
- Anconeus

This is a basic exercise for your triceps, the three heads of which form the bulk of your upper arm. Reversing the grip makes this into a pull-down that also works the muscles of your forearms.

Infraspinatus

Brachioradialis

Anconeus

Trapezius

Deltoids
- Anterior deltoid
- Medial deltoid
- Posterior deltoid

Teres minor

Teres major

Triceps brachii

Latissimus dorsi

Erector spinae

OVERHEAD TRICEPS EXTENSION

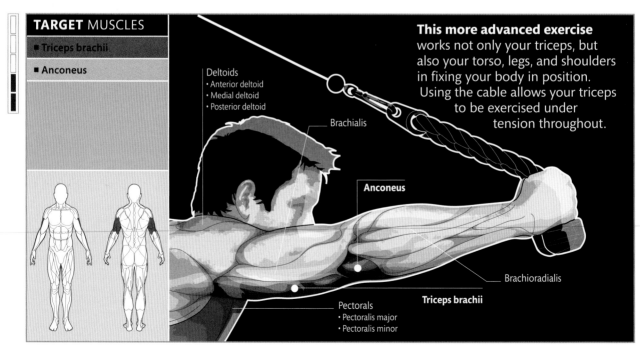

TARGET MUSCLES
- Triceps brachii
- Anconeus

This more advanced exercise works not only your triceps, but also your torso, legs, and shoulders in fixing your body in position. Using the cable allows your triceps to be exercised under tension throughout.

Deltoids
- Anterior deltoid
- Medial deltoid
- Posterior deltoid

Brachialis

Anconeus

Brachioradialis

Triceps brachii

Pectorals
- Pectoralis major
- Pectoralis minor

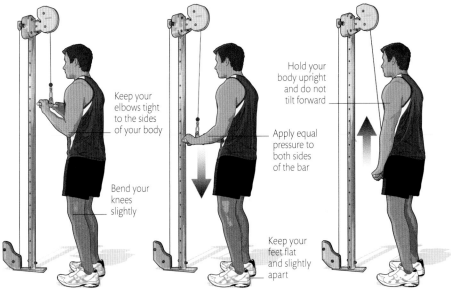

Keep your elbows tight to the sides of your body

Bend your knees slightly

Hold your body upright and do not tilt forward

Apply equal pressure to both sides of the bar

Keep your feet flat and slightly apart

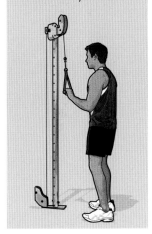

VARIATION

You can perform the triceps push-down with a rope, a V-bar, or a handle (to work one arm at a time if your arms are unevenly developed). In each case, the basic principle remains the same. Your elbow joint acts as a pivot and should not move from your side.

1 Set the pulley to a high position, select your desired weight on the stack, and take an overhand grip on the bar.

2 Push the bar down slowly and under control, using your elbow joints as pivots. Keep your trunk, legs, and hips stationary.

3 Pause at the bottom of the movement with your triceps fully contracted before returning slowly to the start position.

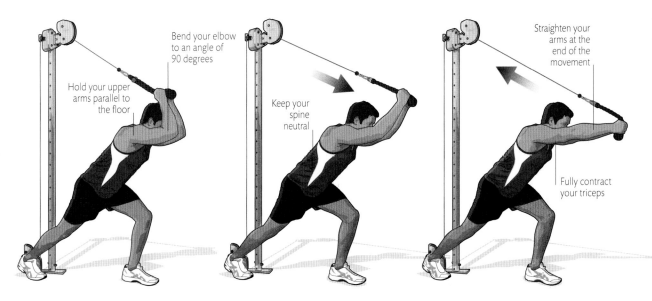

Hold your upper arms parallel to the floor

Bend your elbow to an angle of 90 degrees

Keep your spine neutral

Straighten your arms at the end of the movement

Fully contract your triceps

1 Select your desired weight on the stack and attach a rope to the high pulley cable. Take up a braced split-leg position. Grip the rope so that your elbows point forward and your arms are tight to the sides of your head.

2 From your braced position, with your abs and core muscles tight, extend your arms and contract your triceps in a slow controlled pull. Keep your torso and hips in the same position throughout.

3 Extend your arms until your triceps are fully contracted, exhaling as you go. Return slowly and under control to the start position, with your hands close to the sides of your head and your body well braced.

BARBELL CURL

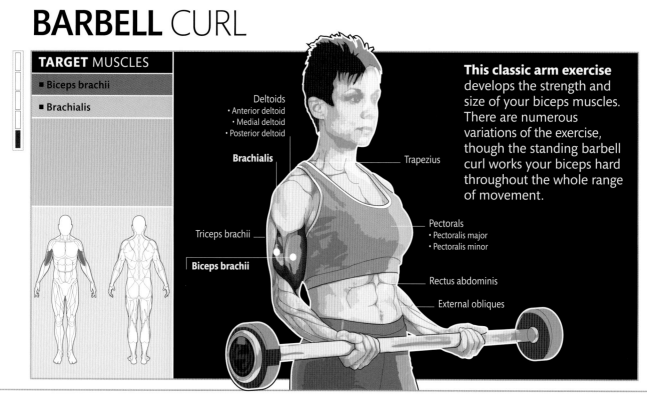

TARGET MUSCLES
- Biceps brachii
- Brachialis

Deltoids
- Anterior deltoid
- Medial deltoid
- Posterior deltoid

Brachialis

Trapezius

Triceps brachii

Biceps brachii

Pectorals
- Pectoralis major
- Pectoralis minor

Rectus abdominis

External obliques

This classic arm exercise develops the strength and size of your biceps muscles. There are numerous variations of the exercise, though the standing barbell curl works your biceps hard throughout the whole range of movement.

HAMMER DUMBBELL CURL

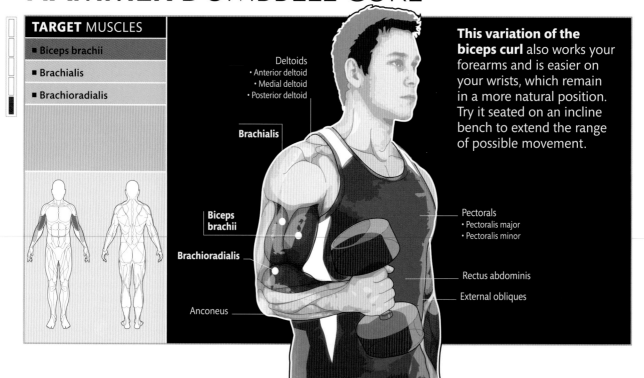

TARGET MUSCLES
- Biceps brachii
- Brachialis
- Brachioradialis

Deltoids
- Anterior deltoid
- Medial deltoid
- Posterior deltoid

Brachialis

Biceps brachii

Brachioradialis

Anconeus

Pectorals
- Pectoralis major
- Pectoralis minor

Rectus abdominis

External obliques

This variation of the biceps curl also works your forearms and is easier on your wrists, which remain in a more natural position. Try it seated on an incline bench to extend the range of possible movement.

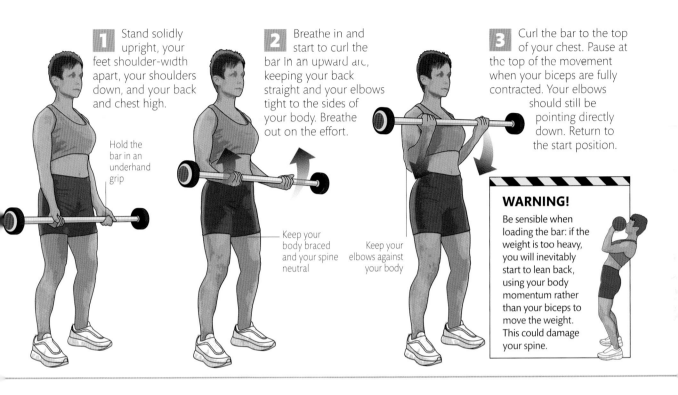

1 Stand solidly upright, your feet shoulder-width apart, your shoulders down, and your back and chest high.

Hold the bar in an underhand grip

2 Breathe in and start to curl the bar in an upward arc, keeping your back straight and your elbows tight to the sides of your body. Breathe out on the effort.

Keep your body braced and your spine neutral

Keep your elbows against your body

3 Curl the bar to the top of your chest. Pause at the top of the movement when your biceps are fully contracted. Your elbows should still be pointing directly down. Return to the start position.

WARNING!
Be sensible when loading the bar: if the weight is too heavy, you will inevitably start to lean back, using your body momentum rather than your biceps to move the weight. This could damage your spine.

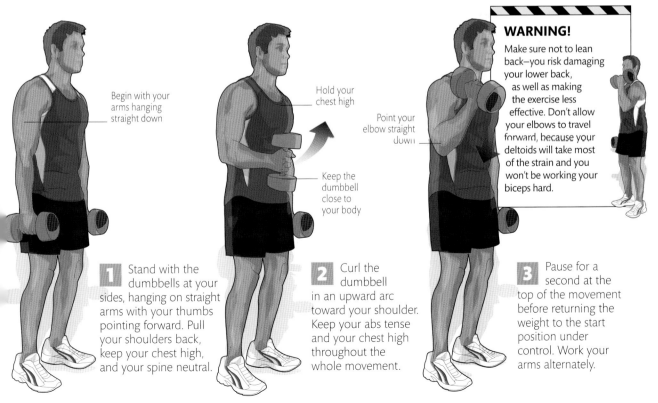

Begin with your arms hanging straight down

Hold your chest high

Keep the dumbbell close to your body

Point your elbow straight down

WARNING!
Make sure not to lean back—you risk damaging your lower back, as well as making the exercise less effective. Don't allow your elbows to travel forward, because your deltoids will take most of the strain and you won't be working your biceps hard.

1 Stand with the dumbbells at your sides, hanging on straight arms with your thumbs pointing forward. Pull your shoulders back, keep your chest high, and your spine neutral.

2 Curl the dumbbell in an upward arc toward your shoulder. Keep your abs tense and your chest high throughout the whole movement.

3 Pause for a second at the top of the movement before returning the weight to the start position under control. Work your arms alternately.

INCLINE DUMBBELL CURL

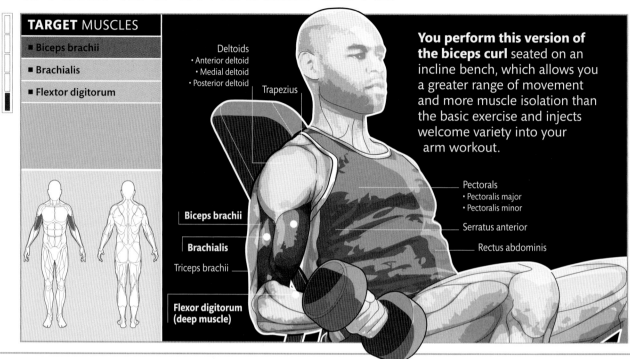

TARGET MUSCLES

- Biceps brachii
- Brachialis
- Flexor digitorum

You perform this version of the biceps curl seated on an incline bench, which allows you a greater range of movement and more muscle isolation than the basic exercise and injects welcome variety into your arm workout.

Deltoids
- Anterior deltoid
- Medial deltoid
- Posterior deltoid

Trapezius

Pectorals
- Pectoralis major
- Pectoralis minor

Serratus anterior

Rectus abdominis

Biceps brachii

Brachialis

Triceps brachii

Flexor digitorum (deep muscle)

CONCENTRATION CURL

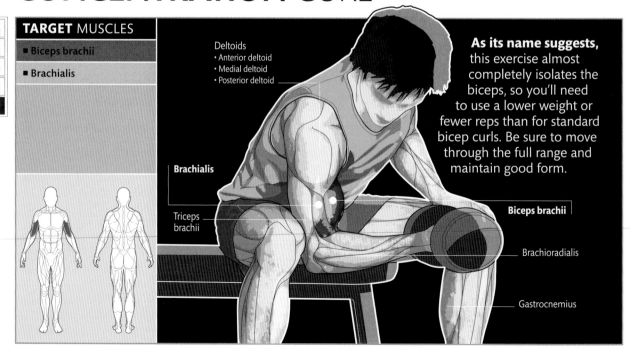

TARGET MUSCLES

- Biceps brachii
- Brachialis

As its name suggests, this exercise almost completely isolates the biceps, so you'll need to use a lower weight or fewer reps than for standard bicep curls. Be sure to move through the full range and maintain good form.

Deltoids
- Anterior deltoid
- Medial deltoid
- Posterior deltoid

Brachialis

Triceps brachii

Biceps brachii

Brachioradialis

Gastrocnemius

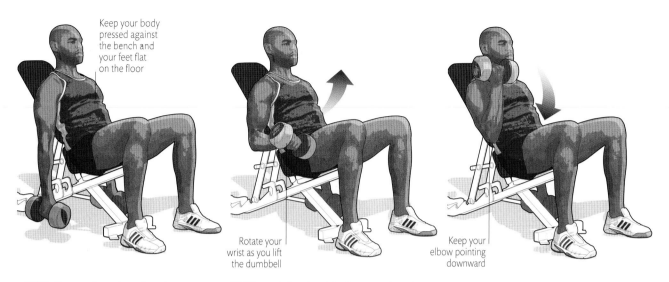

Keep your body pressed against the bench and your feet flat on the floor

Rotate your wrist as you lift the dumbbell

Keep your elbow pointing downward

1 Sit on a bench inclined at a 45-degree angle. Grip a dumbbell in each hand and allow your arms to hang down from your shoulders. Make sure your back is well supported.

2 Curl the dumbbell in one hand in an upward arc toward your shoulder, without allowing it to swing. As you do so, slowly turn your inner wrist toward your upper arm.

3 Pause for a second at the top of the movement before returning to the start position, with your arm hanging straight down. Repeat with your other arm.

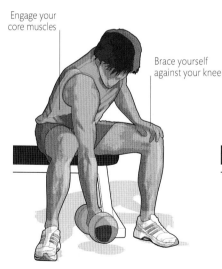

Engage your core muscles

Brace yourself against your knee

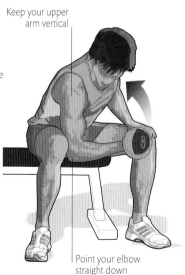

Keep your upper arm vertical

Point your elbow straight down

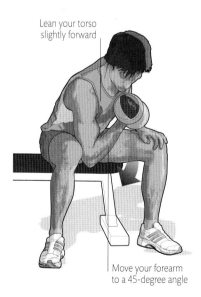

Lean your torso slightly forward

Move your forearm to a 45-degree angle

1 Sit on the end of a bench with your thighs parallel to the floor and your body braced. Hold the back of your upper arm against your inner thigh and let your arm hang down.

2 Curl the weight upward, making sure that your elbow does not move forward and that the back of your upper arm stays in contact with your inner thigh.

3 Pause once you have fully contracted your biceps to take your forearm to a 45-degree angle. Return under control and finish the set before repeating with your other arm.

PREACHER CURL

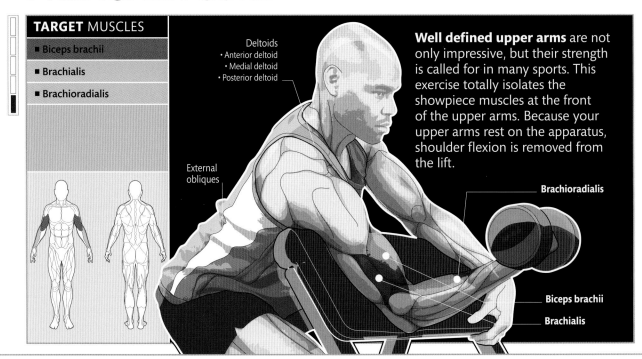

TARGET MUSCLES

- Biceps brachii
- Brachialis
- Brachioradialis

Deltoids
· Anterior deltoid
· Medial deltoid
· Posterior deltoid

External obliques

Brachioradialis

Biceps brachii

Brachialis

Well defined upper arms are not only impressive, but their strength is called for in many sports. This exercise totally isolates the showpiece muscles at the front of the upper arms. Because your upper arms rest on the apparatus, shoulder flexion is removed from the lift.

PULLEY CURL

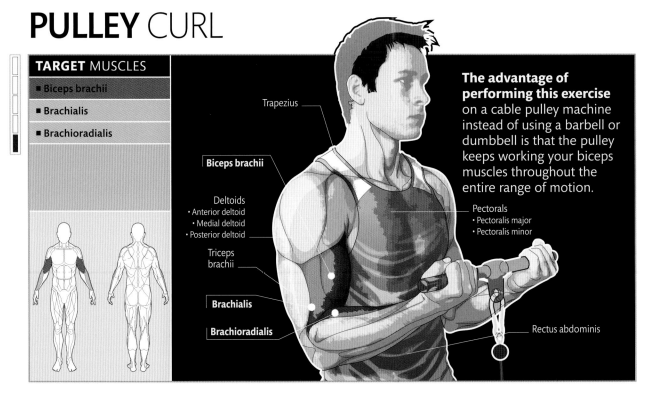

TARGET MUSCLES

- Biceps brachii
- Brachialis
- Brachioradialis

Trapezius

Biceps brachii

Deltoids
· Anterior deltoid
· Medial deltoid
· Posterior deltoid

Triceps brachii

Brachialis

Brachioradialis

Pectorals
· Pectoralis major
· Pectoralis minor

Rectus abdominis

The advantage of performing this exercise on a cable pulley machine instead of using a barbell or dumbbell is that the pulley keeps working your biceps muscles throughout the entire range of motion.

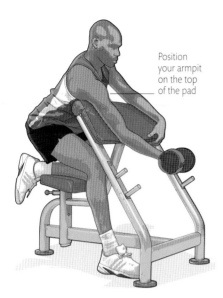

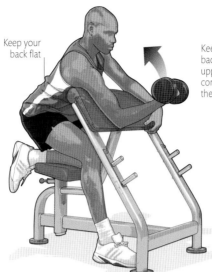

Position your armpit on the top of the pad

Keep your back flat

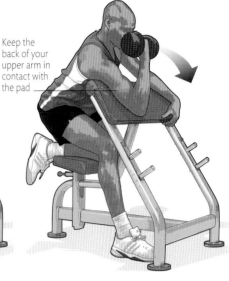

Keep the back of your upper arm in contact with the pad

1 Sit or kneel on the bench with the back of your upper arm on the pad. Grip the dumbbell with your palm facing upward.

2 Raise the dumbbell slowly toward your shoulder through the full range of movement, while inhaling deeply.

3 Lower the dumbbell slowly and under control to the start position. Repeat to complete the set, then change to the other arm.

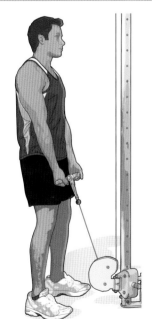

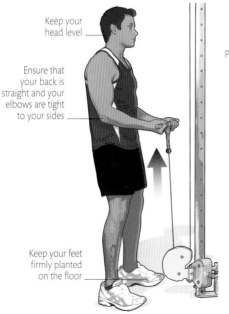

Keep your head level

Ensure that your back is straight and your elbows are tight to your sides

Keep your feet firmly planted on the floor

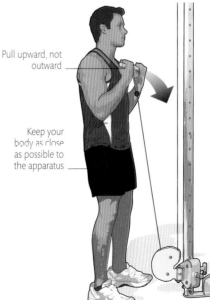

Pull upward, not outward

Keep your body as close as possible to the apparatus

1 Set the pulley to a low position. Stand with your feet hip-width apart and your knees slightly bent. Grip the bar with your palms forward.

2 Raise the bar slowly upward toward your chest by bending your arm at your elbow. Breathe out as you do so. Do not lean back.

3 Pause briefly at the top of the movement, then lower the bar slowly to rest across your thighs in the start position.

REVERSE BARBELL CURL

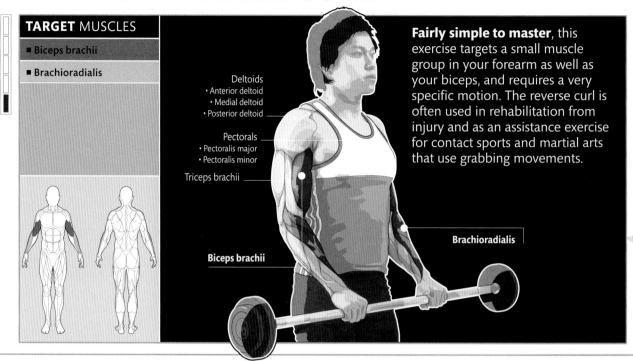

TARGET MUSCLES

- Biceps brachii
- Brachioradialis

Deltoids
· Anterior deltoid
· Medial deltoid
· Posterior deltoid

Pectorals
· Pectoralis major
· Pectoralis minor

Triceps brachii

Biceps brachii

Brachioradialis

Fairly simple to master, this exercise targets a small muscle group in your forearm as well as your biceps, and requires a very specific motion. The reverse curl is often used in rehabilitation from injury and as an assistance exercise for contact sports and martial arts that use grabbing movements.

REVERSE PULLEY CURL

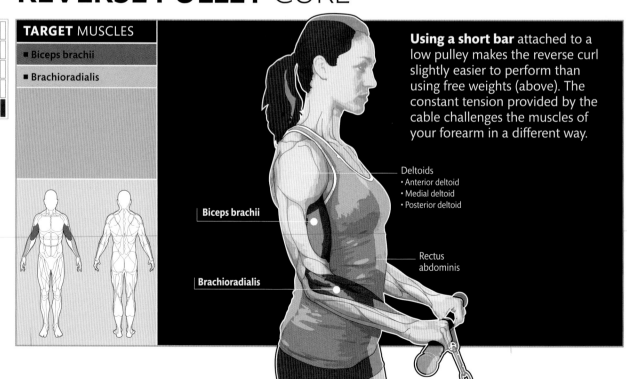

TARGET MUSCLES

- Biceps brachii
- Brachioradialis

Biceps brachii

Deltoids
· Anterior deltoid
· Medial deltoid
· Posterior deltoid

Rectus abdominis

Brachioradialis

Using a short bar attached to a low pulley makes the reverse curl slightly easier to perform than using free weights (above). The constant tension provided by the cable challenges the muscles of your forearm in a different way.

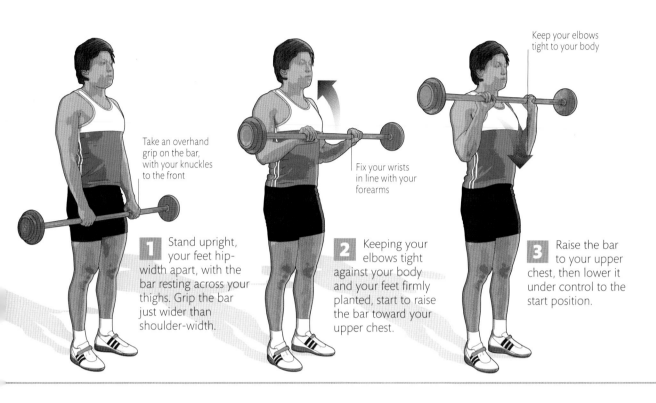

Take an overhand grip on the bar, with your knuckles to the front

1 Stand upright, your feet hip-width apart, with the bar resting across your thighs. Grip the bar just wider than shoulder-width.

Fix your wrists in line with your forearms

2 Keeping your elbows tight against your body and your feet firmly planted, start to raise the bar toward your upper chest.

Keep your elbows tight to your body

3 Raise the bar to your upper chest, then lower it under control to the start position.

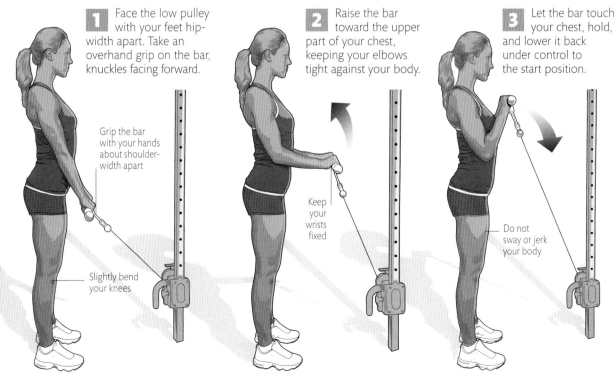

1 Face the low pulley with your feet hip-width apart. Take an overhand grip on the bar, knuckles facing forward.

Grip the bar with your hands about shoulder-width apart

Slightly bend your knees

2 Raise the bar toward the upper part of your chest, keeping your elbows tight against your body.

Keep your wrists fixed

3 Let the bar touch your chest, hold, and lower it back under control to the start position.

Do not sway or jerk your body

WRIST EXTENSION

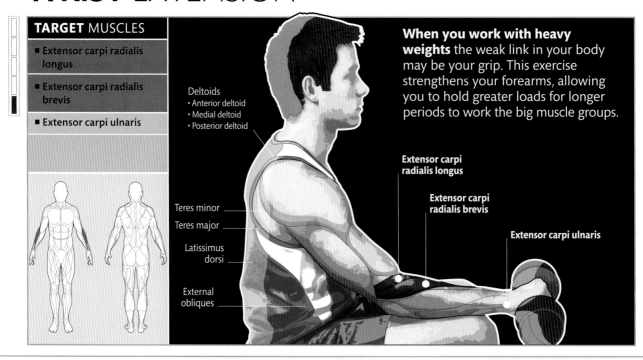

TARGET MUSCLES

- Extensor carpi radialis longus
- Extensor carpi radialis brevis
- Extensor carpi ulnaris

When you work with heavy weights the weak link in your body may be your grip. This exercise strengthens your forearms, allowing you to hold greater loads for longer periods to work the big muscle groups.

Deltoids
- Anterior deltoid
- Medial deltoid
- Posterior deltoid

Teres minor
Teres major
Latissimus dorsi
External obliques

Extensor carpi radialis longus
Extensor carpi radialis brevis
Extensor carpi ulnaris

WRIST FLEXION

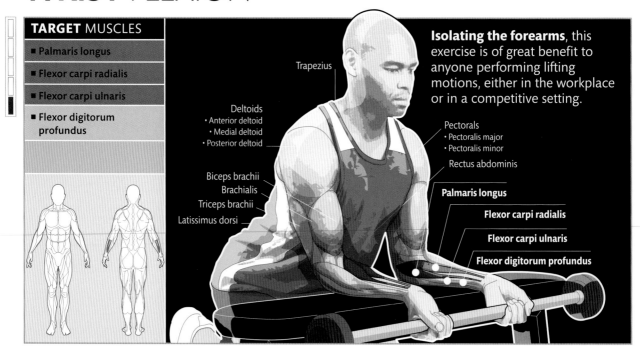

TARGET MUSCLES

- Palmaris longus
- Flexor carpi radialis
- Flexor carpi ulnaris
- Flexor digitorum profundus

Isolating the forearms, this exercise is of great benefit to anyone performing lifting motions, either in the workplace or in a competitive setting.

Trapezius

Deltoids
- Anterior deltoid
- Medial deltoid
- Posterior deltoid

Biceps brachii
Brachialis
Triceps brachii
Latissimus dorsi

Pectorals
- Pectoralis major
- Pectoralis minor
Rectus abdominis

Palmaris longus
Flexor carpi radialis
Flexor carpi ulnaris
Flexor digitorum profundus

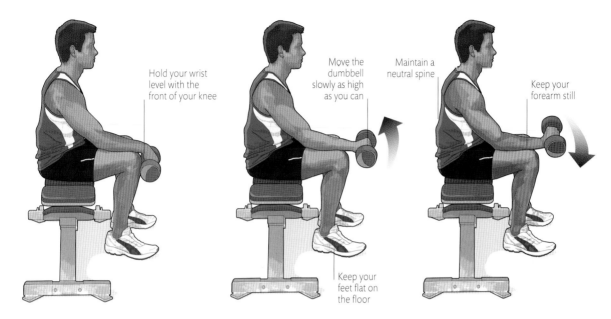

Hold your wrist level with the front of your knee

Move the dumbbell slowly as high as you can

Maintain a neutral spine

Keep your forearm still

Keep your feet flat on the floor

1 Sit on a bench holding one dumbbell in an overhand grip. Rest your forearm along the top of your thigh.

2 Keeping your forearm motionless, use your wrist to raise the dumbbell slowly and under control beyond the horizontal position.

3 Slowly lower the dumbbell to the start position, using your wrist alone. Complete the set before repeating with your other arm.

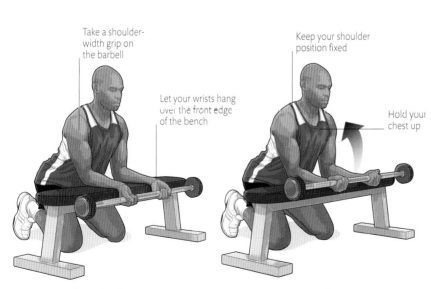

Take a shoulder-width grip on the barbell

Let your wrists hang over the front edge of the bench

Keep your shoulder position fixed

Hold your chest up

Maintain a tight grip on the barbell

WARNING!
Don't let the bar roll toward your fingers in the lowering phase because you risk injuring your wrist or dropping the weight.

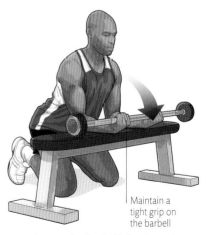

1 Kneel on the floor or on a mat, facing a bench. Holding a barbell with your palms up, rest your forearms across the bench pad.

2 Keeping your forearms motionless, pivot slowly at your wrists to take the barbell up as high as you can manage.

3 Lower the barbell slowly to the start position without extending your arms or leaning forward. Keep a strong grip on the bar throughout.

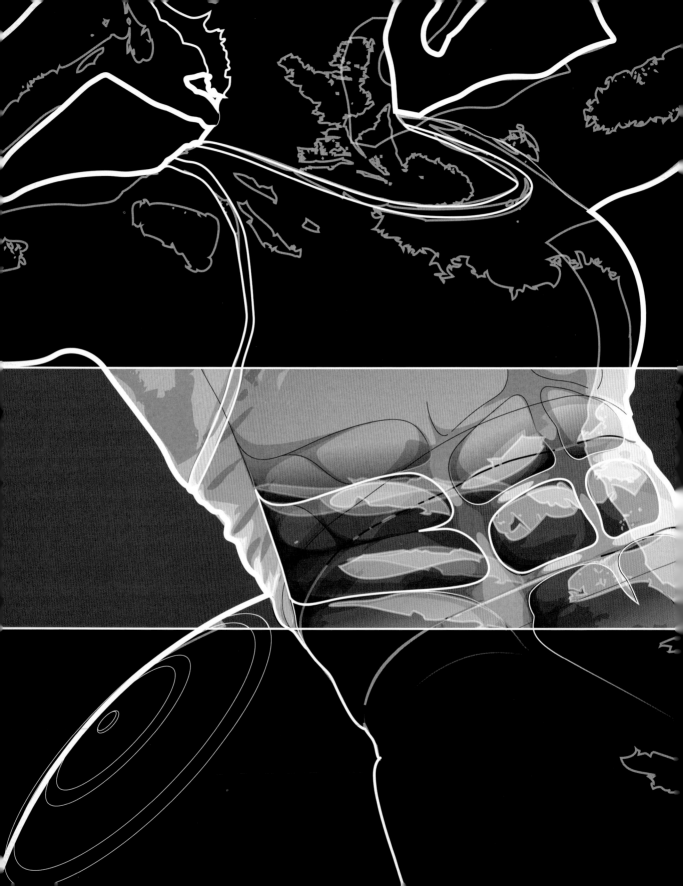

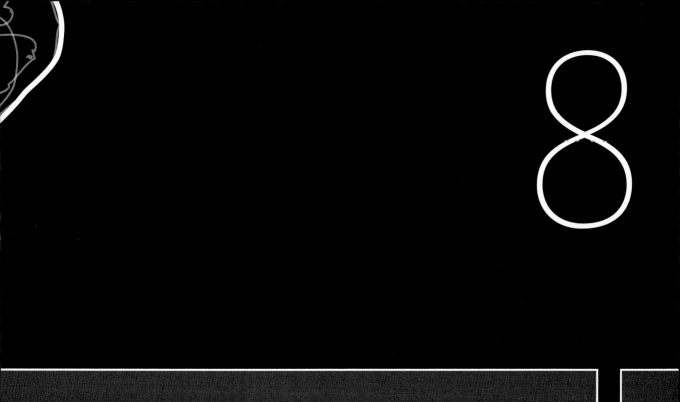

8

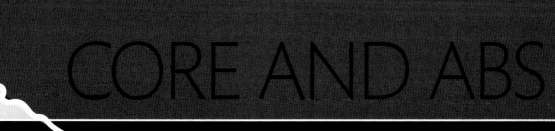

CORE AND ABS

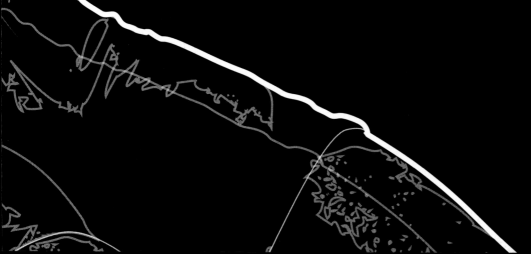

ABDOMINAL CRUNCH

TARGET MUSCLES

- Rectus abdominis
- External obliques

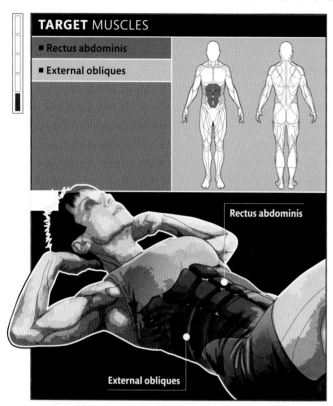

Rectus abdominis

External obliques

The basic abdominal crunch is one of the most simple and popular of all exercises. It helps you to develop a strong core and improves your posture, but you must ensure you have good technique.

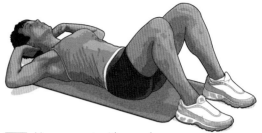

1 Lie on a mat with your knees bent, your feet flat, and your fingers against the sides of your head.

Keep your chin up and your neck extended

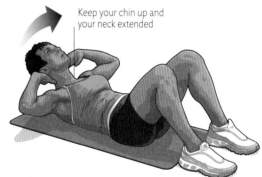

2 Engage your core and raise your shoulders and upper back slightly off the floor. Hold for a moment.

Keep your hips stable throughout

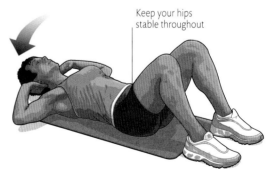

3 Lower your upper body slowly to the floor; don't let gravity or your body's momentum drive your movement.

VARIATION

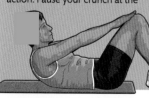

To work your abdominal area more effectively, use a pulsing action. Pause your crunch at the top of the movement and slide your hands up and down your thighs. The movement involved in each pulse is very small, but you should aim to squeeze your abs just a little bit tighter each time. Perform around five "pulses" per crunch repetition.

VARIATION

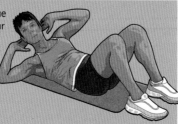

To work the external oblique muscles on the sides of your torso, add a twisting action to your crunches. Alternate your crunches, bringing your left elbow toward your right knee, then your right elbow toward your left knee.

SIT-UP

TARGET MUSCLES

- Rectus abdominis
- External obliques

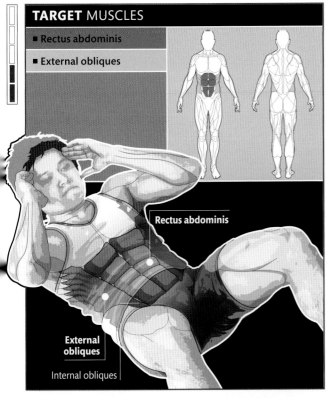

Rectus abdominis

External obliques

Internal obliques

The classic sit-up is still used in many training programs. It is a good abdominal exercise but should be avoided if you have any lower back problems or have a weak core.

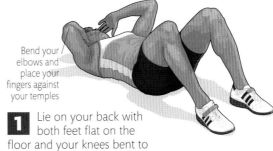

Bend your elbows and place your fingers against your temples

1 Lie on your back with both feet flat on the floor and your knees bent to reduce stress on your spine.

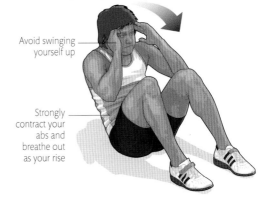

Avoid swinging yourself up

Strongly contract your abs and breathe out as your rise

2 Engage your core muscles and raise your torso upward, leaving just your buttocks and feet on the floor.

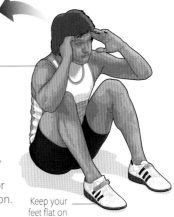

Curl in your shoulders

3 Pause at the upright position, then slowly lower your upper body to the floor back to the start position.

Keep your feet flat on the floor

VARIATION

Changing the position of your arms alters the difficulty of the exercise. Extending your arms ahead of your knees provides the least resistance, while crossing your arms over your chest or holding them by your head increases difficulty. For an advanced workout, hold a weight plate to your chest.

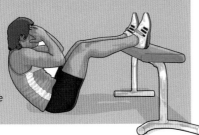

VARIATION

Resting your legs on a bench or other elevated platform isolates your abdominals from the assistance of your hip flexors during the sit-up exercise, providing a more intense abdominal workout.

REVERSE CRUNCH

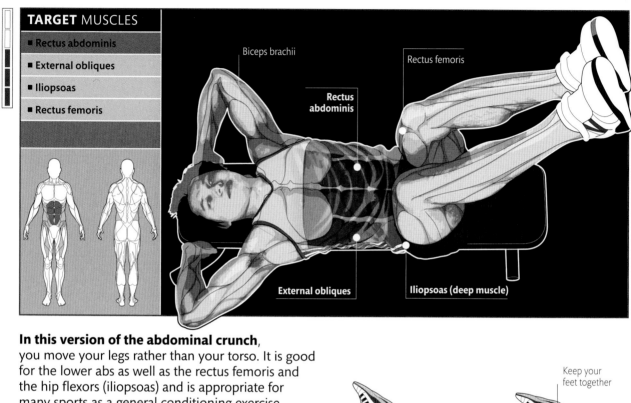

TARGET MUSCLES

- Rectus abdominis
- External obliques
- Iliopsoas
- Rectus femoris

Biceps brachii

Rectus femoris

Rectus abdominis

External obliques

Iliopsoas (deep muscle)

In this version of the abdominal crunch, you move your legs rather than your torso. It is good for the lower abs as well as the rectus femoris and the hip flexors (iliopsoas) and is appropriate for many sports as a general conditioning exercise.

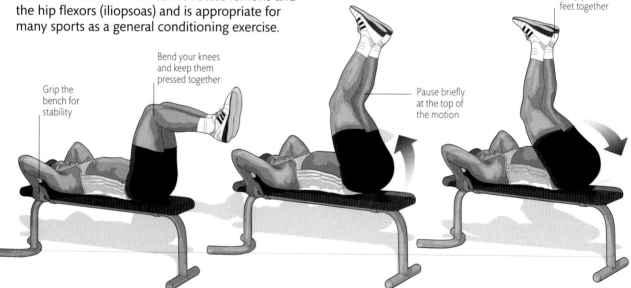

Grip the bench for stability

Bend your knees and keep them pressed together

Pause briefly at the top of the motion

Keep your feet together

1 Lie with your head, shoulders, and buttocks in contact with the surface of a stable bench. Flex your hips and knees to a right angle.

2 Extend your legs and slowly lift your buttocks off the bench. Use your abs to do this, rather than the momentum of your legs.

3 Contract your abs hard and lower your legs slowly to the start position; your buttocks should just make contact with the bench.

FIGURE-4 CRUNCH

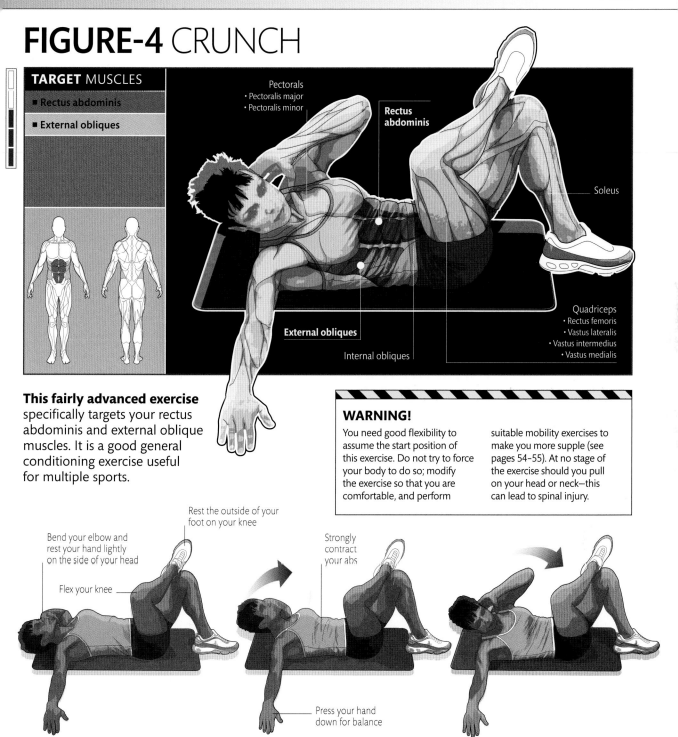

TARGET MUSCLES

- ■ **Rectus abdominis**
- ■ **External obliques**

Pectorals
• Pectoralis major
• Pectoralis minor

Rectus abdominis

Soleus

External obliques

Internal obliques

Quadriceps
• Rectus femoris
• Vastus lateralis
• Vastus intermedius
• Vastus medialis

This fairly advanced exercise specifically targets your rectus abdominis and external oblique muscles. It is a good general conditioning exercise useful for multiple sports.

WARNING!

You need good flexibility to assume the start position of this exercise. Do not try to force your body to do so; modify the exercise so that you are comfortable, and perform suitable mobility exercises to make you more supple (see pages 54–55). At no stage of the exercise should you pull on your head or neck—this can lead to spinal injury.

Bend your elbow and rest your hand lightly on the side of your head

Rest the outside of your foot on your knee

Flex your knee

Strongly contract your abs

Press your hand down for balance

1 Lie on an exercise mat with your knees bent. Extend your right arm on the floor for balance, and cross your right leg over the left.

2 Lift your head and look toward your flexed knee; at the same time, tighten your abs and start bringing your left elbow up.

3 Bring your left elbow and your flexed knee toward one another. Pause and then return under control to the start position.

90-90 CRUNCH

TARGET MUSCLES

- Rectus abdominis
- External obliques
- Transversus abdominis

This fairly easy abdominal crunch puts emphasis on the upper part of your rectus abdominus muscles and takes pressure off your lower back. Perform it with your knees bent and feet fixed.

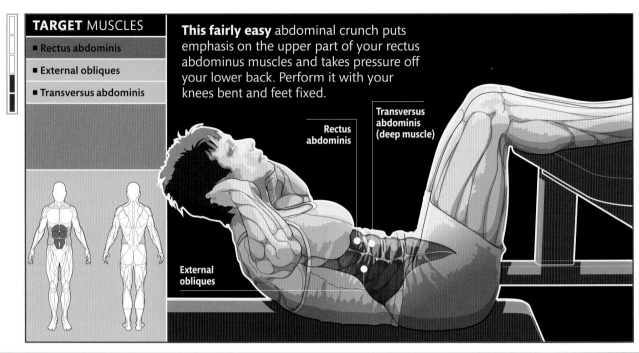

Rectus abdominis

Transversus abdominis (deep muscle)

External obliques

BALL CRUNCH

TARGET MUSCLES

- Rectus abdominis
- External obliques

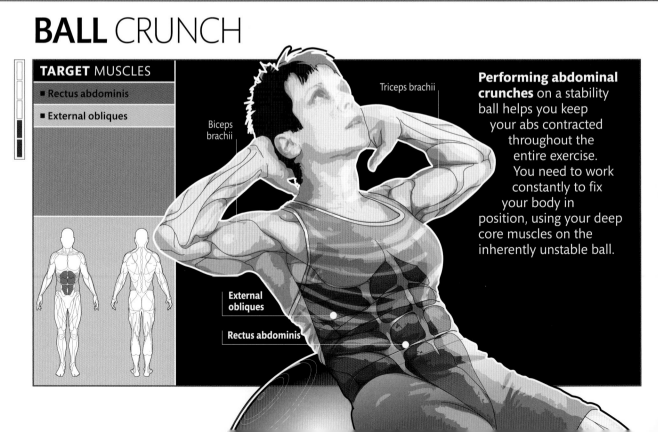

Biceps brachii

Triceps brachii

External obliques

Rectus abdominis

Performing abdominal crunches on a stability ball helps you keep your abs contracted throughout the entire exercise. You need to work constantly to fix your body in position, using your deep core muscles on the inherently unstable ball.

VARIATION

Try this exercise with a twist. Turn your torso slightly to one side as you rise, aiming your left elbow at your right knee. This variation will additionally work your oblique muscles.

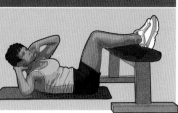

WARNING!

Be sure to place your feet on top of the bench. Do not hook them underneath to provide leverage, this will place great stress on your lower back. Do not pull on your head or neck when performing this exercise and make sure that your lower back and buttocks remain in contact with the floor. Do not fling your head or arms forward when your abdominal muscles start to tire.

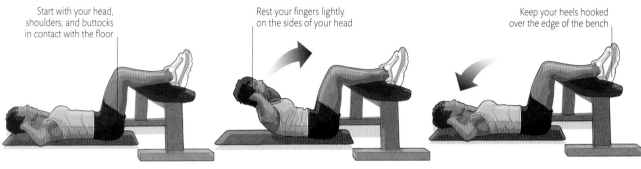

Start with your head, shoulders, and buttocks in contact with the floor

Rest your fingers lightly on the sides of your head

Keep your heels hooked over the edge of the bench

1 Lie flat, with your hips and knees bent at 90 degrees. Rest your calves on a bench, hooking your heels over the edge.

2 Inhale deeply and lift your shoulders off the floor; actively contract your abdominal muscles, curling your torso toward your knees.

3 Exhale, and hold at the top of the movement for a second. Lower your torso back to the starting position under tight control.

WARNING!

Make sure that your body is balanced on the ball. Brace yourself with your feet flat on the floor. Don't pull your head forward as you lift and make sure you lift and lower your body slowly and deliberately, with concentration.

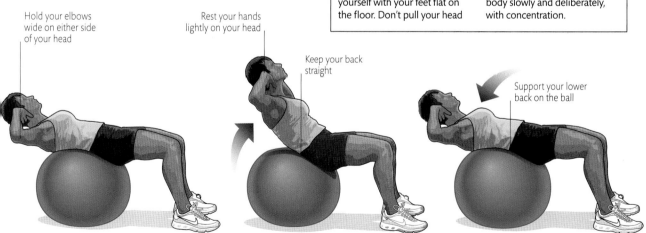

Hold your elbows wide on either side of your head

Rest your hands lightly on your head

Keep your back straight

Support your lower back on the ball

1 Begin with your feet flat on the floor and your knees bent at a 90-degree angle. Rest your hands on the sides of your head.

2 Push your lower back into the ball, contract your abs, and lift your shoulders a few inches, crunching your abs toward your hips.

3 Lower your torso under tight control, still keeping the tension in your abs. Make sure not to "flop" back on to the ball.

BALL TWIST

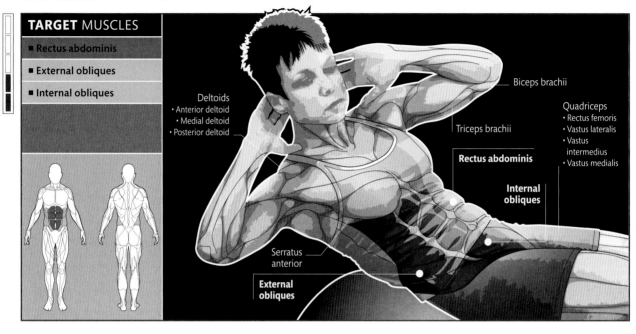

TARGET MUSCLES

- Rectus abdominis
- External obliques
- Internal obliques

Deltoids
• Anterior deltoid
• Medial deltoid
• Posterior deltoid

Biceps brachii

Triceps brachii

Quadriceps
• Rectus femoris
• Vastus lateralis
• Vastus intermedius
• Vastus medialis

Rectus abdominis

Internal obliques

Serratus anterior

External obliques

This exercise not only builds strong abs, but also strengthens the rotational muscles of your torso. Working on the ball also promotes balance, making this a great exercise for activities such as golf and surfing.

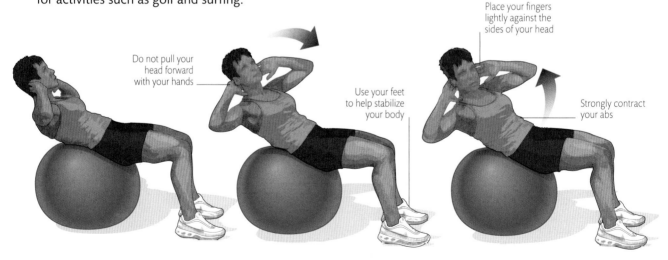

Do not pull your head forward with your hands

Place your fingers lightly against the sides of your head

Use your feet to help stabilize your body

Strongly contract your abs

1 Lie on the stability ball with your lower back well supported, your feet flat on the floor, and your knees at an angle of about 90 degrees. Hold your hands to the sides of your head.

2 Once you feel steady and stable, begin to crunch up. About halfway up, twist your torso to one side—spreading your elbows wide helps you to balance.

3 Hold the top position for around one second, then return to the start position. Keeping your lower body still, lower and untwist your upper body.

BALL PRESS-UP

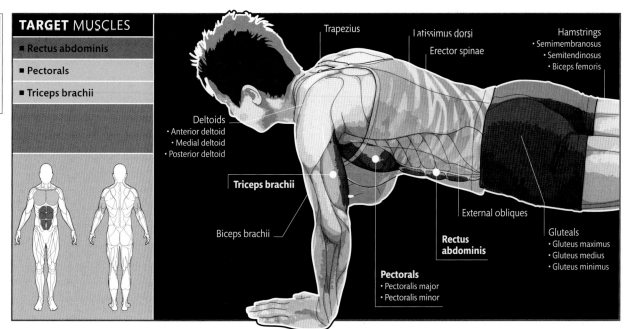

TARGET MUSCLES

- Rectus abdominis
- Pectorals
- Triceps brachii

Trapezius

Latissimus dorsi

Erector spinae

Hamstrings
• Semimembranosus
• Semitendinosus
• Biceps femoris

Deltoids
• Anterior deltoid
• Medial deltoid
• Posterior deltoid

Triceps brachii

Biceps brachii

External obliques

Rectus abdominis

Gluteals
• Gluteus maximus
• Gluteus medius
• Gluteus minimus

Pectorals
• Pectoralis major
• Pectoralis minor

In this exercise, you elevate your feet on to the stability ball to make your chest, shoulders, and upper arms work harder than in a regular push-up (see page 120). The core stabilizers of your torso and hips are also fully engaged, keeping your body in alignment, while your feet are supported on the inherently unstable ball.

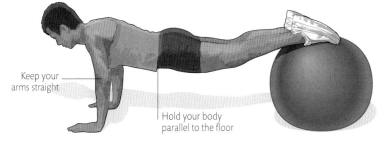

Keep your arms straight

Hold your body parallel to the floor

1 Place your feet on the ball so that your body is supported on your extended toes and on your hands, which should be under your shoulder joints.

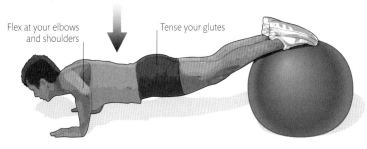

Flex at your elbows and shoulders

Tense your glutes

2 Keeping your core muscles engaged, lower your body slowly as far as you can, before pressing back up to the start position.

WARNING!

Your body should be straight throughout this exercise. Don't allow your midsection to droop toward the floor because you'll place great stress on your back. Exhaling while you push up and inhaling as you lower your torso will help you maintain good form.

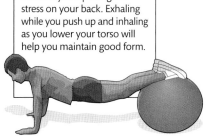

BALL JACK KNIFE

TARGET MUSCLES

- Iliopsoas
- Rectus abdominis

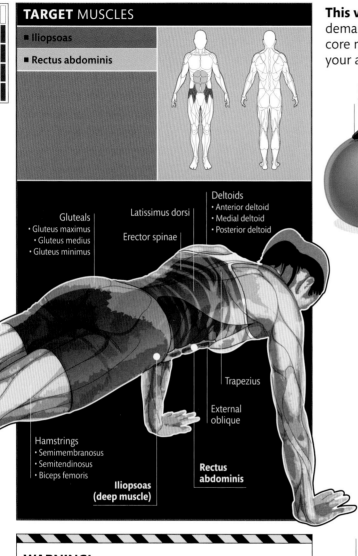

Gluteals
• Gluteus maximus
• Gluteus medius
• Gluteus minimus

Latissimus dorsi

Erector spinae

Deltoids
• Anterior deltoid
• Medial deltoid
• Posterior deltoid

Trapezius

External oblique

Hamstrings
• Semimembranosus
• Semitendinosus
• Biceps femoris

Iliopsoas
(deep muscle)

Rectus
abdominis

This valuable but relatively advanced exercise demands great balance and control. It works the core muscles that flex your hips and also stresses your abdominal muscles.

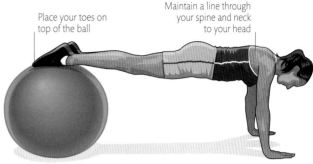

Place your toes on top of the ball

Maintain a line through your spine and neck to your head

1 Start with your body in a push-up position (see page 168). Keep your hands flat on the floor and your feet elevated on the ball. Align your head with your spine.

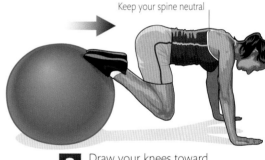

Keep your spine neutral

2 Draw your knees toward your chest, maintaining a neutral spine as the ball rolls forward. Your hips will rise a little as the ball moves.

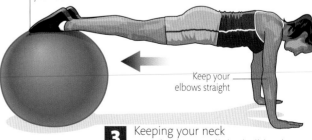

Balance on your toes

Keep your elbows straight

3 Keeping your neck stretched out, roll the ball back by returning your legs to the extended position, with your knees straight.

WARNING!

Make sure that your knees do not drop down and keep from bending your elbows or letting your shoulders rise up toward your ears, because this will place stress on your back.

Choose a ball that has a diameter about the same as the length of your arm; it should allow your back to be parallel to the floor when you assume the push-up position.

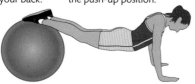

BALL BACK EXTENSION

TARGET MUSCLES

- Erector spinae
- Gluteals
- Hamstrings

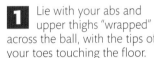

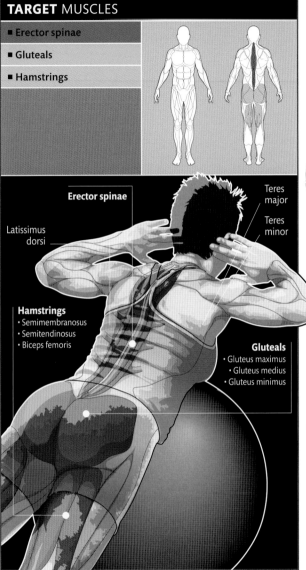

Erector spinae

Latissimus dorsi

Teres major

Teres minor

Hamstrings
- Semimembranosus
- Semitendinosus
- Biceps femoris

Gluteals
- Gluteus maximus
- Gluteus medius
- Gluteus minimus

This exercise helps to balance your trunk by conditioning your lower back muscles that work opposite your abs. A strong trunk provides good protection against back injury.

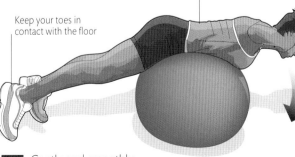

1 Lie with your abs and upper thighs "wrapped" across the ball, with the tips of your toes touching the floor.

Move your elbows back a little on ascent

Keep your knees slightly bent

2 With the tips of your fingers touching the sides of your head, slowly straighten your body while breathing in.

Control your descent by contracting the muscles of your back

Keep your toes in contact with the floor

3 Gently and smoothly lower your upper body to the start position, while breathing out.

WARNING!

Before starting the exercise, check that the ball is the correct size for your limb length. You should be able to touch the floor with straight arms. Keep your movement smooth and controlled; if you straighten your torso too fast you risk compressing the vertebrae in your back and damaging your sciatic nerve. Do not pull your torso above the natural line of your spine—hyperextending your back may be dangerous.

SIDE BEND

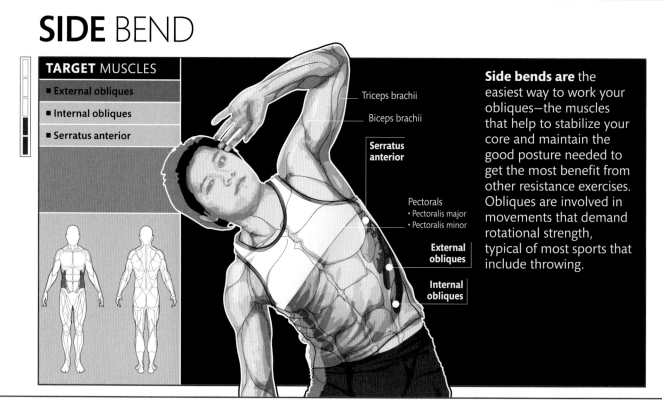

TARGET MUSCLES

- External obliques
- Internal obliques
- Serratus anterior

Triceps brachii

Biceps brachii

Serratus anterior

Pectorals
• Pectoralis major
• Pectoralis minor

External obliques

Internal obliques

Side bends are the easiest way to work your obliques—the muscles that help to stabilize your core and maintain the good posture needed to get the most benefit from other resistance exercises. Obliques are involved in movements that demand rotational strength, typical of most sports that include throwing.

ROMAN CHAIR SIDE BEND

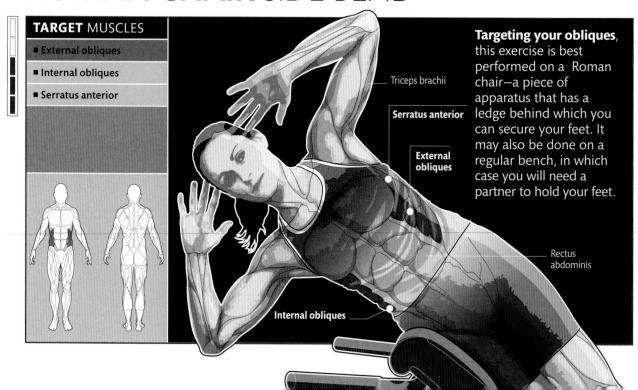

TARGET MUSCLES

- External obliques
- Internal obliques
- Serratus anterior

Triceps brachii

Serratus anterior

External obliques

Internal obliques

Rectus abdominis

Targeting your obliques, this exercise is best performed on a Roman chair—a piece of apparatus that has a ledge behind which you can secure your feet. It may also be done on a regular bench, in which case you will need a partner to hold your feet.

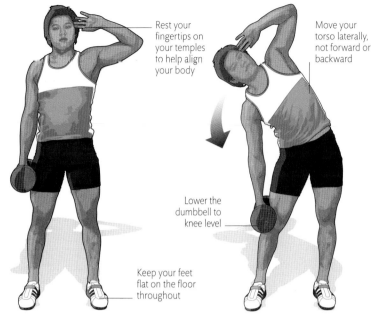
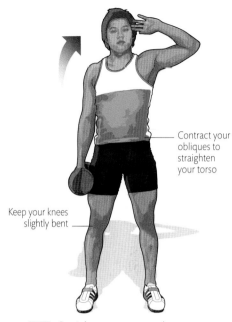

Rest your fingertips on your temples to help align your body

Move your torso laterally, not forward or backward

Contract your obliques to straighten your torso

Lower the dumbbell to knee level

Keep your knees slightly bent

Keep your feet flat on the floor throughout

1 Stand upright with your knees slightly bent and one dumbbell resting on the side of your thigh. Keep your weighted arm straight.

2 Lean slowly sideways and slide the dumbbell down your thigh to knee level, while breathing in. Do not allow the weight to swing.

3 Straighten your torso by contracting your obliques on the side opposite from the weight. Breathe out as you move to the upright position.

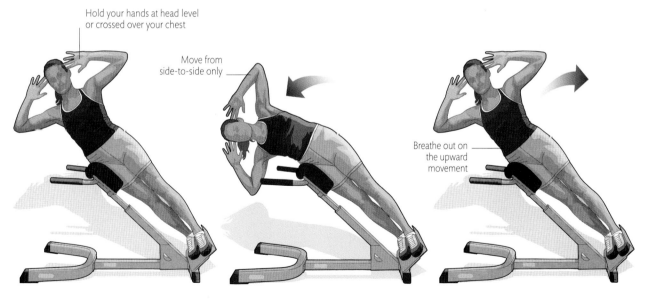

Hold your hands at head level or crossed over your chest

Move from side-to-side only

Breathe out on the upward movement

1 Lie sideways on the Roman chair; adjust it so that your upper body can pivot comfortably at your hips toward the floor.

2 Lean slowly sideways toward the floor, as far as is comfortable. Make sure not to lean forward or back. Breathe in on the descent.

3 Pause at full extension, then gently raise your body to the start position. Complete the set for one side and repeat on the other.

PRONE PLANK

TARGET MUSCLES

- Erector spinae
- External obliques
- Internal obliques
- Rectus abdominis
- Quadriceps

Quadriceps
- Rectus femoris
- Vastus lateralis
- Vastus intermedius
- Vastus medialis

Internal obliques

Gluteals
- Gluteus maximus
- Gluteus medius
- Gluteus minimus

External obliques

Erector spinae

Deltoids
- Anterior deltoid
- Medial deltoid
- Posterior deltoid

Rectus abdominis

Triceps brachii

Biceps brachii

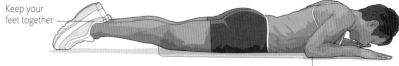

This static floor exercise (also called the bridge) engages your core and many of the major muscle groups of your upper and lower body in maintaining a static position. Use this exercise to help prevent lower back problems.

Keep your feet together

1 Lie face down on an exercise mat with your elbows to your sides and your palms alongside your head, facing down to the floor.

Rest your forearms against the floor

Keep your back flat and tight

Rise up on to your toes

2 Engaging your core and leg muscles, raise your body from the floor, supporting your weight on your forearms and toes while breathing freely.

Keep your hands flat on the floor

VARIATION

You can make the exercise more challenging by simultaneously extending one arm and the opposite leg from the plank position. This position, called the "Superman," demands excellent balance. Conversely, the exercise can be made easier to perform by supporting your lower body on your knees, rather than on your toes.

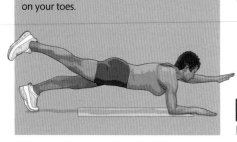

Flex your ankles

Return your body to a prone position

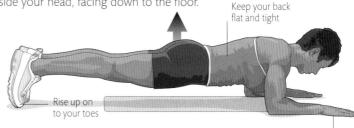

3 Hold the plank position for a short while—try 20 seconds to start with—then gently lower your body back on to the exercise mat.

SIDE PLANK

TARGET MUSCLES

- External obliques
- Internal obliques
- Quadriceps

This is an excellent exercise for developing the muscles located to the sides of your torso; these are vital in maintaining good posture in most activities. This waistline-toning exercise is easy to do at home.

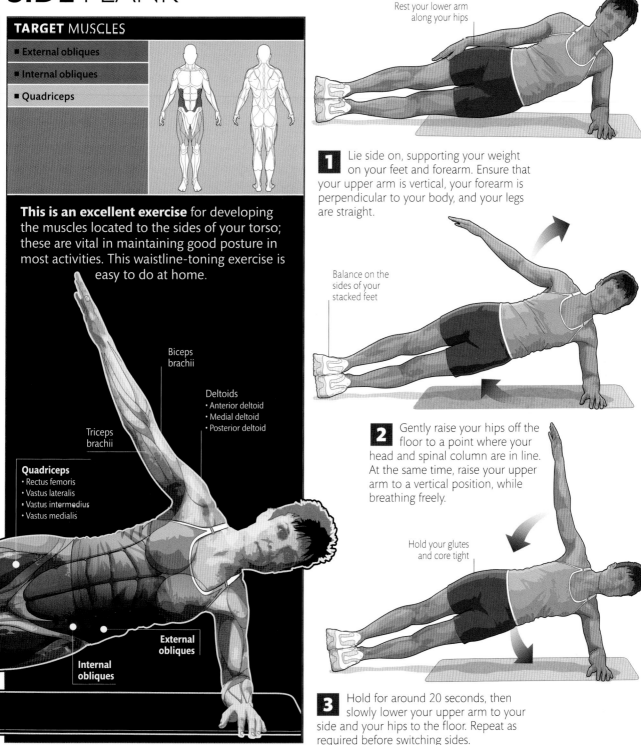

Biceps brachii

Deltoids
- Anterior deltoid
- Medial deltoid
- Posterior deltoid

Triceps brachii

Quadriceps
- Rectus femoris
- Vastus lateralis
- Vastus intermedius
- Vastus medialis

External obliques

Internal obliques

Rest your lower arm along your hips

1 Lie side on, supporting your weight on your feet and forearm. Ensure that your upper arm is vertical, your forearm is perpendicular to your body, and your legs are straight.

Balance on the sides of your stacked feet

2 Gently raise your hips off the floor to a point where your head and spinal column are in line. At the same time, raise your upper arm to a vertical position, while breathing freely.

Hold your glutes and core tight

3 Hold for around 20 seconds, then slowly lower your upper arm to your side and your hips to the floor. Repeat as required before switching sides.

V-LEG RAISE

TARGET MUSCLES

- Rectus abdominis

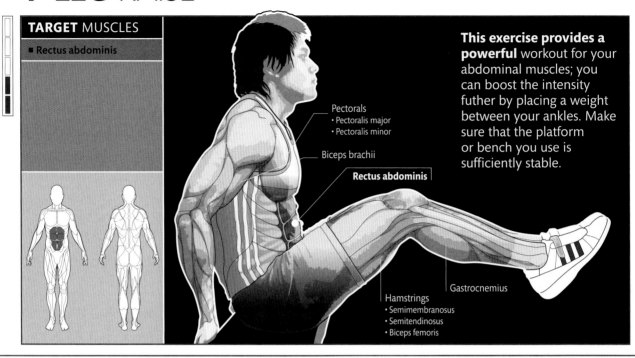

Pectorals
• Pectoralis major
• Pectoralis minor

Biceps brachii

Rectus abdominis

Gastrocnemius

Hamstrings
• Semimembranosus
• Semitendinosus
• Biceps femoris

This exercise provides a powerful workout for your abdominal muscles; you can boost the intensity futher by placing a weight between your ankles. Make sure that the platform or bench you use is sufficiently stable.

SUITCASE DEADLIFT

TARGET MUSCLES

- Quadriceps
- External obliques
- Transversus abdominis
- Hamstrings
- Gluteals

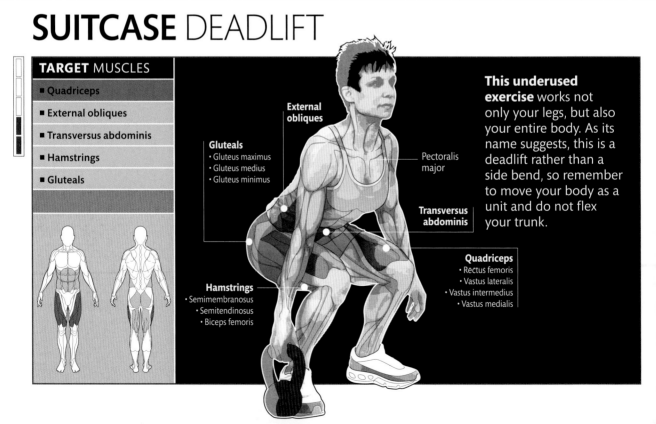

External obliques

Gluteals
• Gluteus maximus
• Gluteus medius
• Gluteus minimus

Pectoralis major

Transversus abdominis

Hamstrings
• Semimembranosus
• Semitendinosus
• Biceps femoris

Quadriceps
• Rectus femoris
• Vastus lateralis
• Vastus intermedius
• Vastus medialis

This underused exercise works not only your legs, but also your entire body. As its name suggests, this is a deadlift rather than a side bend, so remember to move your body as a unit and do not flex your trunk.

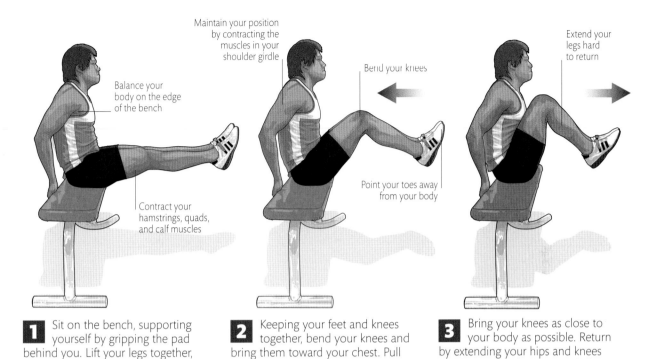

Maintain your position by contracting the muscles in your shoulder girdle

Bend your knees

Balance your body on the edge of the bench

Extend your legs hard to return

Contract your hamstrings, quads, and calf muscles

Point your toes away from your body

1 Sit on the bench, supporting yourself by gripping the pad behind you. Lift your legs together, keeping your toes pointed.

2 Keeping your feet and knees together, bend your knees and bring them toward your chest. Pull your torso forward a little for balance.

3 Bring your knees as close to your body as possible. Return by extending your hips and knees and leaning back to counterbalance.

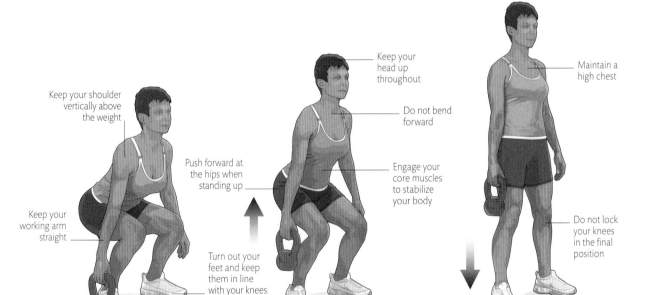

Keep your shoulder vertically above the weight

Push forward at the hips when standing up

Keep your working arm straight

Turn out your feet and keep them in line with your knees

Keep your head up throughout

Do not bend forward

Engage your core muscles to stabilize your body

Maintain a high chest

Do not lock your knees in the final position

1 Adopt the get set position with the kettlebell outside your foot, your hips above your knees, and your back flat and tight.

2 Maintaining good posture throughout, drive up strongly with your legs: imagine that you are pushing your feet into the floor.

3 Stand up straight with the weight by the side of your thigh. Return to the start position and complete the set before switching sides.

WOODCHOP

TARGET MUSCLES

- External obliques
- Pectorals
- Serratus anterior
- Supraspinatus
- Teres major
- Teres minor

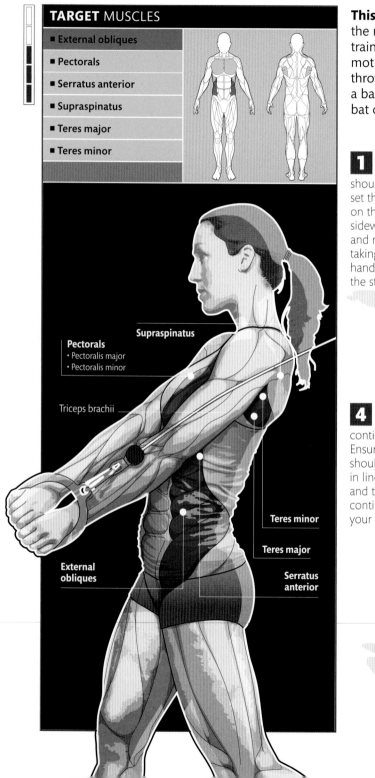

Supraspinatus

Pectorals
• Pectoralis major
• Pectoralis minor

Triceps brachii

Teres minor

Teres major

External obliques

Serratus anterior

This powerful rotational exercise develops the muscles of your trunk, making it ideal for training in sports that involve a twisting motion, such as throwing or hitting a ball with a bat or racket.

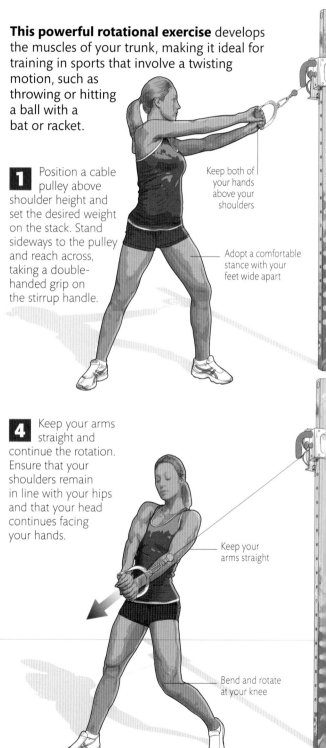

1 Position a cable pulley above shoulder height and set the desired weight on the stack. Stand sideways to the pulley and reach across, taking a double-handed grip on the stirrup handle.

Keep both of your hands above your shoulders

Adopt a comfortable stance with your feet wide apart

4 Keep your arms straight and continue the rotation. Ensure that your shoulders remain in line with your hips and that your head continues facing your hands.

Keep your arms straight

Bend and rotate at your knee

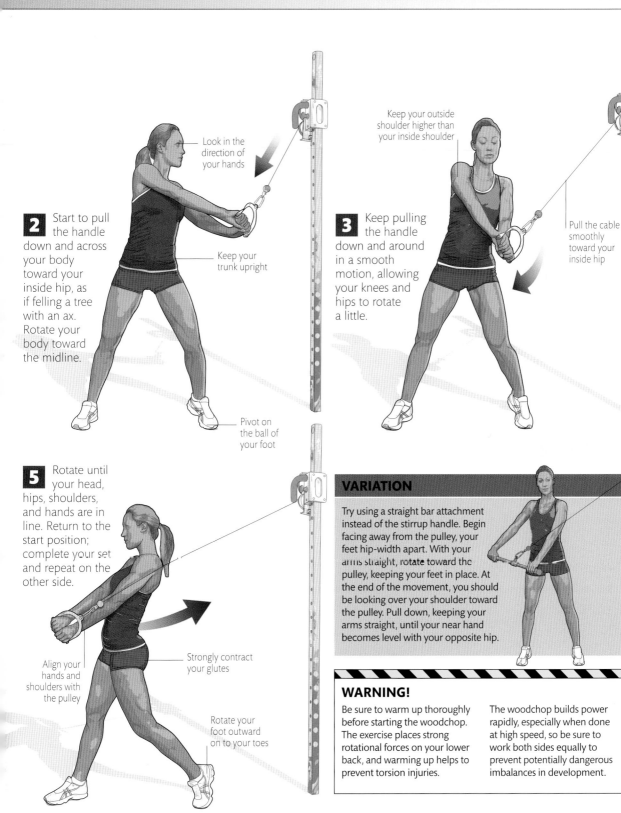

2 Start to pull the handle down and across your body toward your inside hip, as if felling a tree with an ax. Rotate your body toward the midline.

Look in the direction of your hands

Keep your trunk upright

Pivot on the ball of your foot

Keep your outside shoulder higher than your inside shoulder

3 Keep pulling the handle down and around in a smooth motion, allowing your knees and hips to rotate a little.

Pull the cable smoothly toward your inside hip

5 Rotate until your head, hips, shoulders, and hands are in line. Return to the start position; complete your set and repeat on the other side.

Align your hands and shoulders with the pulley

Strongly contract your glutes

Rotate your foot outward on to your toes

VARIATION

Try using a straight bar attachment instead of the stirrup handle. Begin facing away from the pulley, your feet hip-width apart. With your arms straight, rotate toward the pulley, keeping your feet in place. At the end of the movement, you should be looking over your shoulder toward the pulley. Pull down, keeping your arms straight, until your near hand becomes level with your opposite hip.

WARNING!

Be sure to warm up thoroughly before starting the woodchop. The exercise places strong rotational forces on your lower back, and warming up helps to prevent torsion injuries.

The woodchop builds power rapidly, especially when done at high speed, so be sure to work both sides equally to prevent potentially dangerous imbalances in development.

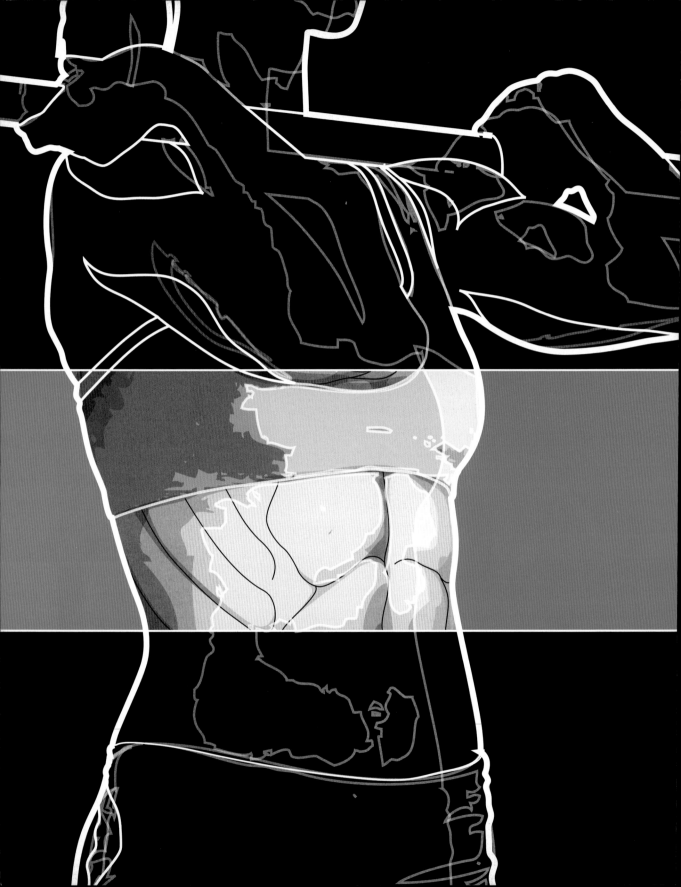

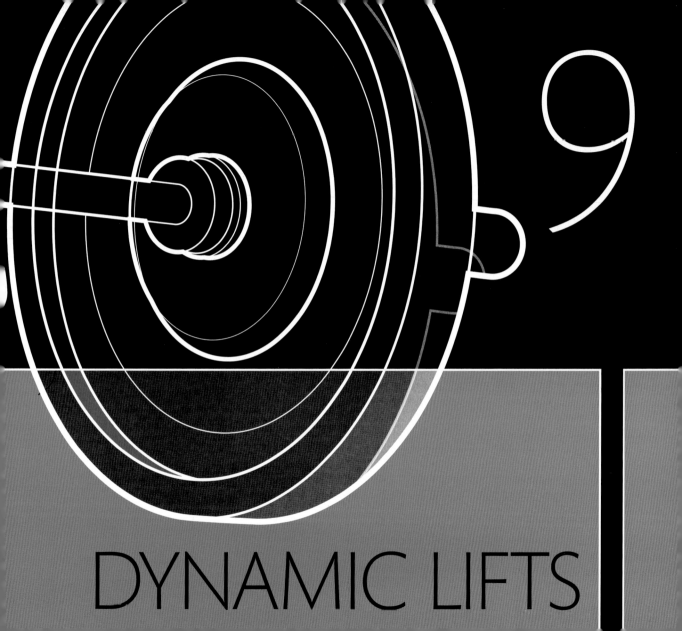

9

DYNAMIC LIFTS

POWER CLEAN

TARGET MUSCLES

■ Quadriceps	■ Gluteals
■ Hamstrings	■ Pectorals
■ Gastrocnemius	■ Deltoids
■ Soleus	

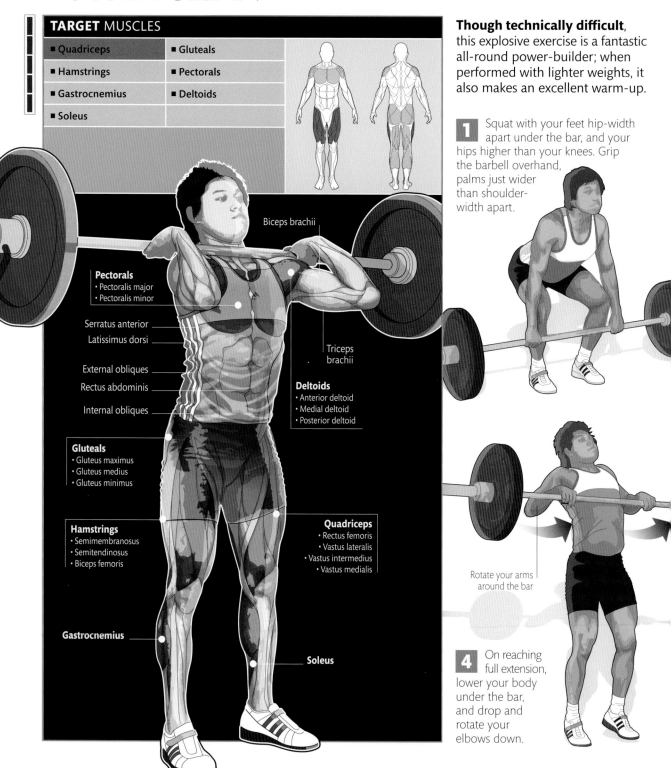

Though technically difficult, this explosive exercise is a fantastic all-round power-builder; when performed with lighter weights, it also makes an excellent warm-up.

1 Squat with your feet hip-width apart under the bar, and your hips higher than your knees. Grip the barbell overhand, palms just wider than shoulder-width apart.

Biceps brachii

Pectorals
• Pectoralis major
• Pectoralis minor

Serratus anterior

Latissimus dorsi

Triceps brachii

External obliques

Rectus abdominis

Deltoids
• Anterior deltoid
• Medial deltoid
• Posterior deltoid

Internal obliques

Gluteals
• Gluteus maximus
• Gluteus medius
• Gluteus minimus

Hamstrings
• Semimembranosus
• Semitendinosus
• Biceps femoris

Quadriceps
• Rectus femoris
• Vastus lateralis
• Vastus intermedius
• Vastus medialis

Gastrocnemius

Soleus

Rotate your arms around the bar

4 On reaching full extension, lower your body under the bar, and drop and rotate your elbows down.

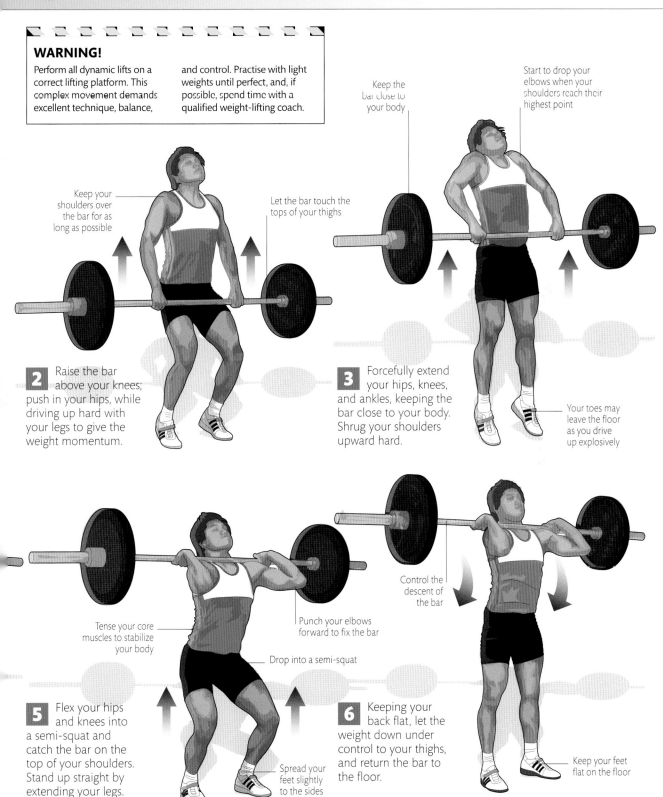

WARNING!

Perform all dynamic lifts on a correct lifting platform. This complex movement demands excellent technique, balance, and control. Practise with light weights until perfect, and, if possible, spend time with a qualified weight-lifting coach.

Keep your shoulders over the bar for as long as possible

Let the bar touch the tops of your thighs

2 Raise the bar above your knees; push in your hips, while driving up hard with your legs to give the weight momentum.

Keep the bar close to your body

Start to drop your elbows when your shoulders reach their highest point

3 Forcefully extend your hips, knees, and ankles, keeping the bar close to your body. Shrug your shoulders upward hard.

Your toes may leave the floor as you drive up explosively

Tense your core muscles to stabilize your body

Punch your elbows forward to fix the bar

Drop into a semi-squat

5 Flex your hips and knees into a semi-squat and catch the bar on the top of your shoulders. Stand up straight by extending your legs.

Spread your feet slightly to the sides

Control the descent of the bar

6 Keeping your back flat, let the weight down under control to your thighs, and return the bar to the floor.

Keep your feet flat on the floor

POWER SNATCH

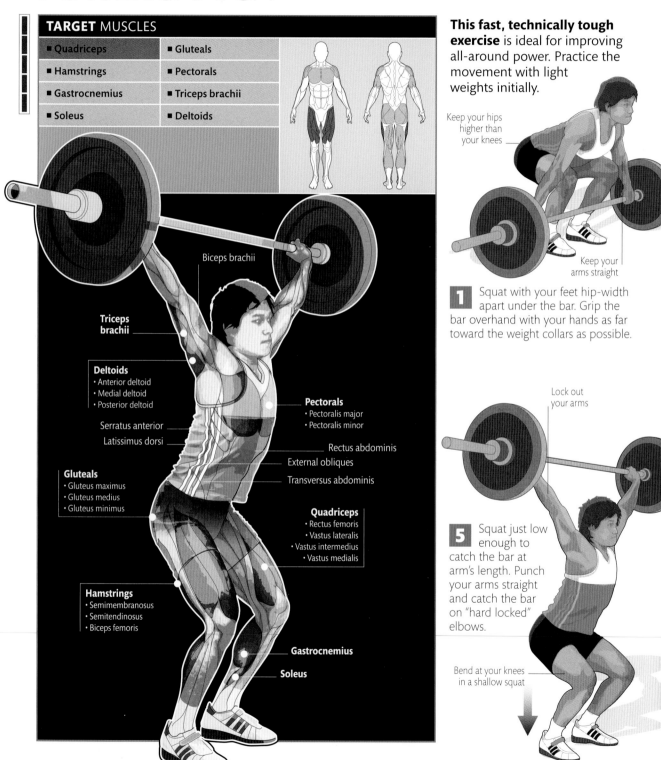

TARGET MUSCLES

▪ Quadriceps	▪ Gluteals
▪ Hamstrings	▪ Pectorals
▪ Gastrocnemius	▪ Triceps brachii
▪ Soleus	▪ Deltoids

This fast, technically tough exercise is ideal for improving all-around power. Practice the movement with light weights initially.

Keep your hips higher than your knees

Keep your arms straight

1 Squat with your feet hip-width apart under the bar. Grip the bar overhand with your hands as far toward the weight collars as possible.

Biceps brachii

Triceps brachii

Deltoids
• Anterior deltoid
• Medial deltoid
• Posterior deltoid

Serratus anterior
Latissimus dorsi

Gluteals
• Gluteus maximus
• Gluteus medius
• Gluteus minimus

Pectorals
• Pectoralis major
• Pectoralis minor

Rectus abdominis
External obliques
Transversus abdominis

Quadriceps
• Rectus femoris
• Vastus lateralis
• Vastus intermedius
• Vastus medialis

Hamstrings
• Semimembranosus
• Semitendinosus
• Biceps femoris

Gastrocnemius

Soleus

Lock out your arms

5 Squat just low enough to catch the bar at arm's length. Punch your arms straight and catch the bar on "hard locked" elbows.

Bend at your knees in a shallow squat

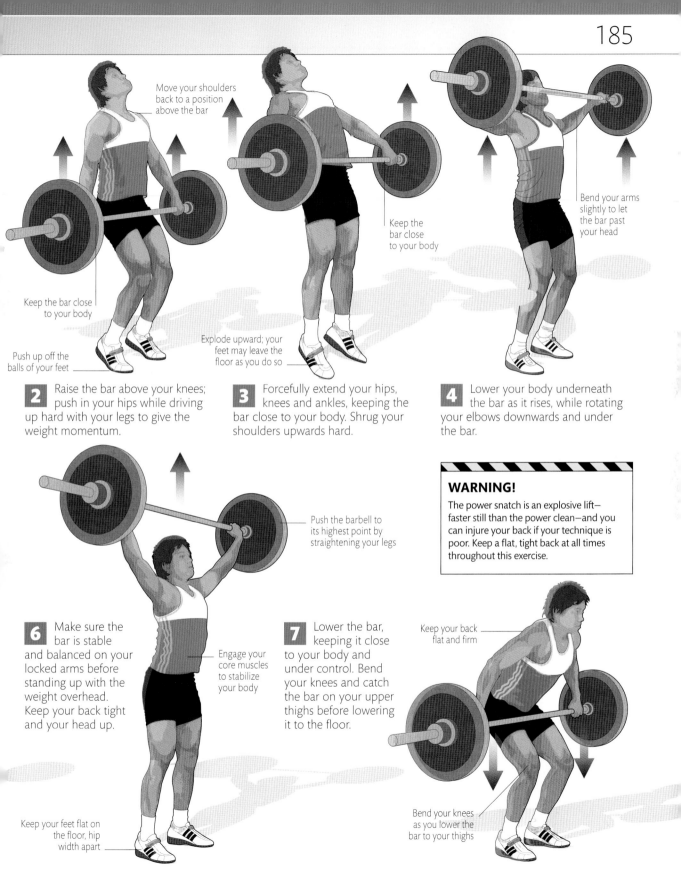

Move your shoulders back to a position above the bar

Keep the bar close to your body

Push up off the balls of your feet

2 Raise the bar above your knees; push in your hips while driving up hard with your legs to give the weight momentum.

Keep the bar close to your body

Explode upward; your feet may leave the floor as you do so

3 Forcefully extend your hips, knees and ankles, keeping the bar close to your body. Shrug your shoulders upwards hard.

Bend your arms slightly to let the bar past your head

4 Lower your body underneath the bar as it rises, while rotating your elbows downwards and under the bar.

Push the barbell to its highest point by straightening your legs

Engage your core muscles to stabilize your body

6 Make sure the bar is stable and balanced on your locked arms before standing up with the weight overhead. Keep your back tight and your head up.

Keep your feet flat on the floor, hip width apart

WARNING!

The power snatch is an explosive lift—faster still than the power clean—and you can injure your back if your technique is poor. Keep a flat, tight back at all times throughout this exercise.

7 Lower the bar, keeping it close to your body and under control. Bend your knees and catch the bar on your upper thighs before lowering it to the floor.

Keep your back flat and firm

Bend your knees as you lower the bar to your thighs

POWER CLEAN FROM HANG

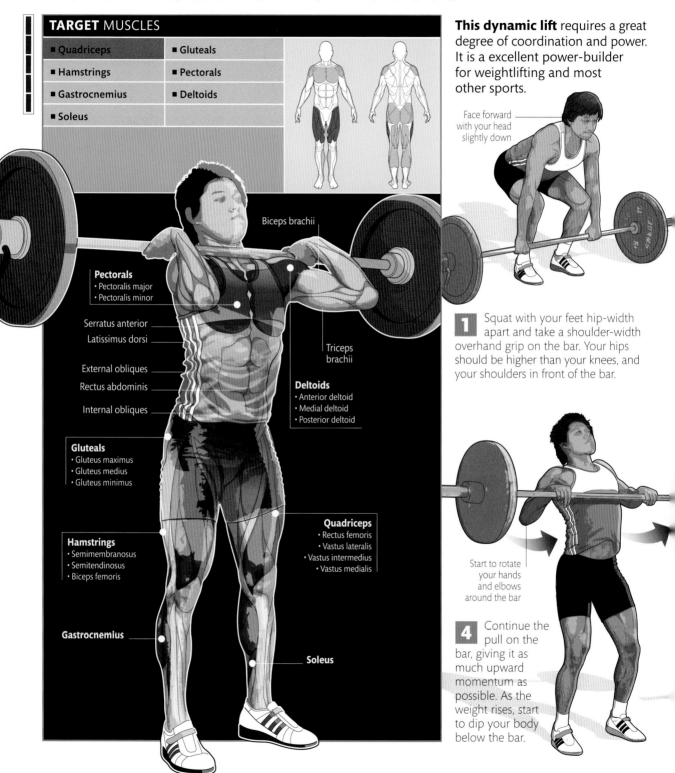

TARGET MUSCLES

■ Quadriceps	■ Gluteals
■ Hamstrings	■ Pectorals
■ Gastrocnemius	■ Deltoids
■ Soleus	

This dynamic lift requires a great degree of coordination and power. It is a excellent power-builder for weightlifting and most other sports.

Face forward with your head slightly down

Biceps brachii

Pectorals
• Pectoralis major
• Pectoralis minor

Serratus anterior

Latissimus dorsi

External obliques

Rectus abdominis

Internal obliques

Triceps brachii

Deltoids
• Anterior deltoid
• Medial deltoid
• Posterior deltoid

Gluteals
• Gluteus maximus
• Gluteus medius
• Gluteus minimus

Quadriceps
• Rectus femoris
• Vastus lateralis
• Vastus intermedius
• Vastus medialis

Hamstrings
• Semimembranosus
• Semitendinosus
• Biceps femoris

Gastrocnemius

Soleus

1 Squat with your feet hip-width apart and take a shoulder-width overhand grip on the bar. Your hips should be higher than your knees, and your shoulders in front of the bar.

Start to rotate your hands and elbows around the bar

4 Continue the pull on the bar, giving it as much upward momentum as possible. As the weight rises, start to dip your body below the bar.

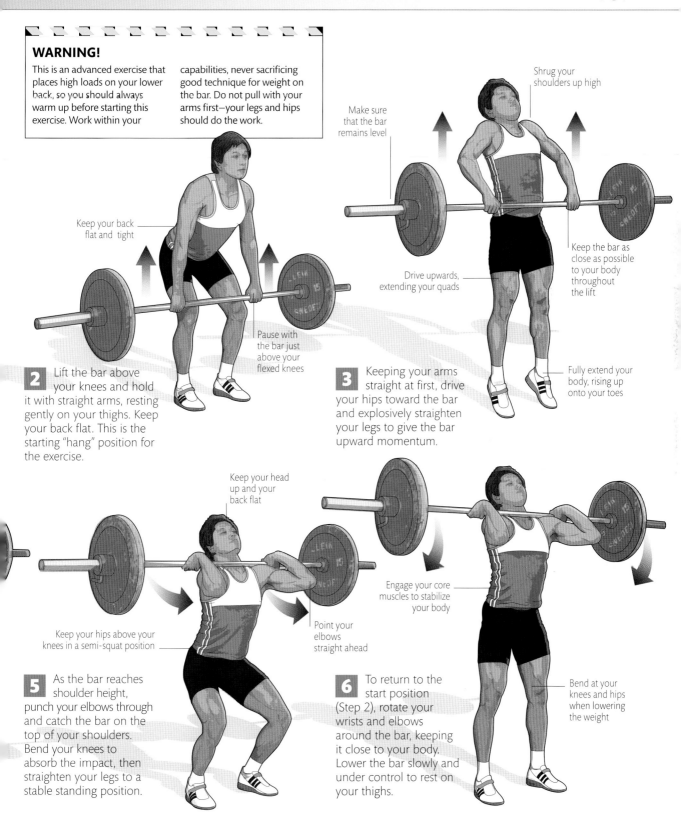

WARNING!

This is an advanced exercise that places high loads on your lower back, so you should always warm up before starting this exercise. Work within your capabilities, never sacrificing good technique for weight on the bar. Do not pull with your arms first—your legs and hips should do the work.

Keep your back flat and tight

Pause with the bar just above your flexed knees

2 Lift the bar above your knees and hold it with straight arms, resting gently on your thighs. Keep your back flat. This is the starting "hang" position for the exercise.

Shrug your shoulders up high

Make sure that the bar remains level

Drive upwards, extending your quads

Keep the bar as close as possible to your body throughout the lift

Fully extend your body, rising up onto your toes

3 Keeping your arms straight at first, drive your hips toward the bar and explosively straighten your legs to give the bar upward momentum.

Keep your head up and your back flat

Keep your hips above your knees in a semi-squat position

Point your elbows straight ahead

5 As the bar reaches shoulder height, punch your elbows through and catch the bar on the top of your shoulders. Bend your knees to absorb the impact, then straighten your legs to a stable standing position.

Engage your core muscles to stabilize your body

Bend at your knees and hips when lowering the weight

6 To return to the start position (Step 2), rotate your wrists and elbows around the bar, keeping it close to your body. Lower the bar slowly and under control to rest on your thighs.

POWER SNATCH FROM HANG

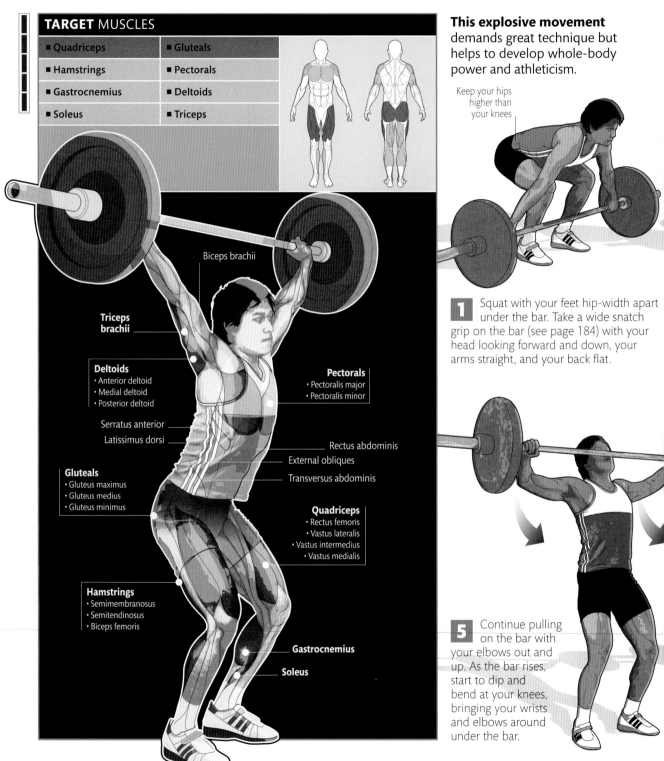

TARGET MUSCLES

■ Quadriceps	■ Gluteals
■ Hamstrings	■ Pectorals
■ Gastrocnemius	■ Deltoids
■ Soleus	■ Triceps

This explosive movement demands great technique but helps to develop whole-body power and athleticism.

Keep your hips higher than your knees

1 Squat with your feet hip-width apart under the bar. Take a wide snatch grip on the bar (see page 184) with your head looking forward and down, your arms straight, and your back flat.

Biceps brachii

Triceps brachii

Deltoids
• Anterior deltoid
• Medial deltoid
• Posterior deltoid

Serratus anterior
Latissimus dorsi

Gluteals
• Gluteus maximus
• Gluteus medius
• Gluteus minimus

Pectorals
• Pectoralis major
• Pectoralis minor

Rectus abdominis
External obliques
Transversus abdominis

Quadriceps
• Rectus femoris
• Vastus lateralis
• Vastus intermedius
• Vastus medialis

Hamstrings
• Semimembranosus
• Semitendinosus
• Biceps femoris

Gastrocnemius

Soleus

5 Continue pulling on the bar with your elbows out and up. As the bar rises, start to dip and bend at your knees, bringing your wrists and elbows around under the bar.

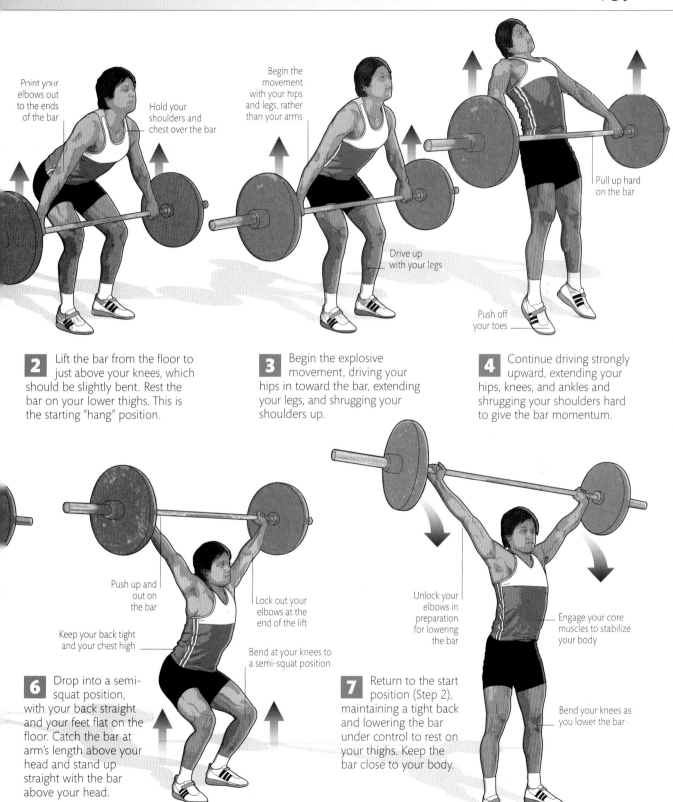

Point your elbows out to the ends of the bar

Hold your shoulders and chest over the bar

2 Lift the bar from the floor to just above your knees, which should be slightly bent. Rest the bar on your lower thighs. This is the starting "hang" position.

Begin the movement with your hips and legs, rather than your arms

3 Begin the explosive movement, driving your hips in toward the bar, extending your legs, and shrugging your shoulders up.

Drive up with your legs

Pull up hard on the bar

Push off your toes

4 Continue driving strongly upward, extending your hips, knees, and ankles and shrugging your shoulders hard to give the bar momentum.

Push up and out on the bar

Lock out your elbows at the end of the lift

Keep your back tight and your chest high

Bend at your knees to a semi-squat position

6 Drop into a semi-squat position, with your back straight and your feet flat on the floor. Catch the bar at arm's length above your head and stand up straight with the bar above your head.

Unlock your elbows in preparation for lowering the bar

Engage your core muscles to stabilize your body

7 Return to the start position (Step 2), maintaining a tight back and lowering the bar under control to rest on your thighs. Keep the bar close to your body.

Bend your knees as you lower the bar

SQUAT CLEAN

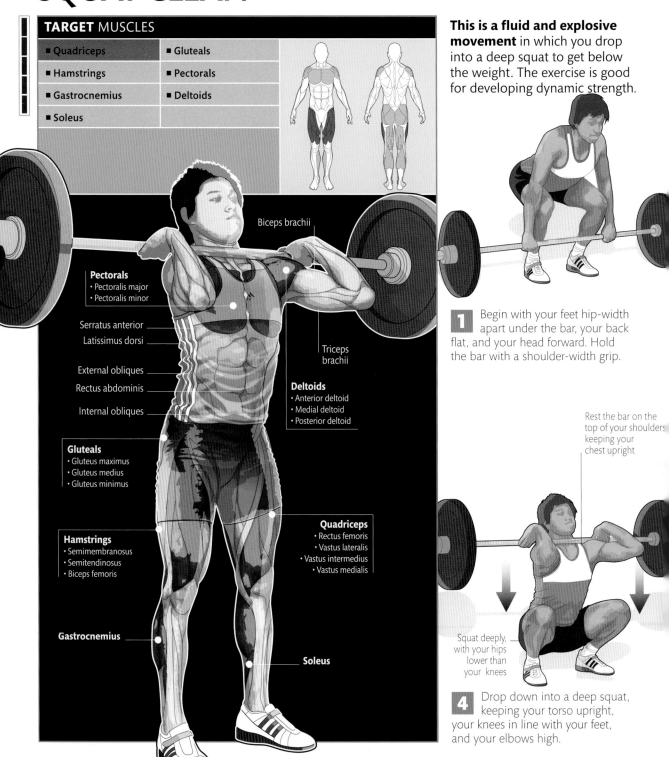

TARGET MUSCLES

- Quadriceps
- Gluteals
- Hamstrings
- Pectorals
- Gastrocnemius
- Deltoids
- Soleus

This is a fluid and explosive movement in which you drop into a deep squat to get below the weight. The exercise is good for developing dynamic strength.

Biceps brachii

Pectorals
• Pectoralis major
• Pectoralis minor

Serratus anterior

Latissimus dorsi

External obliques

Rectus abdominis

Internal obliques

Triceps brachii

Deltoids
• Anterior deltoid
• Medial deltoid
• Posterior deltoid

Gluteals
• Gluteus maximus
• Gluteus medius
• Gluteus minimus

Hamstrings
• Semimembranosus
• Semitendinosus
• Biceps femoris

Quadriceps
• Rectus femoris
• Vastus lateralis
• Vastus intermedius
• Vastus medialis

Gastrocnemius

Soleus

1 Begin with your feet hip-width apart under the bar, your back flat, and your head forward. Hold the bar with a shoulder-width grip.

Rest the bar on the top of your shoulders, keeping your chest upright

Squat deeply, with your hips lower than your knees

4 Drop down into a deep squat, keeping your torso upright, your knees in line with your feet, and your elbows high.

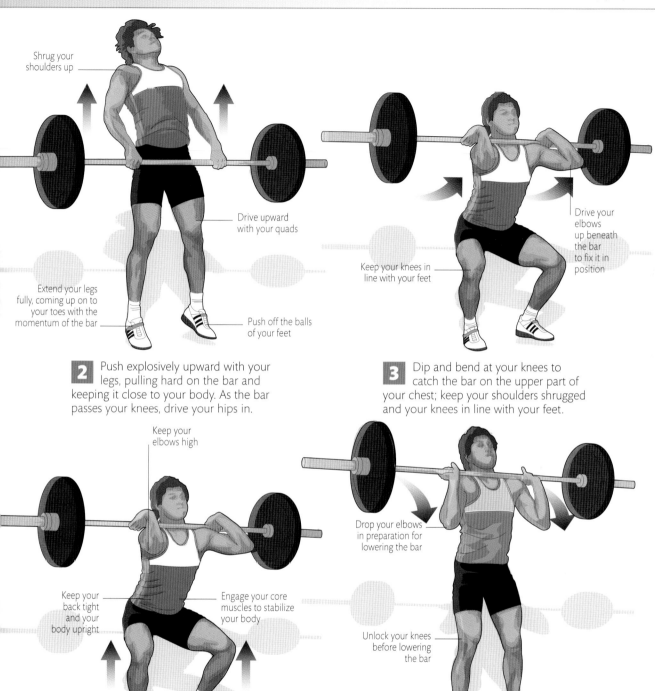

Shrug your shoulders up

Drive upward with your quads

Extend your legs fully, coming up on to your toes with the momentum of the bar

Push off the balls of your feet

Keep your knees in line with your feet

Drive your elbows up beneath the bar to fix it in position

2 Push explosively upward with your legs, pulling hard on the bar and keeping it close to your body. As the bar passes your knees, drive your hips in.

3 Dip and bend at your knees to catch the bar on the upper part of your chest; keep your shoulders shrugged and your knees in line with your feet.

Keep your elbows high

Keep your back tight and your body upright

Engage your core muscles to stabilize your body

Drop your elbows in preparation for lowering the bar

Unlock your knees before lowering the bar

5 Stand up from the deep squatting position. First, raise your buttocks and drive strongly with your legs, keeping your chest high.

6 Lower the bar slowly and under control to rest on your thighs. Keeping a flat back, return the bar to the start position on the floor.

HEAVY FRONT SQUAT

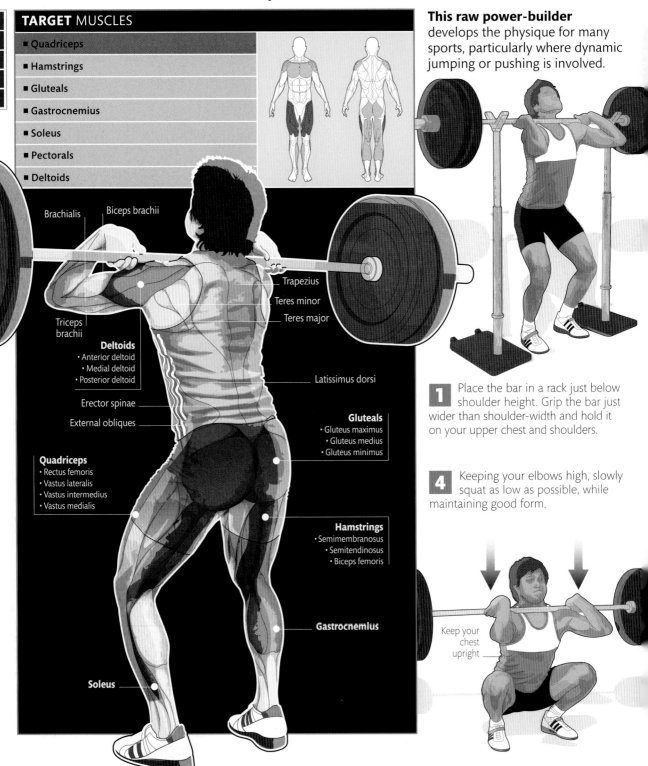

TARGET MUSCLES

- Quadriceps
- Hamstrings
- Gluteals
- Gastrocnemius
- Soleus
- Pectorals
- Deltoids

This raw power-builder develops the physique for many sports, particularly where dynamic jumping or pushing is involved.

Brachialis
Biceps brachii

Triceps brachii

Deltoids
• Anterior deltoid
• Medial deltoid
• Posterior deltoid

Erector spinae

External obliques

Quadriceps
• Rectus femoris
• Vastus lateralis
• Vastus intermedius
• Vastus medialis

Trapezius
Teres minor
Teres major

Latissimus dorsi

Gluteals
• Gluteus maximus
• Gluteus medius
• Gluteus minimus

Hamstrings
• Semimembranosus
• Semitendinosus
• Biceps femoris

Gastrocnemius

Soleus

1 Place the bar in a rack just below shoulder height. Grip the bar just wider than shoulder-width and hold it on your upper chest and shoulders.

4 Keeping your elbows high, slowly squat as low as possible, while maintaining good form.

Keep your chest upright

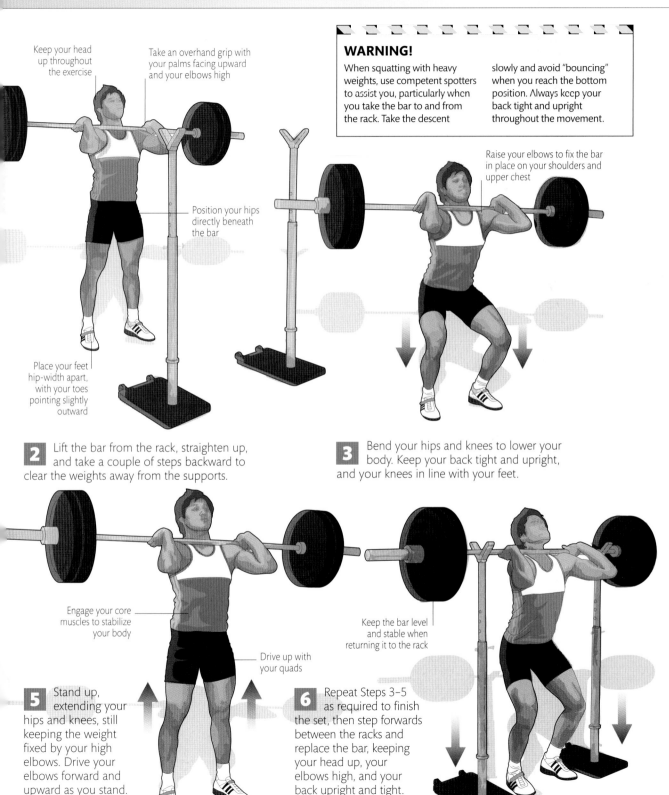

Keep your head up throughout the exercise

Take an overhand grip with your palms facing upward and your elbows high

WARNING!

When squatting with heavy weights, use competent spotters to assist you, particularly when you take the bar to and from the rack. Take the descent slowly and avoid "bouncing" when you reach the bottom position. Always keep your back tight and upright throughout the movement.

Position your hips directly beneath the bar

Place your feet hip-width apart, with your toes pointing slightly outward

Raise your elbows to fix the bar in place on your shoulders and upper chest

2 Lift the bar from the rack, straighten up, and take a couple of steps backward to clear the weights away from the supports.

3 Bend your hips and knees to lower your body. Keep your back tight and upright, and your knees in line with your feet.

Engage your core muscles to stabilize your body

Drive up with your quads

5 Stand up, extending your hips and knees, still keeping the weight fixed by your high elbows. Drive your elbows forward and upward as you stand.

Keep the bar level and stable when returning it to the rack

6 Repeat Steps 3–5 as required to finish the set, then step forwards between the racks and replace the bar, keeping your head up, your elbows high, and your back upright and tight.

OVERHEAD SQUAT

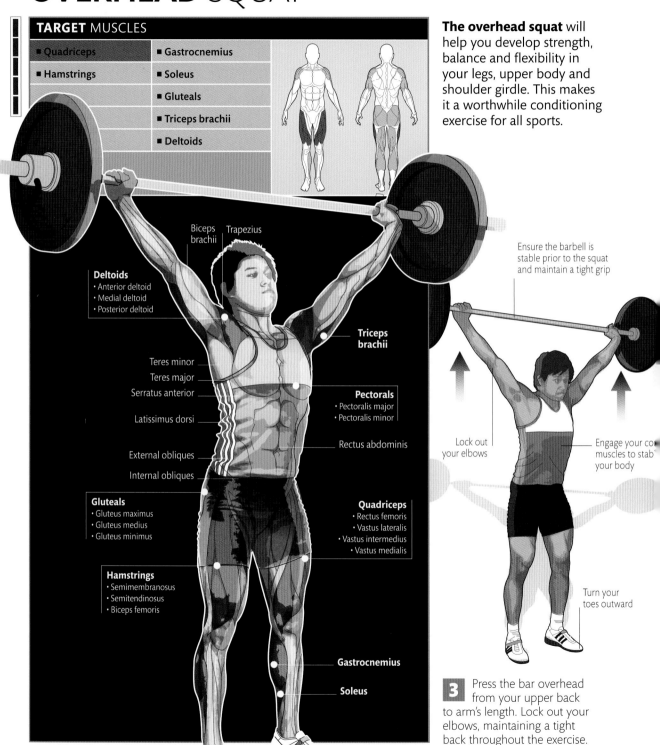

TARGET MUSCLES

- Quadriceps
- Hamstrings
- Gastrocnemius
- Soleus
- Gluteals
- Triceps brachii
- Deltoids

The overhead squat will help you develop strength, balance and flexibility in your legs, upper body and shoulder girdle. This makes it a worthwhile conditioning exercise for all sports.

Biceps brachii

Trapezius

Deltoids
• Anterior deltoid
• Medial deltoid
• Posterior deltoid

Triceps brachii

Teres minor

Teres major

Serratus anterior

Latissimus dorsi

Pectorals
• Pectoralis major
• Pectoralis minor

Rectus abdominis

External obliques

Internal obliques

Gluteals
• Gluteus maximus
• Gluteus medius
• Gluteus minimus

Quadriceps
• Rectus femoris
• Vastus lateralis
• Vastus intermedius
• Vastus medialis

Hamstrings
• Semimembranosus
• Semitendinosus
• Biceps femoris

Gastrocnemius

Soleus

Ensure the barbell is stable prior to the squat and maintain a tight grip

Lock out your elbows

Engage your co muscles to stab your body

Turn your toes outward

3 Press the bar overhead from your upper back to arm's length. Lock out your elbows, maintaining a tight back throughout the exercise.

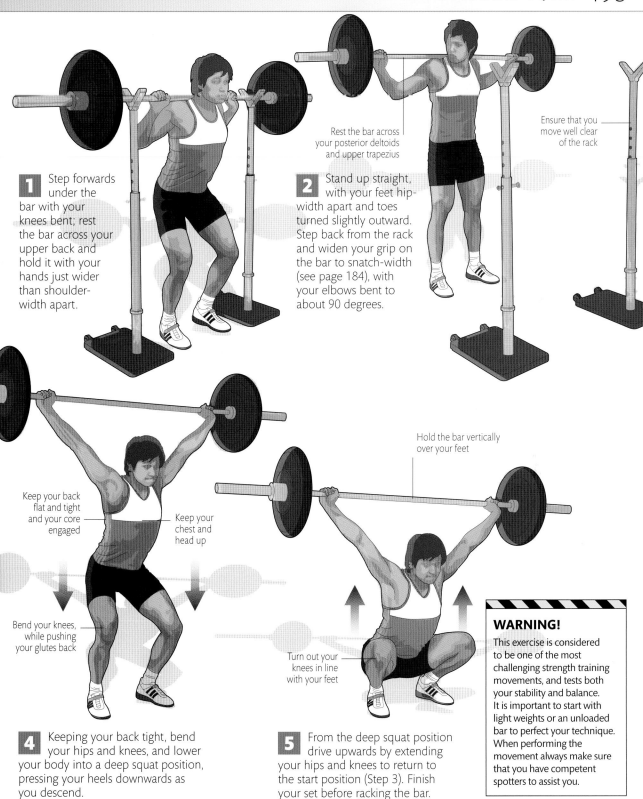

1 Step forwards under the bar with your knees bent; rest the bar across your upper back and hold it with your hands just wider than shoulder-width apart.

Rest the bar across your posterior deltoids and upper trapezius

2 Stand up straight, with your feet hip-width apart and toes turned slightly outward. Step back from the rack and widen your grip on the bar to snatch-width (see page 184), with your elbows bent to about 90 degrees.

Ensure that you move well clear of the rack

Keep your back flat and tight and your core engaged

Keep your chest and head up

Bend your knees, while pushing your glutes back

Hold the bar vertically over your feet

Turn out your knees in line with your feet

4 Keeping your back tight, bend your hips and knees, and lower your body into a deep squat position, pressing your heels downwards as you descend.

5 From the deep squat position drive upwards by extending your hips and knees to return to the start position (Step 3). Finish your set before racking the bar.

WARNING!
This exercise is considered to be one of the most challenging strength training movements, and tests both your stability and balance. It is important to start with light weights or an unloaded bar to perfect your technique. When performing the movement always make sure that you have competent spotters to assist you.

JERK BALANCE

TARGET MUSCLES

- Hamstrings
- Quadriceps
- Gluteals
- Deltoids
- Triceps brachii
- Gastrocnemius
- Soleus

The jerk balance is a compound movement that develops strength in your whole body, in addition to improving your stability and balance.

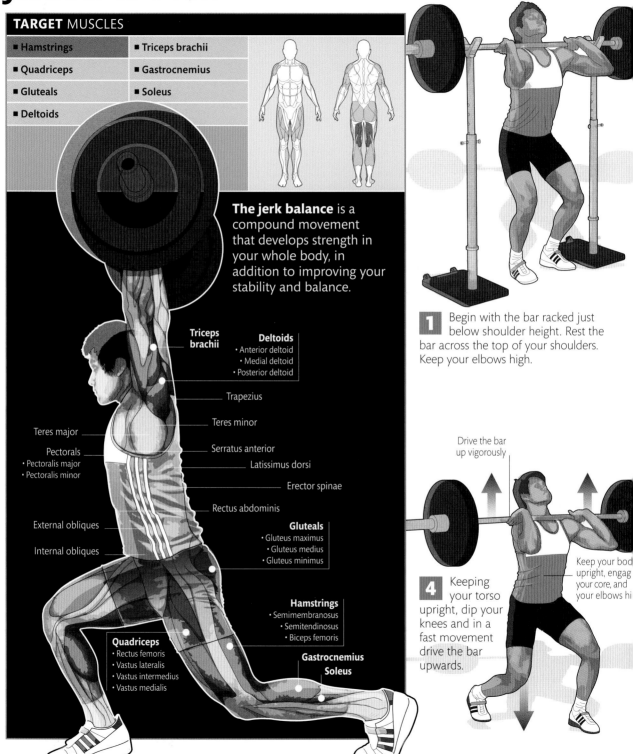

Triceps brachii

Deltoids
· Anterior deltoid
· Medial deltoid
· Posterior deltoid

Trapezius

Teres minor

Teres major

Pectorals
· Pectoralis major
· Pectoralis minor

Serratus anterior

Latissimus dorsi

Erector spinae

Rectus abdominis

External obliques

Internal obliques

Gluteals
· Gluteus maximus
· Gluteus medius
· Gluteus minimus

Hamstrings
· Semimembranosus
· Semitendinosus
· Biceps femoris

Quadriceps
· Rectus femoris
· Vastus lateralis
· Vastus intermedius
· Vastus medialis

**Gastrocnemius
Soleus**

1 Begin with the bar racked just below shoulder height. Rest the bar across the top of your shoulders. Keep your elbows high.

Drive the bar up vigorously

4 Keeping your torso upright, dip your knees and in a fast movement drive the bar upwards.

Keep your bod upright, engag your core, and your elbows hi

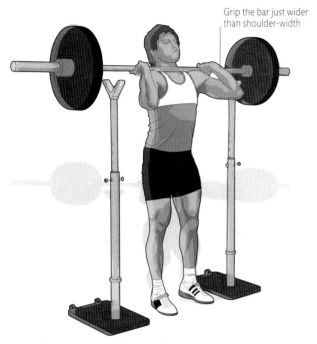

Grip the bar just wider than shoulder-width

2 Stand up with the barbell on top of your shoulders and walk backwards to the back of the platform.

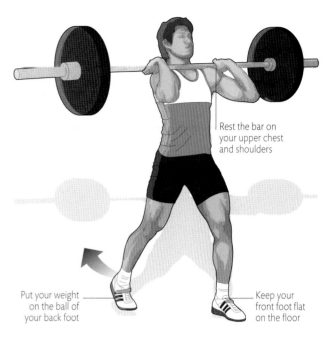

Rest the bar on your upper chest and shoulders

Put your weight on the ball of your back foot

Keep your front foot flat on the floor

3 Assume an upright position with your feet hip-width apart. Keeping your elbows high and your back upright and tight, take a long step forward into the start position for the jerk balance movement.

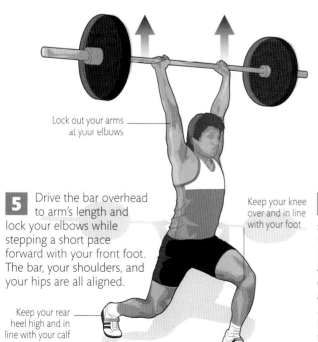

Lock out your arms at your elbows

Keep your knee over and in line with your foot

5 Drive the bar overhead to arm's length and lock your elbows while stepping a short pace forward with your front foot. The bar, your shoulders, and your hips are all aligned.

Keep your rear heel high and in line with your calf

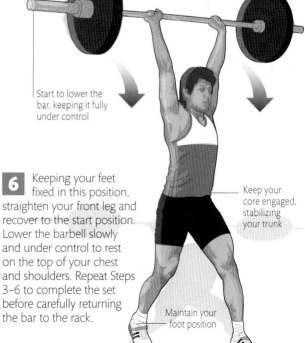

Start to lower the bar, keeping it fully under control

Keep your core engaged, stabilizing your trunk

6 Keeping your feet fixed in this position, straighten your front leg and recover to the start position. Lower the barbell slowly and under control to rest on the top of your chest and shoulders. Repeat Steps 3–6 to complete the set before carefully returning the bar to the rack.

Maintain your foot position

SNATCH BALANCE

TARGET MUSCLES

■ Quadriceps	■ Triceps brachii
■ Hamstrings	■ Gastrocnemius
■ Gluteals	■ Soleus
■ Deltoids	

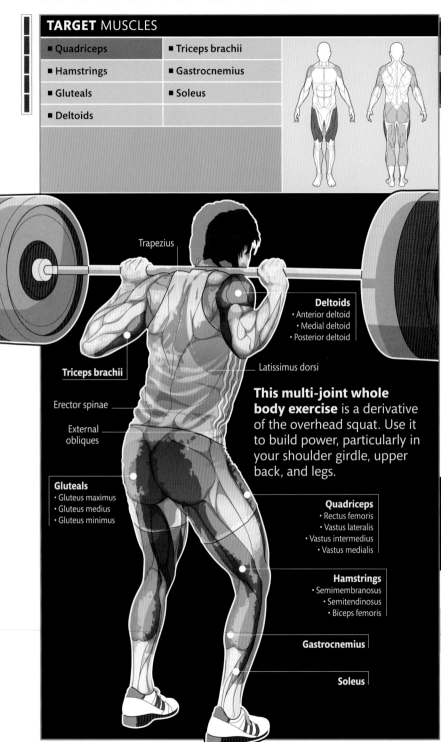

Trapezius

Deltoids
· Anterior deltoid
· Medial deltoid
· Posterior deltoid

Latissimus dorsi

Triceps brachii

Erector spinae

External
obliques

**This multi-joint whole
body exercise** is a derivative
of the overhead squat. Use it
to build power, particularly in
your shoulder girdle, upper
back, and legs.

Gluteals
· Gluteus maximus
· Gluteus medius
· Gluteus minimus

Quadriceps
· Rectus femoris
· Vastus lateralis
· Vastus intermedius
· Vastus medialis

Hamstrings
· Semimembranosus
· Semitendinosus
· Biceps femoris

Gastrocnemius

Soleus

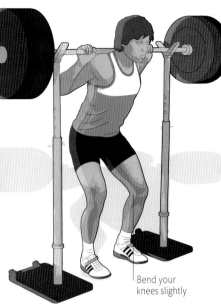

Bend your
knees slightly

1 Place the bar on a rack just
below shoulder height. Rest
the bar across the upper part of
your back.

4 Continue to squat down into a
deep position. Keep your body
upright, your back flat, engaging your
core, and your head upright and in
front of the bar.

Support the bar in line with
your shoulders and feet

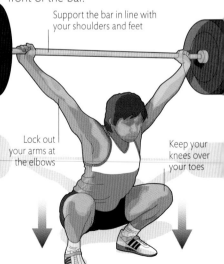

Lock out
your arms at
the elbows

Keep your
knees over
your toes

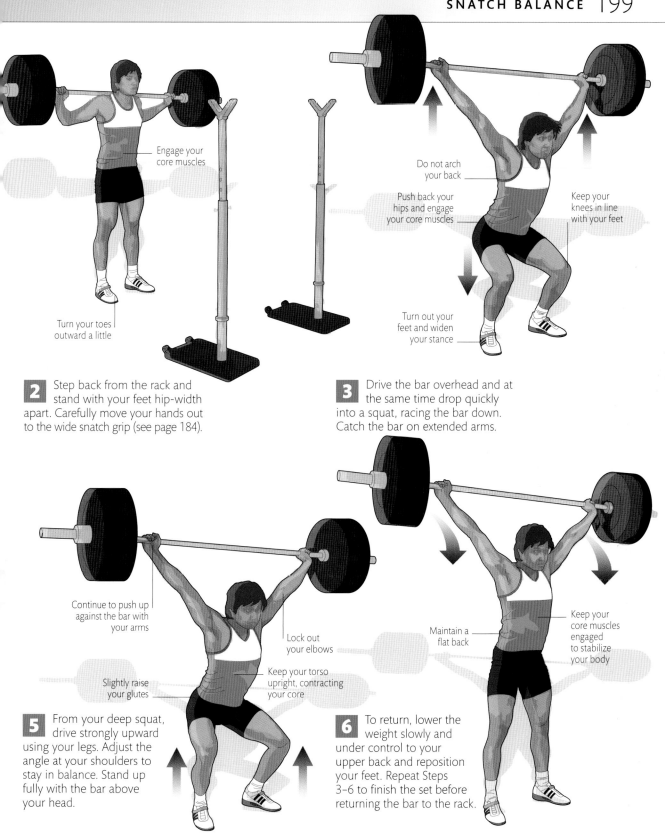

Engage your core muscles

Turn your toes outward a little

Do not arch your back

Push back your hips and engage your core muscles

Keep your knees in line with your feet

Turn out your feet and widen your stance

2 Step back from the rack and stand with your feet hip-width apart. Carefully move your hands out to the wide snatch grip (see page 184).

3 Drive the bar overhead and at the same time drop quickly into a squat, racing the bar down. Catch the bar on extended arms.

Continue to push up against the bar with your arms

Lock out your elbows

Slightly raise your glutes

Keep your torso upright, contracting your core

Maintain a flat back

Keep your core muscles engaged to stabilize your body

5 From your deep squat, drive strongly upward using your legs. Adjust the angle at your shoulders to stay in balance. Stand up fully with the bar above your head.

6 To return, lower the weight slowly and under control to your upper back and reposition your feet. Repeat Steps 3–6 to finish the set before returning the bar to the rack.

SPLIT SNATCH

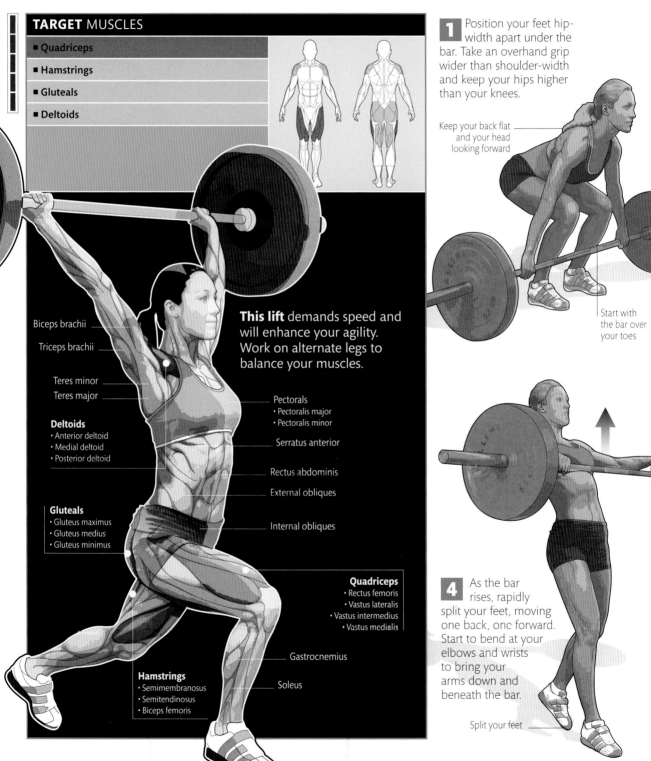

TARGET MUSCLES

- Quadriceps
- Hamstrings
- Gluteals
- Deltoids

1 Position your feet hip-width apart under the bar. Take an overhand grip wider than shoulder-width and keep your hips higher than your knees.

Keep your back flat and your head looking forward

Start with the bar over your toes

This lift demands speed and will enhance your agility. Work on alternate legs to balance your muscles.

Biceps brachii

Triceps brachii

Teres minor
Teres major

Deltoids
· Anterior deltoid
· Medial deltoid
· Posterior deltoid

Gluteals
· Gluteus maximus
· Gluteus medius
· Gluteus minimus

Pectorals
· Pectoralis major
· Pectoralis minor

Serratus anterior

Rectus abdominis

External obliques

Internal obliques

Quadriceps
· Rectus femoris
· Vastus lateralis
· Vastus intermedius
· Vastus medialis

Gastrocnemius

Soleus

Hamstrings
· Semimembranosus
· Semitendinosus
· Biceps femoris

4 As the bar rises, rapidly split your feet, moving one back, one forward. Start to bend at your elbows and wrists to bring your arms down and beneath the bar.

Split your feet

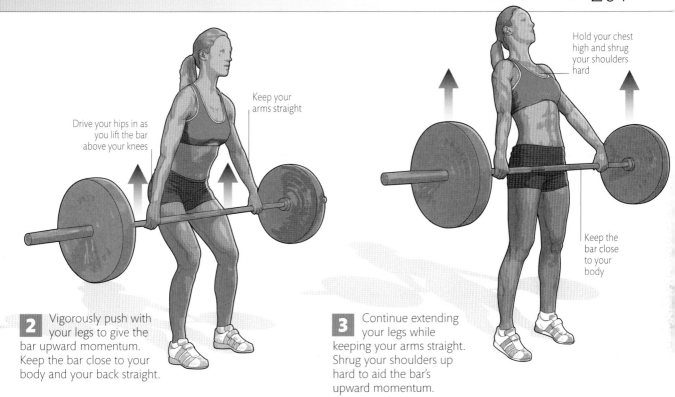

Drive your hips in as you lift the bar above your knees

Keep your arms straight

Hold your chest high and shrug your shoulders hard

Keep the bar close to your body

2 Vigorously push with your legs to give the bar upward momentum. Keep the bar close to your body and your back straight.

3 Continue extending your legs while keeping your arms straight. Shrug your shoulders up hard to aid the bar's upward momentum.

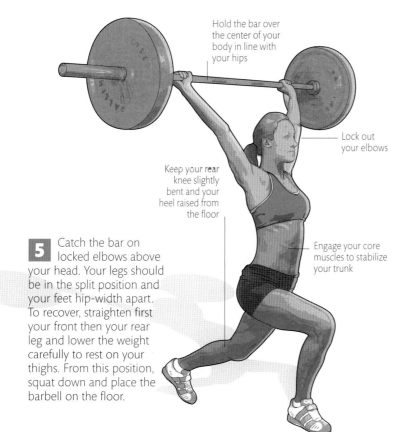

Hold the bar over the center of your body in line with your hips

Lock out your elbows

Keep your rear knee slightly bent and your heel raised from the floor

Engage your core muscles to stabilize your trunk

5 Catch the bar on locked elbows above your head. Your legs should be in the split position and your feet hip-width apart. To recover, straighten first your front then your rear leg and lower the weight carefully to rest on your thighs. From this position, squat down and place the barbell on the floor.

WARNING!

As with all dynamic lifts, the split snatch should be performed on a proper lifting platform with full size 5½- or 11-lb (2.5- or 5-kg) discs. This is because there is always a risk of failing the lift and dropping the bar. In the event of a failed lift, it is important to move your body away from the line of the falling bar. Try to maintain your grip on the bar until it hits the ground. Once on the ground, let go of the bar and allow it to settle on the platform before resetting for the next attempt. Make sure you always work within your capabilities; practise and perfect the move with light weights.

PUSH PRESS

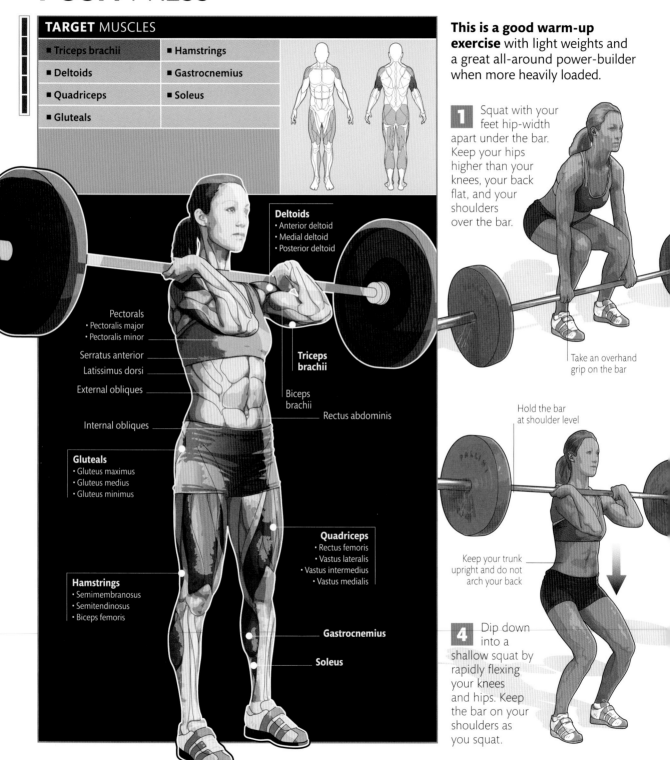

TARGET MUSCLES

■ Triceps brachii	■ Hamstrings
■ Deltoids	■ Gastrocnemius
■ Quadriceps	■ Soleus
■ Gluteals	

Deltoids
• Anterior deltoid
• Medial deltoid
• Posterior deltoid

Pectorals
• Pectoralis major
• Pectoralis minor

Serratus anterior

Latissimus dorsi

External obliques

Internal obliques

Triceps brachii

Biceps brachii

Rectus abdominis

Gluteals
• Gluteus maximus
• Gluteus medius
• Gluteus minimus

Quadriceps
• Rectus femoris
• Vastus lateralis
• Vastus intermedius
• Vastus medialis

Hamstrings
• Semimembranosus
• Semitendinosus
• Biceps femoris

Gastrocnemius

Soleus

This is a good warm-up exercise with light weights and a great all-around power-builder when more heavily loaded.

1 Squat with your feet hip-width apart under the bar. Keep your hips higher than your knees, your back flat, and your shoulders over the bar.

Take an overhand grip on the bar

Hold the bar at shoulder level

Keep your trunk upright and do not arch your back

4 Dip down into a shallow squat by rapidly flexing your knees and hips. Keep the bar on your shoulders as you squat.

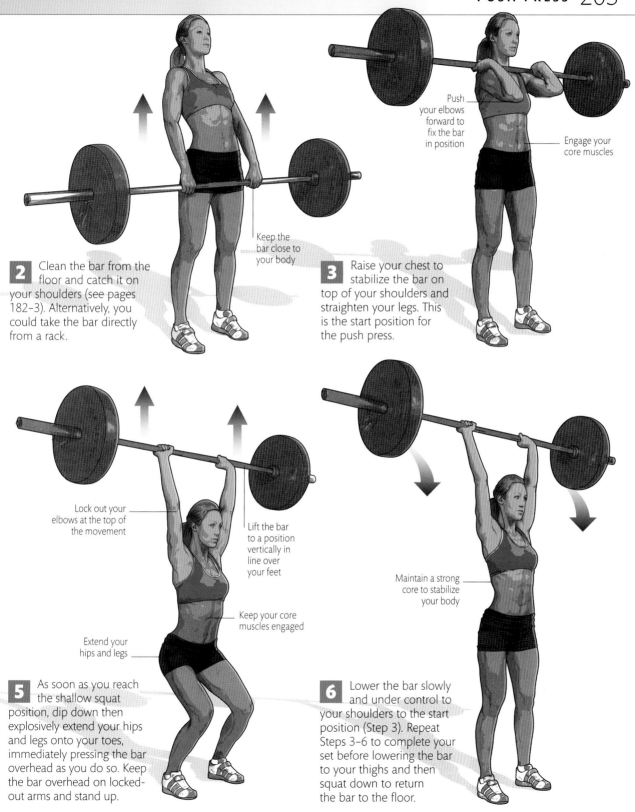

2 Clean the bar from the floor and catch it on your shoulders (see pages 182–3). Alternatively, you could take the bar directly from a rack.

Keep the bar close to your body

Push your elbows forward to fix the bar in position

Engage your core muscles

3 Raise your chest to stabilize the bar on top of your shoulders and straighten your legs. This is the start position for the push press.

Lock out your elbows at the top of the movement

Lift the bar to a position vertically in line over your feet

Keep your core muscles engaged

Extend your hips and legs

5 As soon as you reach the shallow squat position, dip down then explosively extend your hips and legs onto your toes, immediately pressing the bar overhead as you do so. Keep the bar overhead on locked-out arms and stand up.

Maintain a strong core to stabilize your body

6 Lower the bar slowly and under control to your shoulders to the start position (Step 3). Repeat Steps 3–6 to complete your set before lowering the bar to your thighs and then squat down to return the bar to the floor.

KETTLEBELL HIGH-PULL

TARGET MUSCLES

- Quadriceps
- Gluteals
- Trapezius
- Deltoids
- Biceps brachii
- Erector spinae
- Hamstrings
- Gastrocnemius
- Soleus

The kettlebell high-pull is a whole body exercise that builds power. It is great training for explosive movements in sprinting, jumping, boxing, and karate.

1 Squat down with your spine neutral, your shoulders ahead of the weight, your feet shoulder-width apart, and your hips higher than your knees.

Keep your head up and look forward

Ensure that your shoulders are in front of the weight

Keep your arms extended through the first part of the pull

Elevate your elbows above the weight

Keep your back flat

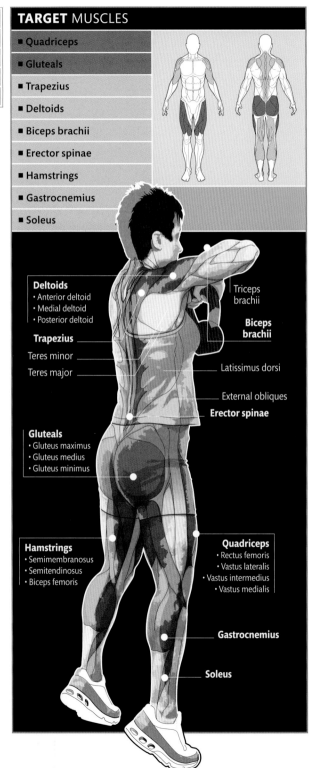

Deltoids
- Anterior deltoid
- Medial deltoid
- Posterior deltoid

Trapezius

Teres minor

Teres major

Triceps brachii

Biceps brachii

Latissimus dorsi

External obliques

Erector spinae

Gluteals
- Gluteus maximus
- Gluteus medius
- Gluteus minimus

Hamstrings
- Semimembranosus
- Semitendinosus
- Biceps femoris

Quadriceps
- Rectus femoris
- Vastus lateralis
- Vastus intermedius
- Vastus medialis

Gastrocnemius

Soleus

2 Begin the pull by pushing down through your feet and driving your hips up and forward.

3 Use the force of the leg drive to extend your body upward. Lift the kettlebell to chest level. Let your momentum carry you up on to your toes then squat down to the start position.

BARBELL JUMP SQUAT

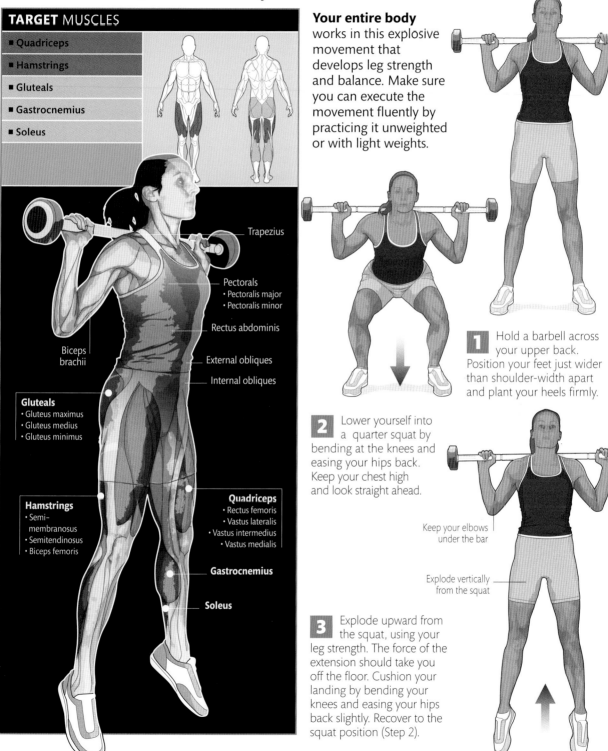

TARGET MUSCLES

- Quadriceps
- Hamstrings
- Gluteals
- Gastrocnemius
- Soleus

Your entire body works in this explosive movement that develops leg strength and balance. Make sure you can execute the movement fluently by practicing it unweighted or with light weights.

Trapezius

Pectorals
• Pectoralis major
• Pectoralis minor

Rectus abdominis

External obliques

Internal obliques

Biceps brachii

Gluteals
• Gluteus maximus
• Gluteus medius
• Gluteus minimus

Hamstrings
• Semi-membranosus
• Semitendinosus
• Biceps femoris

Quadriceps
• Rectus femoris
• Vastus lateralis
• Vastus intermedius
• Vastus medialis

Gastrocnemius

Soleus

1 Hold a barbell across your upper back. Position your feet just wider than shoulder-width apart and plant your heels firmly.

2 Lower yourself into a quarter squat by bending at the knees and easing your hips back. Keep your chest high and look straight ahead.

Keep your elbows under the bar

Explode vertically from the squat

3 Explode upward from the squat, using your leg strength. The force of the extension should take you off the floor. Cushion your landing by bending your knees and easing your hips back slightly. Recover to the squat position (Step 2).

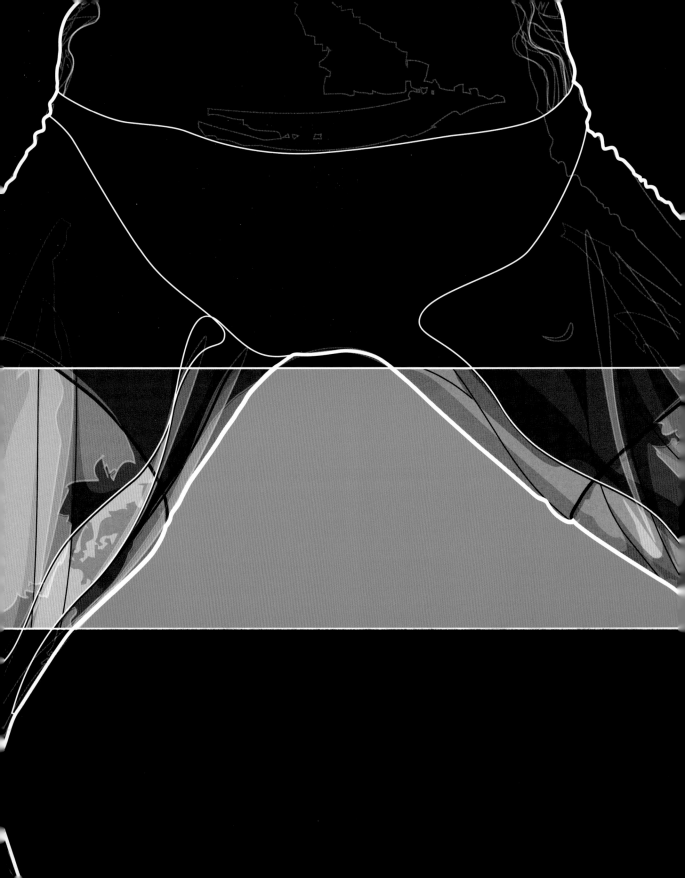

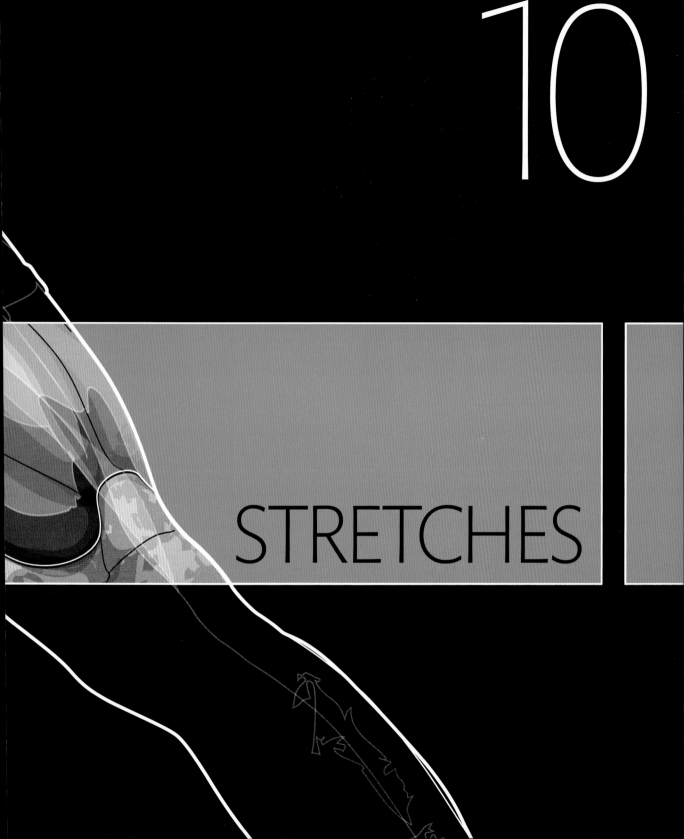

10

STRETCHES

BICEPS STRETCH

Simple to perform, this very specific stretch is particularly useful for gymnasts and swimmers. Move slowly and under control to avoid potential injury.

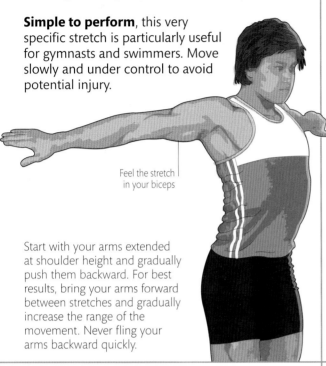

Feel the stretch in your biceps

Start with your arms extended at shoulder height and gradually push them backward. For best results, bring your arms forward between stretches and gradually increase the range of the movement. Never fling your arms backward quickly.

UPPER BACK STRETCH

This easy stretch specifically mobilizes the muscles in your upper back, making it useful across a range of sports, particularly those that involve throwing actions.

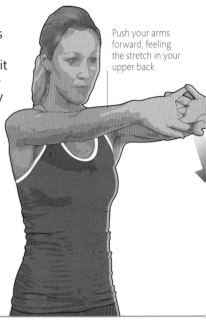

Push your arms forward, feeling the stretch in your upper back

Interlock your fingers, palms facing away from you. Bring your hands to chest level and extend your arms, locking out your elbows and pushing your shoulders forward.

SHOULDER STRETCH

This easy and effective stretch specifically works the muscles around your shoulder joint. It is particularly useful for weightlifters and those engaged in throwing events.

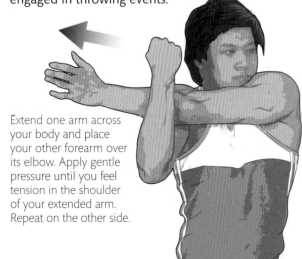

Extend one arm across your body and place your other forearm over its elbow. Apply gentle pressure until you feel tension in the shoulder of your extended arm. Repeat on the other side.

ERECTOR STRETCH

This stretch works the erector spinae muscles that run on either side of your spine from the back of your head to your pelvis.

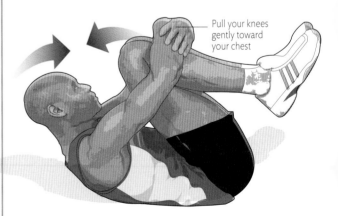

Pull your knees gently toward your chest

Lie back on an exercise mat. Bring your knees toward your chest and wrap your arms around them. Pull gently until you feel the stretch tension in your back.

LAT STRETCH

Specifically targeting the latissimus dorsi muscles, this stretch is useful for weightlifters, rowers, and field athletes.

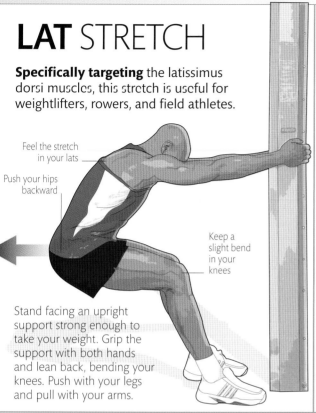

Feel the stretch in your lats

Push your hips backward

Keep a slight bend in your knees

Stand facing an upright support strong enough to take your weight. Grip the support with both hands and lean back, bending your knees. Push with your legs and pull with your arms.

ITB STRETCH 1

The iliotibial band (ITB) is a band of connective tissue that runs down the outside of your thigh. Runners, hikers, gymnasts, and dancers should perform this stretch regularly to help prevent inflammation of the area above the knee—a common cause of pain.

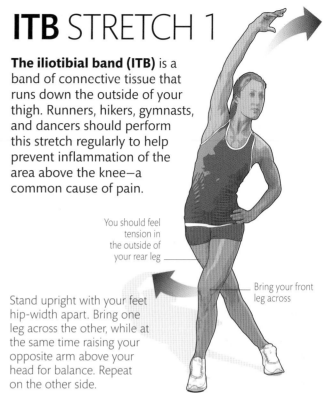

You should feel tension in the outside of your rear leg

Bring your front leg across

Stand upright with your feet hip-width apart. Bring one leg across the other, while at the same time raising your opposite arm above your head for balance. Repeat on the other side.

PEC STRETCH

This stretch targets the pectoral muscles of your upper chest, easing tightness and increasing flexibility. It is also helpful if you train for throwing events.

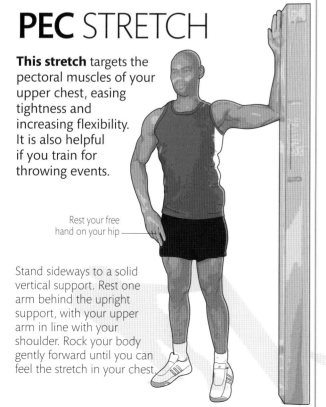

Rest your free hand on your hip

Stand sideways to a solid vertical support. Rest one arm behind the upright support, with your upper arm in line with your shoulder. Rock your body gently forward until you can feel the stretch in your chest.

ITB STRETCH 2

This seated version of the iliotibial band stretch is more advanced than the one shown above because you need greater flexibility in your hip joint to perform it correctly.

Sit on the floor, with your legs extended. Bend one leg and cross it over your extended leg so that your foot is flat on the floor. Supporting yourself with one arm, reach over with your free hand and gently press on the outside of your knee until you can feel the stretch in your ITB.

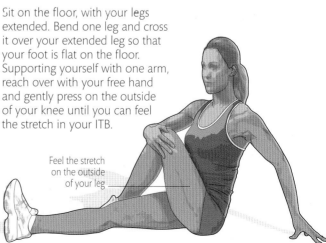

Feel the stretch on the outside of your leg

3-POINT QUAD STRETCH

The purpose of this stretch is to work the quadriceps muscles on the front of your upper thigh and promote flexibility at your knee joint. Relatively simple to perform, it is useful following any type of leg workout.

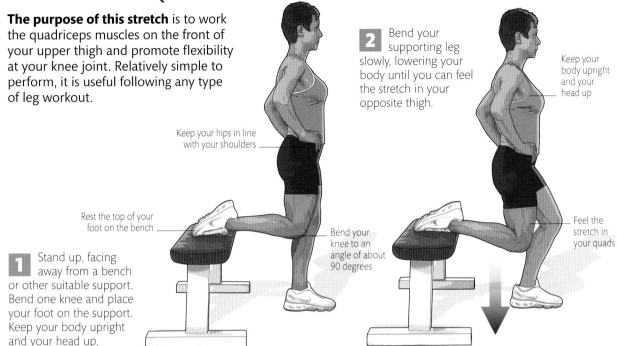

2 Bend your supporting leg slowly, lowering your body until you can feel the stretch in your opposite thigh.

Keep your body upright and your head up

Keep your hips in line with your shoulders

Rest the top of your foot on the bench

Bend your knee to an angle of about 90 degrees

Feel the stretch in your quads

1 Stand up, facing away from a bench or other suitable support. Bend one knee and place your foot on the support. Keep your body upright and your head up.

HAMSTRING
STRETCH 1

Activity that involves repeated knee flexion, such as running or cycling, can cause tightness in your hamstrings. This stretch helps you to protect this vulnerable area.

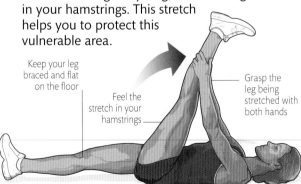

Keep your leg braced and flat on the floor

Feel the stretch in your hamstrings

Grasp the leg being stretched with both hands

Lie on your back with your legs extended. Lift each leg in turn, keeping the knee braced and the toes pulled back toward your body. If you are very flexible, try extending the stretch a little by pulling back on your leg.

HAMSTRING
STRETCH 2

This is a simple all-purpose stretch that works all the muscles in your hamstrings, relieving the tightness that can stress your lower back. Stretch slowly and do not " bounce" at full extension.

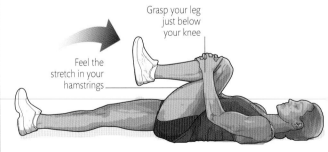

Grasp your leg just below your knee

Feel the stretch in your hamstrings

Lie on your back with your legs extended. Bend one knee. Pull gently on your leg, bringing your knee toward your chest until you feel the stretch. Keep the back of your head against the floor.

3 Push up with your supporting leg to return to the start position. Be sure to repeat the stretch on your other leg.

Flex at the ankle

Push up to return, working your calf muscles strongly

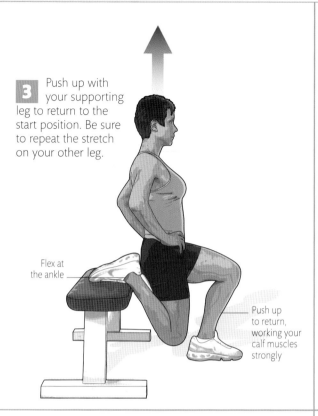

QUAD STRETCH 1

Stretching the large muscles at the front of your thigh will help prevent injuries and reduce soreness. This stretch can be performed one leg at a time, or with both legs together.

Lie face down on a mat and bend one leg at your knee. Reach back with your hand on the same side, grasp your ankle, and pull back gently to feel the stretch in your quads.

Keep your back flat, not arched up

Pull gently on your leg

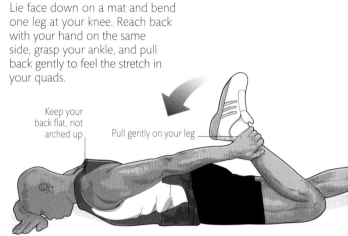

HAMSTRING
STRETCH 3

You can perform this version of the hamstring stretch in a small space, on a track, or at a competition venue.

Start by stepping forward with one foot and then bend your supporting leg. Keep your lead leg braced and both feet flat on the floor. Tilt your pelvis slightly forward. Hold for a few seconds, then switch sides.

Keep your head up, back straight, and abs pulled in

Feel the stretch in your hamstrings

Keep both feet flat on the floor

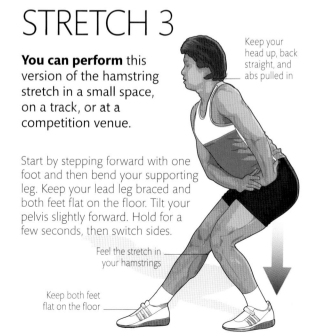

QUAD STRETCH 2

This advanced stretch calls for good hip flexibility. It is a dual-purpose stretch that also works the adductor muscles on the insides of your thighs.

Sit with your trunk upright. Turn your feet in so that their soles touch. Reach forward with your hands and hold your feet together.

Push your knees gently down toward the floor

Feel the stretch in your quads

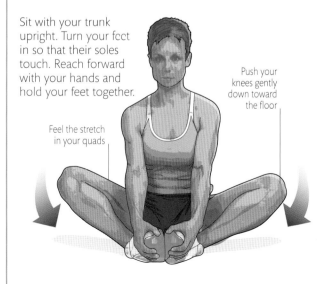

ADDUCTOR
STRETCH 1

Stretching your adductor or groin muscles is key to maintaining hip flexibility for many sports.

Keep your body upright and put your hands on your hips. Bend your lead leg so that your front knee stays over your foot. Keep the trailing leg extended with your foot flat. Rock gently to the side.

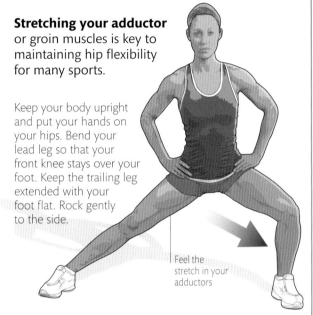

Feel the stretch in your adductors

ADDUCTOR
STRETCH 2

This advanced version of the adductor stretch requires more agility to achieve the extended position: it is ideal for gymnasts and hurdlers.

Squat down on both legs then move one leg out, resting it on the heel of your foot. "Sit in" to apply stretch to your adductors, but do not "bounce."

Pull your toes back toward your body

Feel the stretch in your adductors

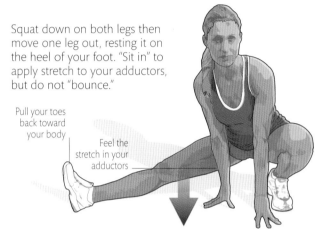

HAMSTRING STRETCH

Tightness in your glutes often manifests itself as lower back pain after a workout. This fairly advanced stretch works your glutes as well as the muscles of your lower back and your hamstrings.

1 Sit on the floor with one leg straight ahead of you and one bent behind, keeping your hips and shoulders in line.

Stabilize your body with your arms

Pull your toes back toward your body

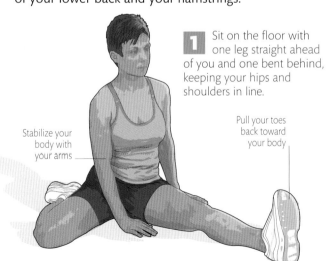

Flex your trunk forward from your hips

Grasp your upper foot

Feel the stretch in your hamstrings

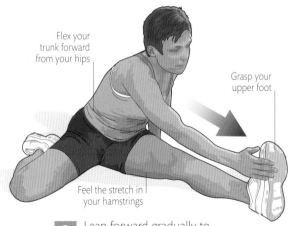

2 Lean forward gradually to your extended foot. If you are able to grab your foot, pull it gently toward you to increase the stretch.

CALF STRETCH

Tight calf muscles are more prone to injury during explosive movements like sprinting, so this easy stretch for your lower legs is a must if you are a runner.

From a standing position, take a good step forward, keeping your feet hip-width apart. Bend the leading leg, keeping your knee over your foot.

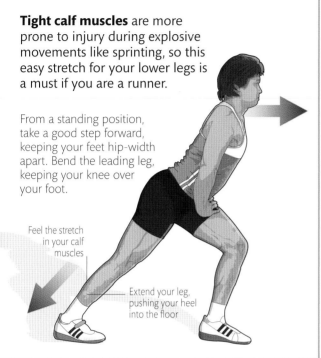

Feel the stretch in your calf muscles

Extend your leg, pushing your heel into the floor

PIKE CALF STRETCH

The muscles of your calf—the gastrocnemius and the deeper soleus—are stretched in this advanced movement.

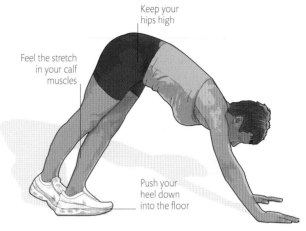

Keep your hips high

Feel the stretch in your calf muscles

Push your heel down into the floor

Take up a pike position, with your body bent forward at your hips and your legs straight. Place your right foot behind your left ankle. Keeping your legs straight, press the heel of your left foot down. Repeat on the other side.

WALKING LUNGE STRETCH

This is a highly effective but simple multipurpose stretching exercise that mobilizes the whole of your hip region.

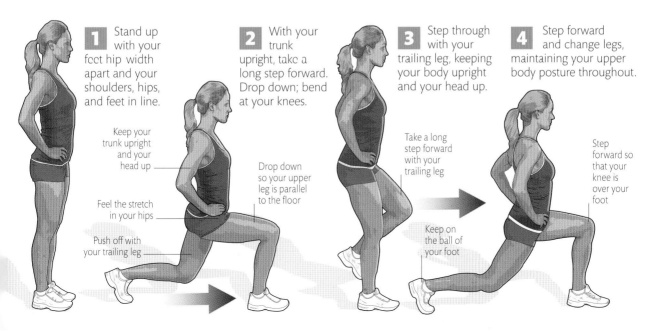

1 Stand up with your feet hip width apart and your shoulders, hips, and feet in line.

2 With your trunk upright, take a long step forward. Drop down; bend at your knees.

3 Step through with your trailing leg, keeping your body upright and your head up.

4 Step forward and change legs, maintaining your upper body posture throughout.

Keep your trunk upright and your head up

Feel the stretch in your hips

Push off with your trailing leg

Drop down so your upper leg is parallel to the floor

Take a long step forward with your trailing leg

Keep on the ball of your foot

Step forward so that your knee is over your foot

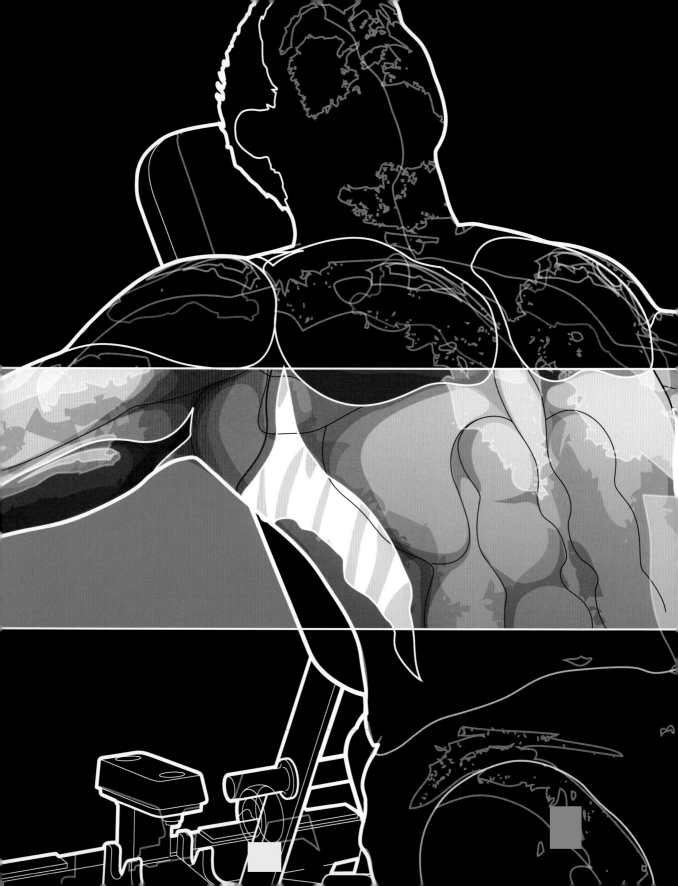

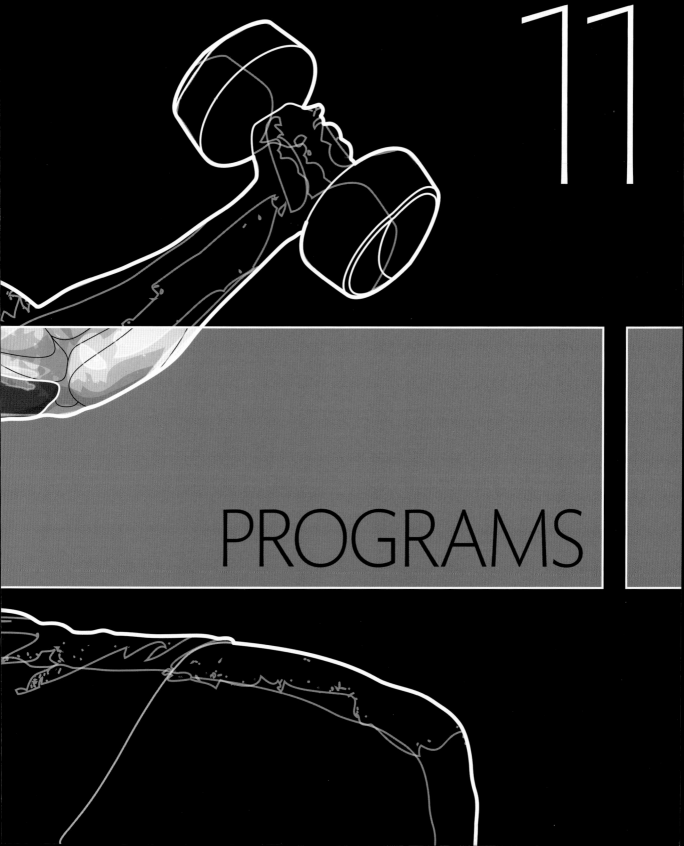

PROGRAMS

INTRODUCTION

The training programs featured in this section have been designed to help you get the very best out of your training, whatever your gender, age, experience, existing strength, or overall goal—be that increasing your strength, developing your physique, bodybuilding, or training for a sport. These tried-and-tested programs cover three main resistance-training goals—strength, body sculpting, and bodybuilding, and a range of basic and advanced programs are provided for each. Using a small number of targeted exercises, each of the programs allows you to complete your resistance training session in around 30–40 minutes, and reduce the chance of you overtraining.

> **WARNING!**
> Never do more than the programs suggest—you may overtrain, which can lead to illness and injury. Always consult your health-care practitioner before starting to train (see page 256).

Q | What can I expect from the programs?
A | The featured programs allow you to tailor your training to help you realize your goals: this approach enables you to achieve the best possible results, and is known as "specificity" (see page 33).

The basic programs in this section provide free-weight, body weight, and resistance machine variants, and none are excessively long. The days of workouts comprising dozens of obscure exercises are gone. Sports scientists recognize that simple, functional programs organized with specificity in mind and performed around 2–3 times per week are a far more effective (and less time-consuming) way to reach your goals.

Where possible, the programs are also designed with high levels of "functionality" (see page 43) in mind—this means that the exercises are applicable to real-life movements, be they at home, work, or in the sports arena, as opposed to working single muscles in isolation. In short, these exercises move your body in the way it was designed to move, meaning that you will get better results, faster.

Q | What are the differences between training with free weights, body weight, and resistance machines?
A | Free weights offer you the highest level of "functionality" of the three. This is because they enable you to perform exercises that closely replicate "real life" movements, without the support and uniformity provided by resistance machines. Unsupported, your body engages additional smaller muscles in order to stabilize you—thus working more muscles than those you are specifically targeting, and offering you "added value" from your workout.

Using your own body weight is another highly functional and effective way of developing strength, especially since it means you can train on the move, with little or no equipment, although this form of training is obviously limited by the weight of your own body. Do not assume, however, that you will find using your body weight easier than other exercise methods.

Resistance machines usually provide you with padded body supports, and enable you to perform exercises in a seated position, meaning that you tend to work targeted muscles in isolation. They can be a useful tool for those starting out, and for those looking to work specific muscles. The machine-based exercises included in these programs have been chosen because they offer as much functionality as possible.

Q | Why should I warm up and cool down?
A | Warming up your muscles is essential because it gets your body ready for your workout while minimizing the risk

BASIC PRINCIPLES

Regardless of the program you follow, some basic training principles always apply:
- **OVERLOAD:** Your training should demand more of your muscles than would normally be the case for everyday activity.
- **RECOVERY:** An essential component in any training regimen, recovery literally means rest. It is while your body is resting that it adapts and strengthens, ready to be overloaded again during the next training session.
- **PROGRESSION:** Your body adapts to the demands being placed on it. If you do not place extra demands on it, your training results will reach a plateau. So you have to gradually (and carefully) increase the number of sets, reps, and weight (or a combination of all three) to see continual progress (see page 33).

of injury and maximizing your potential to learn and improve. Cooling down is equally important, since it returns your body to a resting state in a controlled manner. So do not be tempted to skip your warm-up before your training session or your cool-down at the end of the session, since this will increase your risk of injury and ability to complete your next workout without the restrictions and discomfort caused by tight and aching muscles.

- A good basic warm-up comprises 10 minutes of jumping rope, jogging, or working on the cross-trainer, followed by 10 minutes of dynamic mobility work (see pages 46–47). You can also tailor your warm-up to your training activity if you need something more specific. A certified coach or fitness instructor can advise you.
- Likewise, cooling down can be achieved by 5–10 minutes of gentle jogging or walking, which decreases the body's temperature and heart rate and helps your muscles get rid of waste products, such as lactic acid.
- Finally, perform 5–10 minutes of developmental stretches, which help your muscles to relax and your muscle fibers to realign and reestablish their normal resting length and ranges of movement (see pages 208–13).

Q | Do results differ from person to person?
A | Yes. No two people are the same, and there are a range of factors that will affect how quickly you progress:
- **Your age:** as well as your age in years, age refers to your emotional and biological maturity as well as the number of years of training experience you have—your "training age."
- **Your gender:** men and women have different physiologies and capabilities.
- **Your heredity:** this is your innate ability, genetically determined.
- **Your physical capability:** this is made up of two factors—your heredity and your training history.
- **Your lifestyle:** how well you look after yourself in between training sessions has a major effect on your overall development (see also page 17).

UNDERSTANDING THE CHARTS

These are the terms you need to understand to use the charts effectively:
- **SETS:** A group of repetitions; for example, two sets of five repetitions.
- **REPETITIONS**: The number of times a weight should be lifted—"reps" for short
- **WEIGHT:** the weight to be lifted, expressed as a RM figure. 1RM, for example, means a weight that you can lift only once. 12RM, means a weight that you can lift 12 times before muscular failure.
- **MUSCULAR FAILURE:** This is the point at which you cannot perform another repetition of an exercise within a set.
- **DURATION OF PROGRAM:** A range is given for the number of weeks the program should be followed. You should not exceed this number.
- **FREQUENCY OF PROGRAM:** This is the number of workouts you should do per week, with the number of rest days you should take between workouts.
- **RECOVERY TIME:** This is the amount of rest time in seconds or minutes that you should take between exercises.
- **APPLICATION OF SPLIT PROGRAM:** This information applies to the split programs and details the days of the week that each half of the split should be performed, indicated by an A or a B. The splits are performed on an alternating two-week basis.

Q | How long do I follow a program?
A | Each of the programs has a predetermined duration (6–14 weeks). You should follow the program for the specified time, adhering to the program guidelines. If you follow a program for longer than stated, your body will adapt to it and your results will be less than expected. In fact, you can actually regress and get weaker if you follow a program for longer than prescribed.

66 **The featured programs allow you to tailor your training to help you realize your goals: this approach enables you to achieve the best possible results** 99

EXERCISE FUNCTIONALITY MATRIX

Exercises can be graded by "functionality." A "functional" exercise is one that carries over into real-life movements—the repetitive pulls, pushes, lifts, and standing—or stepping-up actions—needed for everyday life (and most sports movements) by working several muscles at once rather than in isolation, one at a time.

Q | What does the matrix show?
A | The matrix below and on pages 220–21 lists all the exercises in the book (including their page number and any variations) and places them on a scale of functionality. On the far right are the most functional exercises—the ones that require you to work several muscles simultaneously. On the far left are the most isolated exercises—these are the ones

EXERCISE GROUP	MOST ISOLATED
LEGS	■ Machine leg curl (pp. 80–81) ■ Pulley leg curl (p. 81 var.) ■ Machine leg extension (pp. 80–81) ■ Hip abductor (pp. 82–83) ■ Hip adductor (pp. 82–83) ■ 45-degree leg press (pp. 78–79) ■ One-leg 45-degree leg press (p. 79 var.) ■ Machine calf raise (p. 84 var.)
BACK	■ Lat pull-down (p. 93) ■ Seated pulley row (pp. 96–97) ■ Back extension (pp. 104–05) ■ Prone row (pp. 106–07) ■ Straight arm pulley (pp. 106–07)
CHEST	■ Pulley cross-over (pp. 116–17) ■ Low pulley cross-over (p. 116 var.) ■ Mid pulley cross-over (p. 116 var.) ■ Machine fly (p. 119) ■ Incline fly (pp. 114–15) ■ Flat fly (p. 114 var.) ■ Machine bench press (pp. 118–19) ■ Ball push-up (p. 120 var.)

that focus primarily on working one muscle in isolation. As you can see, many exercises fall in between these two extremes and are placed on the scale accordingly.

The most functional exercises are the most effective for integrated strength training, whereas the most isolated are useful when the goal is to strengthen a weakness or to develop the muscle for aesthetic purposes, as in the case of body sculpting or bodybuilding. Both functional and isolated exercises are used throughout the programs.

For ease of reference, all the exercises are grouped by body part—six in total—followed by a section on dynamic lifts. Since they work a high number of muscles simultaneously throughout the entire body they are all listed at the most functional end of the scale.

MOST FUNCTIONAL

- Bulgarian barbell split squat (p. 70)
- Bulgarian dumbbell split squat (p. 71)
- Barbell step-up (pp. 76–77)
- Dumbbell step-up (p. 76 var.)
- Calf raise (p. 84)
- Straight leg deadlift (p. 85)
- Romanian deadlift (pp. 88–89)
- Romanian deadlift using rack (p. 88 var.)

- Sumo squat (p. 64 var.)
- Barbell hack squat (p. 67)

- Back squat (pp. 64–65)
- Front squat (p. 66)
- Dumbbell split squat (p. 68)
- Overhead split squat (p. 69)
- Barbell lunge (pp. 72–73)
- Overhead barbell lunge (p. 73)
- Forward lunge (p. 74)
- Lateral lunge (p. 75)
- Deadlift (pp. 86–87)
- Dumbbell deadlift (p. 87 var.)

- Standing pulley row (pp. 98–99)
- One-arm row (pp. 98–99)
- Barbell pull-over (pp. 102–03)
- E-Z bar pull-over (p. 102 var.)
- Dumbbell pull-over (p. 102 var.)
- Good morning barbell (pp. 104–05)

- Assisted chin-up (p. 92)
- Chin-up (pp. 94–95)
- Chin-up var. grip (p. 94)
- Bent-over row (pp. 100–01)

- Barbell bench press (pp. 110–11)
- Dumbbell bench press (pp. 110–11)
- Incline barbell bench press (p. 112)
- Incline dumbbell bench press (p. 113)

- Push-up (p. 120)
- Frame-supported push-up (p. 121)
- Raised frame-supported push-up (p. 121 var.)

EXERCISE GROUP	MOST ISOLATED
SHOULDERS	■ Prone lateral raise (p. 133 var.) ■ Scarecrow rotation (pp. 134–35) ■ Prone scarecrow rotation (p. 135 var.)	■ Dumbbell shoulder shrug (p. 128) ■ Shoulder shrug from hang (p. 129) ■ Front dumbbell raise (p. 130) ■ Lateral dumbbell raise (p. 131) ■ Rear lateral raise (pp. 132–33) ■ Machine shoulder press (p. 125 var.)
ARMS	■ Incline bicep curl (pp. 152–53) ■ Concentration curl (pp. 152–53) ■ Preacher curl (pp. 154–55) ■ Wrist flexion (pp. 158–59) ■ Wrist extension (pp. 158–59) ■ Dumbbell triceps extension (p. 142) ■ Triceps kickback (pp. 144–45)	■ Triceps push-down (pp. 148–49) ■ Overhead triceps extension (pp. 148–49) ■ Barbell curl (pp. 150–51) ■ Dumbbell hammer curl (pp. 150–51) ■ Pulley curl (pp. 154–55) ■ Reverse barbell curl (pp. 156–57) ■ Reverse pulley curl (pp. 156–57) ■ Barbell triceps extension (p. 143) ■ Prone triceps extension (pp. 144–45)
ABS AND CORE	■ Abdominal crunch (p. 162) ■ Abdominal crunch var. (p. 162 var. 1) ■ 90-90 crunch (pp. 166–67) ■ 90-90 crunch with twist (p. 167) ■ Ball crunch (pp. 166–67)	■ Figure-4 crunch (p. 165) ■ Ball twist (p. 168) ■ Ball push-up (p. 169) ■ Ball jack knife (p. 170) ■ Ball back extension (p. 171) ■ Roman chair side bend (pp. 172–73) ■ Abdominal crunch crunch with twist (p. 162 var. 2) ■ Sit-up (p. 163) ■ Sit-up var. 2 (p. 163)
DYNAMIC LIFTS		

MOST FUNCTIONAL ▷

- **Upright row** (pp. 126–27)
- **Upright dumbbell row** (p. 126 var.)
- **Upright pulley row** (p. 126 var.)
- **External dumbbell rotation** (p. 135)
- **Internal pulley rotation** (pp. 136–37)
- **External pulley rotation** (pp. 136–37)
- **Seated barbell military press** (p. 124 var.)

- **Barbell military press** (p. 124)
- **Dumbbell shoulder press** (p. 125)

- **Bench dip** (p. 140)
- **Close-grip bench press** (p. 146–147)
- **Close-grip barbell bench press** (p. 147 var.)

- **Bar dip** (p. 141)
- **Close-grip push-up** (p. 146 var.)

- **Prone plank** (p. 174)
- **Prone plank var.** (p. 174 var.)
- **Side plank** (p. 175)
- **V-leg raise** (pp. 176–77)

- **Side bend** (pp. 172–73)

- **Suitcase deadlift** (pp. 176–77)
- **Woodchop** (pp. 178–79)
- **Low pulley woodchop** (p. 179)

- **Kettlebell high-pull** (p. 204)

- **Power clean** (pp. 182–83)
- **Power snatch** (pp. 184–85)
- **Power clean from hang** (pp. 186–87)
- **Power snatch from hang** (pp. 188–89)
- **Squat clean** (pp. 190–91)
- **Heavy front squat** (pp. 192–93)
- **Overhead squat** (pp. 194–95)
- **Jerk balance** (pp. 196–97)
- **Snatch balance** (pp. 198–99)
- **Split snatch** (pp. 200–01)
- **Push press** (pp. 202–03)
- **Barbell jump squat** (p. 205)

MUSCULAR ENDURANCE

At a basic level, strength training is about making sure that we are strong enough to cope with the demands of daily life—the repetitive pulls, pushes, lifts, and standing- or stepping-up actions—without undue fatigue or any injury.

Q | What will I achieve?
A | The programs are designed to develop your strength endurance—the ability to move a relatively small weight through a specific range of motion lots of times.

Q | What do the charts show?
A | The charts feature three different training programs, using either resistance machines, body weight, or free weights. Choose one type of training only, depending on your personal preference, your experience, and what equipment you have available. Do not attempt more than one program in a single training session, and do not be tempted to do exercises on an ad hoc basis.

Q | How do I follow the charts?
A | You should work through each training program from the top down, after you have warmed up your muscles. Each of the featured exercises includes a page reference to its step-by-step instruction in the main part of the book. This is followed by the number of sets, reps, and amount of weight you should use, followed by a cool down routine. The weight you should use for each exercise is expressed either in terms of your personal RM (Rep Maximum) for the machines and free weights, or as NMF (Near Muscular Failure) when you are using your own body weight. The approximate duration, the frequency of each program, and the recovery time between each set of exercises is provided at the bottom of the chart.

Q | How will I progress?
A | Two of the key concepts in resistance training are overload and progression. Once you reach a point at which you complete a set easily you can either increase the weight you are using by a small amount, such as 2–5 lb (1–2 kg) for the upper body and 4–9 lb (2–4 kg) for the lower body, or add another rep for each set, up to a maximum of 20 reps. Alternatively, reduce your recovery time by five seconds if starting at one minute rest between exercises or sets. Do not go below 30 seconds rest. At the end of the six-week period, review your progress and decide whether you should move on to one of the other programs.

MACHINE				
Mobilization warm-up (pp. 46–47) 10 mins				
EXERCISE	**PAGE**	**SETS**	**REPS**	**WEIGHT** (RM)
Machine bench press	118–19	2–3	12+	12
Seated pulley row or **Machine shoulder press**	96–97 118–119	2–3 2–3	12+ 12+	12 12
Upright pulley row	127	2–3	12+	12
Lat pull-down	92–93	2–3	12+	12
45-degree leg press	78–79	2–3	12+	12
Smith machine calf raise	84	2–3	12+	12
COOL DOWN ROUTINE				
Warm down 5 mins				
Developmental stretching (pp. 208–13) 15 mins				

■ **DURATION OF PROGRAM**
6 weeks

■ **FREQUENCY OF PROGRAM**
3 workouts/week, 1–2 days' rest between workouts

■ **RECOVERY TIME**
30 secs–1 min between exercises

BASIC PROGRAMS

BODY WEIGHT				FREE WEIGHT				
Mobilization warm-up (pp. 46–47) 10 mins				Mobilization warm-up (pp. 46–47) 10 mins				
EXERCISE	PAGE	SETS	WEIGHT	EXERCISE	PAGE	SETS	REPS	WEIGHT (RM)
Push-up	120	2–3	NMF*	Back squat	64–65	2–3	12+	12
Chin-up or Assisted chin-up	92–93 94–95	2–3	NMF*	Dumbbell bench press	110–11	2–3	12+	12
Body weight squat	58	2–3	NMF*	Chin-up	94 (Var.)	2–3	12+	12
Reverse crunch	164	2–3	NMF*	Dumbbell shoulder press	125	2–3	12+	12
Prone plank	174	2–3	NMF*	One-arm row	98–99	2–3	12+	12
Side plank	175	2–3	NMF*	Barbell deadlift	86–87	2–3	12+	12
Sit-up	163	2–3	NMF*					

*NMF—Near Muscular Failure

COOL DOWN ROUTINE	COOL DOWN ROUTINE
Warm down 5 mins	Warm down 5 mins
Developmental stretching (pp. 208–13) 15 mins	Developmental stretching (pp. 208–13) 15 mins

■ **DURATION OF PROGRAM**
6 weeks

■ **FREQUENCY OF PROGRAM**
3 workouts/week, 1–2 days' rest between workouts

■ **RECOVERY TIME**
30 secs–1 min between exercises

■ **DURATION OF PROGRAM**
6 weeks

■ **FREQUENCY OF PROGRAM**
3 workouts/week, 1–2 days' rest between workouts

■ **RECOVERY TIME**
30 secs–1 min between exercises

BODY SCULPTING

Many people who take up resistance training want a better "physique." By this, they imagine more muscle and better muscle definition provided not only by larger muscles but also by reduced body fat levels. A good analogy is to image the difference between a golf ball under a comforter and a soccer ball under a sheet. Aiming for that "beach" body is the purpose of the physique training programs.

Q | What do the charts show?
A | There are three programs here—a basic routine that uses resistance machines, body weight, and free weights (pp. 224–27), then two split routines (pp. 228–29) that enable you to split your training over different days and different types of exercises.

Q | How do I use the basic programs?
A | Work through each training program from the top down, after you have warmed up your muscles. Each of the featured exercises includes a page reference to its step-by-step instruction in the main part of the book. This is followed by the number of sets, reps, and amount of weight you should use, followed by a cool down routine. The weight you should use for each exercise is expressed either in terms of your personal RM (Rep Maximum) for the machines and free weights, or as NMF (Near Muscular Failure) when you are using your own body weight. The approximate duration, the frequency of each program, and the recovery time between each set of exercises is provided at the bottom of the chart.

Q | What is the free weight "mix and match" chart?
A | The "mix and match" chart divides the exercises by body part, starting with the chest then finishing with the biceps. You can create your own exercise program by choosing one exercise from each body part section, and perform the stated number of sets and reps. Program duration, frequency, and recovery time is given at the end. You can swap exercises for each training session as you require. As always, the chart starts with a warm-up and finishes with a cool down.

Q | What is a split program?
A | A split program enables you to break up your training over more than one day, the theory being that you can train more intensively—for example, on Day 1 you

exercise your chest, shoulders and arms, and on Day 2 you train your back and legs, while your chest, shoulders and arms are in their recovery phase. There are two split programs provided on pp. 226–27.

Q | How do I use the split program (option 1)?
A | Option 1 provides a program that runs over two days (a "two-day split"). The information is arranged in the same way as for the basic programs but the days of the week on which you train or rest are provided over an alternating two-week period in the box at the bottom. The letters A or B indicate which body parts are being trained. Once you reach the end of the two-week period, simply repeat it all over again for the duration of the program.

Q | How do I use the split program (option 2)?
A | Option 2 provides a split that is broken up into functional exercises and isolation exercises. Functional exercises work more than one muscle at a time. Isolation exercises work only one muscle at a time. So this split program allows adequate recovery time by working your body in different ways. The information is arranged in the same way as for the Option 1 split program—the days of the week on which you train or rest are provided over an alternating two-week period in the box at the bottom. The letters A or B indicate whether you are on a functional or isolation day. Once you have completed the two-week period, simply repeat it for the duration of the program.

Q | What will I achieve?
A | The programs are designed to increase your muscle mass and will help to reducing your body fat.

Q | Are the physique training exercises functional?
A | As far as possible, yes. More often than not it is better to perform exercises that enhance the functional performance of the body and mimimise the risk of developing postural, muscular imbalances. Generally speaking, the more "isolated"—focused on one individual muscle—an exercise is, the less functional it will be. By their nature, resistance machines also provide a far less functional form of training. The compound, multijoint exercises, the pushes, pulls, squats and so on can be seen as more functional. The isolation exercises have, however, been included in some of the accompanying programs—these are fine to use as long as their limited nature is recognized.

BASIC PROGRAMS

MACHINE					BODY WEIGHT			
Mobilization warm-up (pp. 46–47) 10 mins					Mobilization warm-up (pp. 46–47) 10 mins			
EXERCISE	**PAGE**	**SETS**	**REPS**	**WEIGHT** (RM)	**EXERCISE**	**PAGE**	**SETS**	**WEIGHT**
Machine bench press or Machine fly*	118–19	3–6	6–12	12	Push-up	120	3–6	NMF*
Seated pulley row	96–97	3–6	6–12	12	Chin-up or Assisted chin-up	94–95 92	3–6 3–6	NMF* NMF*
Machine shoulder press or Upright pulley row*	1 25 127	3–6 3–6	6–12 6–12	12 12	Body weight squat	58	3–6	NMF*
Lat pull-down	93	3–6	6–12	12	Bar dip	141	3–6	NMF*
Machine leg extension or 45-degree leg press*	80–81 78–79	3–6	6–12	12	Reverse crunch	164	3–6	NMF*
Machine calf raise	84–85	3–6	6–12	12	Prone plank	174	3–6	NMF*
Pulley curl or Reverse pulley curl*	154–55 156–57	3–6	6–12	12	Side plank	175	3–6	NMF*
Triceps push-down	148–49	3–6	6–12	12	Sit-up	163	3–6	NMF*

*Alternate every session

*NMF—Near Muscular Failure

COOL DOWN ROUTINE

COOL DOWN ROUTINE

Warm down 5 mins	Warm down 5 mins
Developmental stretching (pp. 208–13) 15 mins	Developmental stretching (pp. 208–13) 15 mins

■ **DURATION OF PROGRAM**
6–8 weeks

■ **FREQUENCY OF PROGRAM**
3 workouts/week, 2 days' rest between workouts

■ **RECOVERY TIME**
30 secs–1 min 30 secs between exercises

■ **DURATION OF PROGRAM**
6–8 weeks

■ **FREQUENCY OF PROGRAM**
3 workouts/week, 2 days' rest between workouts

■ **RECOVERY TIME**
30 secs–1 min 30 secs between exercises

CONTINUED ▶

BASIC PROGRAMS (CONTINUED)

Mobilization warm-up (pp. 46–47) 10 mins

EXERCISE	PAGE	SETS	REPS	WEIGHT (RM)
CHEST EXERCISES (CHOOSE ONE...)				
Dumbbell bench press	110–11	3–6	6–12	12–14
Barbell bench press	110–11	3–6	6–12	12–14
Flat dumbbell fly	114 (Var.)	3–6	6–12	12–14
Incline fly	114–15	3–6	6–12	12–14
BACK EXERCISES (CHOOSE ONE...)				
One-arm row	98–99	3–6	6–12	12–14
Bend forward barbell row	100–01	3–6	6–12	12–14
Lat pull down	93	3–6	6–12	12–14
Barbell pull-over	102–03	3–6	6–12	12–14
SHOULDER EXERCISES (CHOOSE ONE...)				
Dumbbell shoulder press	125	3–6	6–12	12–14
Military barbell press	124	3–6	6–12	12–14
Upright row var	126–27	3–6	6–12	12–14
Any shoulder raise	130–33	3–6	6–12	12–14

FREEWEIGHT "Mix and match" continued

EXERCISE	PAGE	SETS	REPS	WEIGHT (RM)
LEG EXERCISES (CHOOSE ONE...)				
Back squat	64–65	3–6	6–12	12–14
Front barbell squat	66–67	3–6	6–12	12–14
Forward lunge or Dumbbell split squat	74 68	3–6	6–12	12–14
Barbell step-up	76–77	3–6	6–12	12–14
LOWER BACK EXERCISES (CHOOSE ONE...)				
Good morning barbell	104–05	3–6	6–12	12–14
Back extension	104–05	3–6	6–12	12–14
Straight-leg deadlift	85	3–6	6–12	12–14
Ball back extension	171	3–6	6–12	12–14
TRUNK EXERCISES (CHOOSE ONE...)				
Abs crunch or sit-up	162–63	3–6	6–12	12–14
Prone pank	174	3–6	6–12	12–14
Side plank	175	3–6	6–12	12–14
V leg raise	176	3–6	6–12	12–14

FREEWEIGHT "Mix and match" continued

EXERCISE	PAGE	SETS	REPS	WEIGHT (RM)
TRICEP EXERCISES (CHOOSE ONE...)				
Dumbbell triceps extension or **Barbell triceps extension**	142–43	3–6	10–12	12–14
Close-grip bench press	146–47	3–6	10–12	12–14
Triceps push-down	148–49	3–6	10–12	12–14
Bench or **bar dip**	140–41	3–6	10–12	12–14
BICEP EXERCISES (CHOOSE ONE...)				
Any bicep curl exercise	150–57	3–6	10–12	12–14

COOL DOWN ROUTINE

Warm down 5 mins

Developmental stretching (pp. 208–13) 15 mins

■ **DURATION OF PROGRAM**
8 weeks

■ **FREQUENCY OF PROGRAM**
3 workouts/week, 2 days' rest between workouts

■ **RECOVERY TIME**
30 secs–1 min 30 secs between exercises

Q | Are training for physique and a "toned" appearance the same thing?
A | No. Often people see training for physique as a less extreme version of bodybuilding. In most cases the goal is to enhance muscle mass and reduce body fat levels. This results in the elusive "toned" appearance, where muscle definition is visible. However, muscle "tone" is increased with all forms of resistance training, and so to call a defined, low body fat look as "toned" is technically misleading. Sumo wrestlers, for example, will have very high levels of muscle tone but few would describe them using the colloquial term "toned."

Q | Will I get too bulky?
A | Many people are afraid of becoming overly muscular as a result of engaging in resistance training. The reality is that very few individuals are genetically capable of gaining significant muscle mass, and so it is unlikely to be a problem for the majority of those following a training program. It is an issue that is even less of a problem for women than men, as females have much lower levels of the muscle-building hormones, such as testosterone.

Q | How much body fat will I lose?
A | Increasing muscle mass through resistance training will raise metabolism significantly, which has valuable knock-on benefits to keeping your body fat levels low. If a person is currently holding more body fat than they like, then resistance training will help resolve this.

Q | How can I vary the workout?
A | The beauty of this workout is in its flexibility. As long as you exercise each of the listed body parts in each training session, you can vary the specific exercise. This stops your muscles from becoming too familiar with any one movement, and, arguably, helps you delevop faster—especially on a functional basis.

ADVANCED—SPLIT PROGRAMS

SPLIT PROGRAM (OPTION 1)

SESSION A—CHEST, SHOULDERS, AND ARMS

Mobilization warm-up (pp. 46–47) 10 mins

EXERCISE	PAGE	SETS	REPS	WEIGHT (RM)
Dumbbell bench press	110–11	3–6	6–12	12–14
Incline fly	114–15	3–6	6–12	12–14
Dumbbell shoulder press	125	3–6	6–12	12–14
Rear lat raise	132–33	3–6	6–12	12–14
Good morning barbell	104–05	3–6	6–12	12–14
Barbell biceps curl	150–51	3–6	6–12	12–14
Bench or bar dip	140–41	3–6	6–12	12–14

COOL DOWN ROUTINE

Warm down 5 mins

Developmental stretching (pp. 208–13) 15 mins

SESSION B—LEGS AND BACK

Mobilization warm-up (pp. 46–47) 10 mins

EXERCISE	PAGE	SETS	REPS	WEIGHT (RM)
Back squat	64–65	3–6	6–12	12–14
Lat pull down	93	3–6	6–12	12–14
Straight leg deadlift	85	3–6	6–12	12–14
Seated pulley row	96–97	3–6	6–12	12–14
Calf raise	84	3–6	6–12	12–14
Barbell pullover	102–03	3–6	10–12	12–14
Back extension	104–05	3–6	6–12	12–14

COOL DOWN ROUTINE

Warm down 5 mins

Developmental stretching (pp. 208–13) 15 mins

■ **DURATION OF PROGRAM**
6–8 weeks

■ **RECOVERY TIME**
30 secs–1 min 30 secs between exercises

APPLICATION OF SPLIT PROGRAMS

DAY OF WEEK	MON	TUES	WED	THUR	FRI	SAT	SUN
WEEK 1,3,5…etc.	A	B	Rest	A	B	Rest	A
WEEK 2,4,6…etc.	B	A	Rest	B	A	Rest	B

SPLIT PROGRAM (OPTION 2)

SESSION A–FUNCTIONAL DAY

Mobilization warm-up (pp. 46–47) 10 mins

EXERCISE	PAGE	SETS	REPS	WEIGHT (RM)
Barbell bench press	110–11	2	10–12	12–14
Chin-up	94–95	2	10–12	12–14
Dumbbell shoulder press	125	2	10–12	12–14
Back squat	64–65	2	10–12	12–14
Straight-leg deadlift	85	2	10–12	12–14
Any upright row	126–27	2	10–12	12–14

SESSION B–ISOLATION DAY

Mobilization warm-up (pp. 46–47) 10 mins

EXERCISE	PAGE	SETS	REPS	WEIGHT (RM)
Pulley cross-over	116–17	2	10–12	12–14
Straight-arm pull-down	106–07	2	10–12	12–14
Any shoulder raise	130–33	2	10–12	12–14
Machine leg extension	81	2	10–12	12–14
Machine leg curl	80	2	10–12	12–14
Dumbbell shoulder shrug	128–29	2	10–12	12–14
Any bicep curl	150–57	2	10–12	12–14
Triceps push-down	148–49	2	10–12	12–14
Calf raise	84	2	10–12	12–14

COOL DOWN ROUTINE

Warm down 5 mins

Developmental stretching (pp. 208–13) 15 mins

COOL DOWN ROUTINE

Warm down 5 mins

Developmental stretching (pp. 208–13) 15 mins

■ **DURATION OF PROGRAM**
6–8 weeks

■ **RECOVERY TIME**
30 secs–1 min 30 secs between exercises

APPLICATION OF SPLIT PROGRAMS

DAY OF WEEK	MON	TUES	WED	THUR	FRI	SAT	SUN
WEEK 1,3,5...etc	A	B	Rest	A	B	Rest	A
WEEK 2,4,6...etc.	B	A	Rest	B	A	Rest	B

BODYBUILDING

Bodybuilding is the process of enhancing muscle mass to the greatest possible extent. It is also about reducing body fat so that the muscle clearly shows through the skin. Bodybuilding is both a method of improving physical appearance as well as a competitive sport—its most famous champion being the former Mr. Universe and Mr. Olympia, Arnold Schwarzenegger.

Q | What do the charts show?
A | The programs outlined here and on the next page are founded on high-intensity, abbreviated bodybuilding training. The basic programs offer a choice of highly effective programs that use either resistance machines or free weights. Two split versions then follow.

Q | How do I use the basic programs?
A | The basic programs provide whole-body workouts. You should work through each training program from the top down, after you have warmed up your muscles. Each of the featured exercises include a page reference to its step-by-step instruction in the main part of the book. This is followed by the number of sets, reps, and amount of weight you should use, followed by a cool down routine. The weight you should use for each exercise is expressed in terms of your personal RM (Rep Maximum) for the machines and free weights. The approximate duration, the frequency of each program, and the recovery time between each set of exercises is provided at the bottom of the chart.

Q | What are the split programs?
A | The split routines are a progression from the basic routines on p. 231 and provide more focused and advanced exercise technique sessions. You will notice that the total volume of work does not increase although targeting specific muscle groups is a more advanced training method. You should complete the basic bodybuilding program before attempting the split routines.

Q | What does the split program (option 1) do?
A | Option 1 provides a strong focus on muscle groups as intended by a split routine but using more isolated exercises. The information is arranged in the same way as for the basic programs but the days of the week on which you train or rest are provided over an alternating two-week period in the box at the bottom. The letters A or B indicate which body parts are being trained. Once you reach the end of the two-week period, simply repeat it all over again for the duration of the program.

Q | What does the split routine (option 2) do?
A | Option 2 provides a more challenging split routine than option 1 through the use of more functional exercises.

Q | Should I train harder to build more muscle?
A | No. The key to successful bodybuilding is to train smarter, not harder. It is more common to see well-meaning, passionate bodybuilding trainees doing too much, rather than too little.

Q | Why are there no body weight exercises?
A | There are no body weight exercises included in any of the bodybuilding programs because it is very difficult to increase the amount of weight you are lifting—you are limited to the weight of your own body, which is not sufficient for this type of resistance training.

WARNING!

You need to be realistic about how much muscle mass you can develop, as only a few people are genetically suited to seriously bulking up. In fact, a genetically average individual, training naturally, would severely overtrain if they attempted to follow the programs of elite bodybuilders. Even if they could cope with the training without physiologically breaking down, they would still struggle to gain muscle mass. This is because most people's muscles simply can't recover quickly enough between overly frequent and intense sessions, let alone grow in size.

BASIC PROGRAMS

MACHINE					FREE WEIGHT				
Mobilization warm-up (pp. 46–47) 10 mins					Mobilization warm-up (pp. 46–47) 10 mins				
EXERCISE	PAGE	SETS	REPS	WEIGHT (RM)	EXERCISE	PAGE	SETS	REPS	WEIGHT (RM)
Machine bench press	118–19	3–6	6–12	12	Close-grip bench press	146–47	3–6	6–12	12
Seated pulley row	96–97	3–6	6–12	12	Back squats	64–65	3–6	6–12	12
Machine shoulder press or Upright pulley row	125 127	3–6 3–6	6–12 6–12	12 12	Bent-over row	100–01	3–6	6–12	12
Lat pull-down	92–93	3–6	6–12	12	Incline fly	114–15	3–6	6–12	12
45-degree leg press	78–79	3–6	6–12	12	Chin-up (wide grip)	94 (Var.)	3–6	6–12	12
Calf raise	84	3–6	6–12	12	Military barbell press	124	3–6	6–12	12
Pulley curl	154–5	3–6	6–12	12	Calf raise	84	3–6	6–12	12
Triceps push-down or Assisted bar dip	148–49 141	3–6 3–6	6–12 6–12	12 12	Barbell curl	150–51	3–6	6–12	12
COOL DOWN ROUTINE					COOL DOWN ROUTINE				
Warm down 5 mins					Warm down 5 mins				
Developmental stretching (pp. 208–13) 15 mins					Developmental stretching (pp. 208–13) 15 mins				

- **DURATION OF PROGRAM**
  6–8 weeks

- **FREQUENCY OF PROGRAM**
  2–3 workouts/week, 1–2 days' rest between workouts

- **RECOVERY TIME**
  30 secs–1 min 30 secs between exercises

- **DURATION OF PROGRAM**
  6–8 weeks

- **FREQUENCY OF PROGRAM**
  2–3 workouts/week, 1–2 days' rest between workouts

- **RECOVERY TIME**
  30 secs–1 min 30 secs between exercises

SPLIT PROGRAMS

BASIC SPLIT PROGRAM (OPTION 1)

SESSION A: CHEST, SHOULDERS, AND ARMS

Mobilization warm-up (pp. 46–47) 10 mins

EXERCISE	PAGE	SETS	REPS	WEIGHT (RM)
Machine bench press	118–19	3–6	6–12	10–12
Machine shoulder press	125 (Var.)	3–6	6–12	10–12
Pulley cross-over	116–17	3–6	6–12	10–12
Any lateral raise	131–33	3–6	6–12	10–12
Preacher curl	154–55	3–6	6–12	10–12
Tricep kickback	150–51	3–6	6–12	10–12

COOL DOWN ROUTINE

Warm-down 5 mins

Developmental stretching (pp. 208–13) 15 mins

SESSION B: LEGS AND BACK

Mobilization warm-up (pp. 46–47) 10 mins

EXERCISE	PAGE	SETS	REPS	WEIGHT (RM)
Machine leg extension	80–81	3–6	6–12	10–12
Seated pulley row	96–97	3–6	6–12	10–12
Machine leg curl	80–81	3–6	6–12	10–12
Dumbbell pull-over	104–05 (Var.)	3–6	6–12	10–12
Calf raise	125	3–6	6–12	10–12
One-arm row	98–99	3–6	6–12	10–12

COOL DOWN ROUTINE

Warm-down 5 mins

Developmental stretching (pp. 208–13) 15 mins

■ **DURATION OF PROGRAM**
6–8 weeks

■ **RECOVERY TIME**
30 secs–1 min 30 secs between exercises

APPLICATION OF SPLIT PROGRAMS

DAY OF WEEK	MON	TUES	WED	THUR	FRI	SAT	SUN
WEEK 1,3,5…etc.	A	B	Rest	A	B	Rest	A
WEEK 2,4,6…etc.	B	A	Rest	B	A	Rest	B

ADVANCED SPLIT PROGRAM (OPTION 2)

SESSION A: CHEST, SHOULDERS, AND ARMS

Mobilization warm-up (pp. 46–47) 10 mins

EXERCISE	PAGE	SETS	REPS	WEIGHT (RM)
Barbell bench press	110–11	3–6	6–12	10–12
Military barbell press	124	3–6	6–12	10–12
Incline fly	114–15	3–6	6–12	10–12
Upright barbell row	126–27	3–6	6–12	10–12
Concentration curl	152–53	3–6	6–12	10–12
Barbell curl	150–51	3–6	6–12	10–12

COOL DOWN ROUTINE

Warm-down 5 mins

Developmental stretching (pp. 208–13) 15 mins

SESSION B: LEGS AND BACK

Mobilization warm-up (pp. 46–47) 10 mins

EXERCISE	PAGE	SETS	REPS	WEIGHT (RM)
Back squat	64–65	3–6	6–12	10–12
Barbell pull-over	102–03	3–6	6–12	10–12
Romanian deadlift	88–89	3–6	6–12	10–12
Bent-over row	100–01	3–6	6–12	10–12
Calf raise	125	3–6	6–12	10–12

COOL DOWN ROUTINE

Warm-down 5 mins

Developmental stretching (pp. 208–13) 15 mins

■ **DURATION OF PROGRAM**
6–8 Weeks

■ **RECOVERY TIME**
30 secs–1 min 30 secs between exercises

APPLICATION OF SPLIT PROGRAMS

DAY OF WEEK	MON	TUES	WED	THUR	FRI	SAT	SUN
WEEK 1,3,5...etc	A	B	Rest	A	B	Rest	A
WEEK 2,4,6...etc	B	A	Rest	B	A	Rest	B

MAXIMAL STRENGTH

The following programs will help you to develop a high level of strength from head to toe—enabling you to perform any real-world movement that may ever be asked of you—through a series of functional exercises. They build on the strength endurance program given on pages 222–223 and will build your strength over a 14-week period.

Q | What do the charts show?
A | There are two separate programs to follow. The first is a basic, but highly effective whole-body program, and the second a more advanced split program. The programs are equally effective in achieving your strength goals, but the split program allows you to focus specifically on a group of muscles during a training session, allowing a more targeted approach. The information is arranged in the same way as for the basic programs but the days of the week on which you train or rest are provided over an alternating two-week period in the box at the bottom. The letters A or B indicate which body parts are being trained. Once you reach the end of the two-week period, simply repeat it all over again for the duration of the program.

Q | How do I follow the programs?
A | Begin the cycle by lifting a weight that is challenging for six repetitions, but that allows comfortable completion of all sets. The goal of the program is to progress toward lifting the largest weight you can, once only. Every two weeks, the number of repetitions decreases, but with a weekly increase of weight: 2 lb–5½ lb (1–2.5 kg) upper body; 4½ lb–9 lb (2–4 kg) lower body. You should be aiming to lift the largest amount of weight once in the final week—week 14.

WHOLE-BODY PROGRAM

Mobilization warm-up (pp. 46–47) 10 mins

EXERCISE	PAGE	SETS	REPS	WEIGHT (RM)
Dumbbell bench press	110–11	3	6	6
Back squat	64–65	3	6	6
Lat pull-down	93	3	6	
Military barbell press	124	3	6	6
Bent-over row	100–01	3	6	6

LOADS AND INTENSITIES

WEEK	SETS	REPS	WEIGHT (RM)
Weeks 1–2	3	6	6
Weeks 3–4	3	4	4
Weeks 6–5	4	3	3
Weeks 7–8	4	1–2	2

COOL DOWN ROUTINE

Warm down 5 mins

Developmental stretching (pp. 208–13) 15 mins

■ **DURATION OF PROGRAM**
8 weeks

■ **FREQUENCY OF PROGRAM**
3 workouts/week, 2 days' rest between workouts

■ **RECOVERY TIME**
2–5 minutes between exercises

ADVANCED SPLIT PROGRAM

SESSION A: CHEST, SHOULDERS, AND ARMS

Mobilization warm-up (pp. 46–47) 10 mins

EXERCISE	PAGE	SETS	REPS	WEIGHT (RM)
Dumbbell bench press	110–11	3	6	6
Shoulder shrug fom hang	129	3	6	6
Incline fly	114–15	3	6	6
Incline bicep curl	152	3	6	6
Prone triceps extension	144	3	6	6

LOADS AND INTENSITIES

WEEK	SETS	REPS	WEIGHT (RM)
Weeks 1–2	3	6	6
Weeks 3–4	3	4	4
Weeks 6–5	4	3	3
Weeks 7–8	4	1–2	2

COOL DOWN ROUTINE

Warm down 5 mins

Developmental stretching (pp. 208–13) 15 mins

SESSION B: LEGS AND BACK

Mobilization warm-up (pp. 46–47) 10 mins

EXERCISE	PAGE	SETS	REPS	WEIGHT (RM)
Straight arm pull down	106–07	3	6	6
Front barbell squat	66	3	6	6
Good morning barbell	104–05	3	6	6
Barbell step-up	76	3	6	6
Prone row	106–07	3	6	6

LOADS AND INTENSITIES

WEEK	SETS	REPS	WEIGHT (RM)
Weeks 1–2	3	6	6
Weeks 3–4	3	4	4
Weeks 6–5	4	3	3
Weeks 7–8	4	2	2

COOL DOWN ROUTINE

Warm down 5 mins

Developmental stretching (pp. 208–13) 15 mins

■ **DURATION OF PROGRAM**
8 weeks

■ **RECOVERY TIME**
2–5 minutes between exercises

APPLICATION OF SPLIT PROGRAMS

DAY OF WEEK	MON	TUES	WED	THUR	FRI	SAT	SUN
WEEK 1,3,5...etc.	A	B	Rest	A	B	Rest	A
WEEK 2,4,6...etc.	B	A	Rest	B	A	Rest	B

CORE STRENGTH

The "core" (or "trunk") refers to the muscles found in your midsection. For many people, this is the sought-after "six pack" of abdominal muscles, but the reality is more complex than this. In effect, there are two layers of core muscles; the superficial ones (such as your Rectus abdominus) that are visible in a lean individual, and the deep stabilizers, which are buried deeper in your trunk and which we cannot see.

Q | What do the charts show?
A | The charts show two different types of programs—the first works the core muscles in isolation, the second adopts a more integrated approach and gives you two equally effective but different program options.

Q | What does the isolated core conditioning program do?
A | In this approach, the core is seen almost as a separate area, which must be trained and strengthened using specific exercises. Start by completing 1–2 sets of 10 reps for each exercise. As long as good technique is maintained, add 2 reps to each exercise, every session, until you are completing 2 sets of 50 reps. Do not add additional reps if you are not ready—a quality over quantity approach is best.

Q | What do the functional core programs do?
A | Favored by many elite coaches, these types of program are an integrated method of training. Integrated core conditioning is the training of the core through other movements with the goal being to enhance the overall performance of that key movement, and not just to develop a strong core as an end in itself.

Q | Which one should I choose?
A | The functional core programs are the best overall. Weightlifters, for example, achieve their phenomenal core strength by performing functional, challenging movements on their feet. But this should not be seen as the preserve of the athletes—everyone can learn to perform exercises such as squats, cleans, snatches, and deadlifts. By its nature, the isolated core program approach is less functional and at first glance less useful, but is good for physique development or bodybuilding where isolating a muscle and making it grow is the desired result.

ISOLATED CORE PROGRAM

Mobilization warm-up (pp. 46–47) 10 mins

EXERCISE	PAGE	SETS	REPS
Abs crunch or sit-up (floor or stability ball)	162–63 167	1–2	10–50
Reverse crunch	164	1–2	10–50
Figure 4 crunch	165	1–2	10–50
Ball jack knife	170	1–2	10–50
Side bend	172	1–2	10–50
V leg raise	176–77	1–2	10–50
Prone plank	174	1	NMF*
Side plank	175	1	NMF*

*NMF—Near Muscular Failure

COOL DOWN ROUTINE

Warm-down 5 mins

Developmental stretching (pp. 208–13) 15 mins

■ **DURATION OF PROGRAM**
4–6 weeks

■ **FREQUENCY OF PROGRAM**
2–3 workouts/week, 1–2 days' rest between workouts

■ **RECOVERY TIME**
30 secs–1 minute between exercises

FUNCTIONAL CORE PROGRAMS

OPTION 1

Mobilization warm-up (pp. 46–47) 10 mins

EXERCISE	PAGE	SETS	REPS	WEIGHT (RM)
Power clean	182–83	2–6	6	6
Standing pulley row	98–99	2–6	6	6
Barbell bench press	110–11	2–6	6	6
Bent-over row	100–01	2–6	6	6
Military barbell press	124–25	2–6	6	6
Overhead squat	194–95	2–6	6	6
Front barbell squat	66–67	2–6	6	6
Barbell deadlift	86–87	2–6	6	6

COOL DOWN ROUTINE

Warm-down 5 mins

Developmental stretching (pp. 208–13) 15 mins

OPTION 2

Mobilization warm-up (pp. 46–47) 10 mins

EXERCISE	PAGE	SETS	REPS	WEIGHT (RM)
Power snatch	184–85	2–6	6	6
Frame-supported push-up	121	2–6	6	6
One-arm row	98–99	2–6	6	6
Suitcase deadlift	177	2–6	6	6
Back squat	64–65	2–6	6	6
Overhead barbell lunge	73	2–6	6	6
Straight-leg deadlift	85	2–6	6	6

COOL DOWN ROUTINE

Warm-down 5 mins

Developmental stretching (pp. 208–13) 15 mins

■ **DURATION OF PROGRAMS**
4–6 weeks

■ **FREQUENCY OF PROGRAMS**
2–3 workouts/week, 1–2 days' rest between workouts

■ **RECOVERY TIME**
2–5 minutes between exercises

LOAD AND VOLUME INCREASES
As long as good technique is maintained at all times you can either add:
2–4 lb (1–2 kg) for upper body
4–9 lb (2–4 kg) for lower body
or add additional sets, up to a maximum of 6 sets.

SPORTS-SPECIFIC EXERCISES

All the exercises in this book provide great strength training in themselves. However, a large proportion are also of great benefit for training for specific sports. Almost all athletes, regardless of their chosen sport, will spend time in the gym performing specific strengthening and conditioning exercises that will help them excel in their chosen field.

Q | How do I read the charts?
A | Each of the most sports-specific exercises featured in the book are grouped together into "exercise groups." The "types" of exercise within each group are then listed beneath, with the corresponding page number to help you navigate around the book. Each exercise group is then discussed, reading across the page. Find out what each exercise group does for

---

EXERCISE GROUP:
SQUATS

Types
Back squat (pp. 64–65)
Sumo squat (p. 64 var.)
Front barbell squat (pp. 66–67)
Hack barbell squat (pp. 66–67)
Heavy front squat (pp. 192–93)
Overhead squat (pp. 194–95)

Q | What do squats do?
A | Squats are the key strength builder for the entire core of the body. Often squats are seen as a leg exercise or more specifically a quadriceps exercise, but they actually train the muscles of the feet, ankle stabilizers, muscles of the lower leg, knee stabilizers, hamstrings, abductors and adductors, groin, glutes, and almost every muscle of the core region.

EXERCISE GROUP:
SPLIT SQUATS AND LUNGES

Types
Dumbbell split squat (p. 68)
Overhead split squat (p. 69)
Bulgarian barbell split squat (p. 70)
Bulgarian dumbbell split squat (p. 71)
Barbell lunge (p. 72)
Overhead barbell lunge (p. 73)
Forward lunge (p. 74)
Lateral lunge (p. 75)
Barbell step-up (pp. 76–77)

Q | What do split squats and lunges do?
A | Split squats and lunges develop single leg strength. Most sports involve movements in which body weight is thrown onto the outside leg, which decelerates the athlete, who then has to accelerate rapidly in the opposite direction ("cutting"). This requires enormous strength and power in a single leg, so training to develop this strength is vital.

EXERCISE GROUP:
DEADLIFTS (BENT LEG)

Types
Barbell deadlift (pp. 86–87)
Dumbbell deadlift (p. 87 var.)
Suitcase deadlift (pp. 176–77)

Q | What do deadlifts (bent leg) do?
A | The deadlifts (bent leg) are similar to squats (see above) but differ in terms of bar position. With the bar being lifted from the floor the mechanics of the exercise differs from squats in terms of how deeply the knees are bent and how much the torso leans forward. In the deadlift the bar is positioned forward on the athlete's center of balance.

the various muscles, why is it important for sports ability, and which sports the exercise is specifically useful for.

Q | Are these exercises only relevant to athletes?
A | No. These exercises are useful for anyone interested in enhancing their sports performance, from beginner right through to high-level athletes.

Q | Why are these exercises termed sports-specific?
A | Functional exercises that mirror the joint actions and forces experienced by athletes are also known as sports-specific. This is particularly the case when referring to dynamic lifts, favored by many elite coaches and athletes who work in sports that require highly explosive movements, such as football players and track and field athletes.

Q | Why are squats important?
A | Squats are vital for developing sports-specific leg strength, which is useful in its own right but is also the foundation for explosive jumping and sprinting power. Squats will make you stronger and more powerful, and improve your posture. They are also one of the best core strength exercises you can do.
  There are numerous variations of the squat. Which one you choose will depend on the exact demands of your sport.

Q | Which sports do squats apply to?
A | The list of sports that benefit from squats is almost a comprehensive list of every sport ever invented. If you are a sportsperson you must include squats in your training program. (See pp. 246–47 for a full list of relevant sports.)

Q | Why are split squats and lunges important?
A | In any sort of running action, an athlete is only ever on one leg, so strength and stability in a single leg is essential. For example, the potential for inefficiency, energy wastage, and injury in a sprinter (in track and field or on the wing in a team sport) who has not developed strength and stability in the ankle, knee, and hip joints is high. If your sport involves movement in multiple directions, as most do, practice lunging in multiple directions in training.

Q | Which sports do split squats and lunges apply to?
A | There are very few sports where single leg strength is of little relevance—rowing and powerlifting are perhaps the key examples. So these exercises apply to lots of sports including soccer, rugby, basketball, tennis, and Australian rules football. Hockey players, wide receivers, cornerbacks, or running backs in football who are regularly required to perform cutting movements will all benefit as well. (See pp. 246–47 for a full list of relevant sports.)

Q | Why are deadlifts (bent leg) important?
A | As with the squats, deadlifts (bent leg) are important for all athletes but particularly those whose sports require high levels of gripping, lifting, and pulling.
  In addition, deadlifts variants, such as the suitcase deadlift, are highly effective core exercises, since in most sports, loads are rarely perfectly balanced. The suitcase deadlift is a very effective exercise for training the core to cope with lifting an uneven load.

Q | Which sports do deadlifts (bent leg) apply to?
A | Deadlifts have been prescribed to judo players and hammer throwers and are of benefit to rowers, in terms of developing a base level of pulling strength, and rugby players, who are often expected to pull and lift opposition players physically. (See pp. 246–47 for a full list of relevant sports.)

EXERCISE GROUP:
DEADLIFTS (STRAIGHT LEG)

Types
Straight-leg deadlift (p. 85)
Romanian deadlift (pp. 88–89)
Good Morning barbell (pp. 104–05)

Q | What do deadlifts (straight leg) do?
A | The straight-leg versions of the deadlift (the "Good Morning" is a cross between a squat and a straight-leg deadlift) strengthen the hamstrings, lower back, and glutes. However, they are less functional than squats or deadlifts (bent leg), since the knees do not bend.

EXERCISE GROUP:
PULL- AND CHIN-UPS

Types
Assisted chin-up (pp. 92)
Lat pull-down (p. 93)
Wide-grip lat pull-down (p. 93 var.)
Chin-up (pp. 94–95)
Chin-up variable grip (p. 94 var.)

Q | What do pull- and chin-ups do?
A | Pull- and chin-ups are excellent exercises for developing general strength in the pulling muscles of the arms and back as well as enhancing grip strength.

EXERCISE GROUP:
SEATED PULLEY ROWS

Types
Seated pulley row (pp. 96–97)
Standing pulley row (pp. 98–99)
Prone row (pp. 106–07)

Q | What do seated pulley rows do?
A | Seated pulley rows work the upper body, particularly the back, and grip strength.

EXERCISE GROUP:
STANDING ROWS

Types
Standing pulley row (pp. 98–99)
One-arm row (pp. 98–99)
Bent-over row (pp. 100–01)
Upright row (pp. 126–27)
Upright dumbbell row (p. 126 var.)

Q | What do standing rows do?
A | The standing versions of the rowing exercises challenge and train the linkage of the upper body pulling movements to the lower body, via the core. Standing rows also develop grip strength.

Q | Why are deadlifts (straight leg) important?
A | The main importance for the deadlifts (straight leg) comes in enhancing hamstring strength to help prevent knee injuries, often in female athletes. Bodybuilders also use them for developing the hamstring muscle for aesthetic purposes.

Q | Which sports do deadlifts (straight leg) apply to?
A | Aside from bodybuilding for aesthetic purposes, straight leg deadlifts are performed by MMA, judo, and hammer throwers, where superior hamstring strength and knee stability are required. (See pp. 246–47 for a full list of relevant sports.)

Q | Why are pull- and chin-ups important?
A | Athough they are not particularly sports-specific (few sports require an athlete to lift their own body weight) they are important for climbers and gymnasts who need strength in these areas. They can also be useful in countering the development of muscular imbalances in athletes who place great emphasis on the development of chest exercises.

Q | Which sports do pull- and chin-ups apply to?
A | Climbers and gymnasts, who constantly have to lift their own body weight, benefit most from these exercises. They are also useful for any sport that demands a high ability to grip and pull. Examples include hammer throwing, wrestling, judo, rowing, and rugby. Most other sports are also likely to benefit from these exercises during general conditioning phases of training. (See pp. 246–47 for a full list of relevant sports.)

Q | Why are seated pulley rows important?
A | Developing strength in your back and upper body, especially for pulling movements, is very important for any athlete.

Q | Which sports do seated pulley rows apply to?
A | Rowing benefits most from seated pulley rows. As with pull- and chin-ups, these exercises may also benefit sports that require a high ability to grip and pull, such as hammer throwing, wrestling, judo, rowing, and rugby. However, the linkage of the pulling mechanics of the upper body, through the core and to the lower body will need to be trained separately. (See pp. 246–47 for a full list of relevant sports.)

Q | Why are standing rows important?
A | In many sports, athletes attempt to lift and pull in a standing position. The standing row is very useful for training this action.
   The one-arm row is even more useful if performed without knee and hand support, which artificially helps support the body—in the real world, the body has to provide its own foundation internally.

Q | Which sports do standing rows apply to?
A | Many sports benefit from the general, whole-body strength foundation that standing rows provide. Specifically, those sports which require pulling and lifting movements, executed in a standing position, such as hammer throwing, judo, MMA, rowing, and rugby. Standing rows are useful for most sports during foundation strength training. (See pp. 246–47 for a full list of relevant sports.)

EXERCISE GROUP:
STRAIGHT-ARM PULLS

Types
Barbell pull-over (pp. 102–03)
E-Z bar pull-over (p. 102 var.)
Dumbbell pull-over (p. 102 var.)
Straight-arm pull-down (pp. 106–07)

Q | What do straight-arm pulls do?
A | Straight-arm pulls strengthen the muscles used in bringing the arm down from an overhead postion through the sagital plane (head to toe direction) of the body.

EXERCISE GROUP:
PRESSING MOVEMENTS: THE CHEST

Types
Barbell bench press (pp. 110–11)
Dumbbell bench press (pp. 110–11)
Bench press incline barbell (p. 112)
Bench press incline dumbell (p. 113)
Push-up (p. 120)
Ball push-up (p. 120 var.)
Frame-supported push-up (p. 121)
Close-grip bench press (p. 146–47)
Close-grip bench press (p. 147)
Close-grip push-up (p. 146 var.)

Q | What do pressing movements do?
A | Pressing movements from a lying position, such as the ever-popular bench press, strengthen the chest, shoulders, and triceps.

EXERCISE GROUP:
SHOULDER/OVERHEAD PRESSES

Types
Military barbell press (p. 124)
Dumbbell shoulder press (p. 125)
Push press (pp. 204–05)

Q | What do shoulder/overhead presses do?
A | Overhead presses are similar to bench presses but with a different shoulder angle. They are excellent exercises for developing basic strength in overhead lifts and general shoulder strength and stability.
   These exercises are much better done in a standing position—the seated version is a bodybuilding variation.

Q | Why are straight-arm pulls important?
A | Training the arms for sports where force is applied through a straight arm is important. As well as this, straight arm pulls are useful for injury prevention.

Q | Which sports do straight-arm pulls apply to?
A | Sports that straight arm pulls apply to include swimming (butterfly and front crawl), fast bowling in cricket, and perhaps the tennis serve. However, the arm action in these sports is complex and needs other exercises for full strength conditioning. (See pp. 246–47 for a full list of relevant sports.)

Q | Why are pressing movements important?
A | Developing the strength provided by pressing movements is useful in sports where competitors are required to perform one- or two-arm pressing movements such as pushing off from the floor or against an opponent.

Q | Which sports do pressing movements apply to?
A | There is some benefit to wrestling, MMA, soccer (goalkeepers), and rugby, whose players need to apply pressing movements. There is also some carryover to sports such as boxing and shot-putting and to many other sports that require general shoulder strength, stability, and injury prevention. (See pp. 246–47 for a full list of relevant sports.)

Q | Why are shoulder/overhead presses important?
A | When performed standing, shoulder/overhead presses involve the entire body from toe to finger tip. Unlike the pressing movements (above), the weight can be explosively driven up overhead. Exercises such as the push press are explosive versions of an overhead press and train almost every muscle, including legs, trunk, shoulders, and arms.

Q | Which sports do shoulder/overhead presses apply to?
A | Most sports will benefit from overhead pressing for general conditioning purposes. Punching in combat sports and shot-putting derive the greatest direct benefits. In rugby, the forward responsible for lifting in the line-out would also do well to press overhead. (See pp. 246–47 for a full list of relevant sports.)

EXERCISE GROUP:
SHOULDER ROTATIONS

Types
External dumbbell rotation (p. 135)
Internal rotation (pp. 136–37)
External rotation (pp. 136–37)

Q | What do shoulder rotations do?
A | The shoulder is a very mobile joint but because of this tends to be prone to injury, especially in the rotator cuff—the group of four muscles responsible for holding the ball and socket joint together and controlling all shoulder movements, such as internal and external rotations.

EXERCISE GROUP:
CABLE CHOPS/ROTATIONS

Types
Woodchop (p. 178)
Low pulley woodchop (p. 178 var.)

Q | What do cable chops/rotations do?
A | Cable chops, such as the woodchop type exercises, help develop explosive rotational force and power, or conversely, help to train resisting rotational forces. Cable machines are very useful and versatile for this type of exercise so should be used to train almost any form of rotational exercise.

EXERCISE GROUP:
DYNAMIC LIFTS

Types
Power clean (pp. 182–83)
Power snatch (pp. 184–85)
Power clean from hang (pp. 186–87)
Power snatch from hang (pp. 188–89)
Squat clean (pp. 190–91)
Split snatch (pp. 200–01)
Kettleball high pull (p. 204)

Q | What do dynamic lifts do?
A | The dynamic lifts are designed to develop maximum power, which is perhaps the key determinant of sporting success. The dynamic lifts involve explosive, powerful, near simultaneous extension of the ankle, knee, and hip joints—the "triple extension."

EXERCISE GROUP:
JUMP SQUAT

Q | What does the jump squat do?
A | The jump squat delivers many of the benefits of the dynamic lifts, but without having to learn technical lifts.

Q | Why are shoulder rotations important?
A | Strengthening the muscles in the shoulder is very important for sports performance and injury prevention, so many strength coaches and physical therapists prescribe shoulder rotations for this reason. Be aware that other functional free weight exercises such as the snatch (see pp. 202–03) are also very useful for strengthening the rotator cuff.

Q | Which sports do shoulder rotations apply to?
A | Almost all sports involving the shoulder joint will benefit from these exercises as a means of preventing shoulder injury. Even where other shoulder exercises are used it is still worth including shoulder rotations. Arm wrestling and perhaps racket sports may benefit from these exercises directly. (See pp. 246–47 for a full list of relevant sports.)

Q | Why are cable chops/rotations important?
A | There are very few sports that do not require the development of rotational power—it is an essential part of any training program. If explosive rotation is desired the chop can be performed explosively in rotation. If stability and resistance is required the exercise can be performed with only the arms moving and the pillar (legs and core) fixed.

Q | Which sports do cable chops/rotations apply to?
A | Almost every sport involves some movement in the transverse (rotational) plane. Some, such as golf, boxing, baseball, and shot-putting, are wholly reliant upon it. Sports which involve little rotation, such as powerlifting, are not likely to benefit much. Even in running, athletes are required to resist rotational forces which develop as a natural consequence of running mechanics. (See pp. 246–47 for a full list of relevant sports.)

Q | Why are dynamic lifts important?
A | Many sporting movements, such as jumping and sprinting, rely on the triple extension developed by dynamic lifts. As well as the lifting part of these exercises, the "catch" part is important, too, where the bar is decelerated. This can have a very important training effect, since in almost all sports the athlete is forced to decelerate; any change of direction or landing of a jump are key examples.

Q | Which sports do dynamic lifts apply to?
A | Clearly dynamic weightlifters benefit from these exercises but almost every other sport that requires speed, power, stability, balance, and control will also benefit greatly. Something as simple as training the rapid splitting of the feet in the split versions of these lifts could have important impact on foot speed and agility. (See pp. 246–47 for a full list of relevant sports.)

Q | Why is the jump squat important?
A | The dynamic lifts (above) are very important exercises but they are also take time to learn. Many athletes find that they spend so long trying to perfect the lifts that they never manage to handle any significant load in them. The jump squat is, however, simpler to perform but delivers similar benefits to the development of triple extension.

Q | Which sports does the jump squat apply to?
A | As for the dynamic lifts, the jump squat is suitable for any sport that require speed, power, stability, balance, and control. (See pp. 246–47 for a full list of relevant sports.)

SPORTS-SPECIFIC MATRIX

The term "sports-specific" is applied to exercises that mirror the particular movements of an athlete in their chosen sport. This allows you to break different sports down into their general movement types and train those movements to improve your overall level of performance.

Q | What does the chart show?
A | The chart has been developed by analyzing the movement patterns of each of the listed sports and categorizing each of the exercise groups in this book by their relevance to those specfic sports, as follows: "direct relevance" (black square), "partial/general relevance" (clear square), or no

Key
On the right are all the exercise groups, as detailed on pp. 238–45. Below are the sports they are relevant to. The key is:
■ Directly relevant
□ Partial/general relevance

	Squats	Split squats and lunges	Deadlifts (bent leg)	Deadlifts (straight leg)	Pull- and chin-ups	Seated pulley rows	Standing rows	Straight-arms pulls	Pressing movements: the chest	Shoulder/overhead presses	Shoulder rotations	Cable chops/rotations	Olympic lifts	Jump squat
American/Canadian Football	■	■	□	□	□	□	■		□	■	□	□	■	■
Australian Rules Football	■	■	□	□	□	□	■		□	□	□	□	■	■
Badminton	□	■			□	□	□	□		□	■	□	□	□
Baseball / Softball	■	■			□	□	□			□	■	■	■	■
Basketball	■	■		□	□	□	□				■	□	■	■
Boxing	■	■			□	□	□		■	■	□	■	■	■
Canoeing			□		□	■	■	□			□	■		
Climbing	□	□	□		■						□	□		
Cricket	■	■			□	□	□	□			■	■	■	■
Cycling	■	□	□										■	■
Distance Running	■	■	□									□	□	□
Fencing	□	■										□	□	□
Field Hockey	■	■		□								■	■	■
Gaelic Football	■	■			□	□	■		□	□	□	□	■	■
Golf	□	□			□	□	□				□	■	□	□
Gymnastics	■	□	□		■			□		□	■	□	■	■
Hammer	■	□	■	■	□	□	■			□	□	■	■	□
Hurling	■	■			□		□			□	□	■	■	■
Ice Hockey	■	■										■	□	□
Ice Skating	□	□										□	□	□
Javelin	■	■			□	□	□	□		□	■	■	■	■
Judo	■	■	■	■	□	□	■		□	□	□	■	■	■
Jumping Sports	■	■		□								□	■	■
Kayaking			□		□	■	■	□			□	■		

relevance (blank). In the case of squash/racketball, squats are of partial/general relevance, whereas split squats and lunges are of direct relevance. Although it is still important to develop your two-legged leg strength in squash/racketball at a foundation level (and hence the general relevance) single-leg strength is arguably more important and directly related, due to the explosive multidirectional movements you would make when accelerating or lunging for the ball. Squats are typically associated with sports that require two-legged stability, such as skiing and windsurfing, or have skill-specific two-legged movements, such as scrimmaging in football or jumping to shoot a hoop in basketball.

Key

On the right are all the exercise groups, as detailed on pp. 238–45. Below are the sports they are relevant to. The key is:

■ Directly relevant
□ Partialy/general relevance

Sport	Squats	Split squats and lunges	Deadlifts (bent leg)	Deadlifts (straight leg)	Pull- and chin-ups	Seated pulley rows	Standing rows	Straight-arms pulls	Pressing movements: the chest	Shoulder/overhead presses	Shoulder rotations	Cable chops/rotations	Olympic lifts	Jump squat
Lacrosse	■	■			□	□	□					■	■	■
Middle Distance Running	■	■		□								□	■	■
Mixed Martial Arts	■	■	■	■	□	□	■		■	■	■	■	■	■
Netball	□	■								□	□	□	□	□
Powerlifting	■		■	■	□	□	□		■	□			□	□
Rowing	■		■	□	□	■	■				□	■	■	□
Rugby League	■	■	□	□	□	□	■		■	□	□	■	■	■
Rugby Union	■	■	■	□	□	□	■		■	■	□	■	■	■
Skiing	■	□										□	□	□
Soccer	■	■		□								□	■	■
Squash/Racketball	□	■			□	□	□	□			□	■	□	□
Striking Martial Arts	■	■			□	□	□		■	■	□	■	■	■
Surfing	■	■										□	□	□
Swimming	□	□		□	□	□	□	□		□		■	□	■
Table tennis		■										■	■	
Tennis	■	■			□	□	□	□		□	■	■	■	■
Shot Putt & Discus	■	■	□	□	□	□	□		■	■	■	■	■	□
Sprints	■	■		□								□	■	■
Volleyball	■	■			□	□	□	□		□	■	■	■	■
Waterskiing	■			□	□	□	□	■				□		
Water Polo	□				□	□	□	□		□	■	□	□	□
Weightlifting	■	■	■	□	□		□			■	□		■	■
Windsurfing	■		□		□	□	□					□		
Wrestling	■	■	■		□	□	■		■	□		■	■	■

GLOSSARY

%1RM The load lifted in an exercise as a percentage of your *1RM* (*one repetition maximum*).

1RM (One Repetition Maximum) The maximum amount of weight that you can lift in a single repetition for a specific training exercise.

Abductor A muscle that functions to pull a limb away from your body.

Achilles tendon A long *tendon* in your body that attaches your calf muscles to your heel bone.

Adductor A muscle that functions to pull a limb toward your body.

Aerobic A process that requires oxygen. Aerobic *metabolism* occurs during long-duration, low-intensity exercises, such as long-distance running and swimming.

Alternating grip A grip taken on a bar in which one palm faces toward your body, the other away. This form of grip prevents a loaded bar from rolling in your hands and is recommended when working with very heavy weights, especially when performing deadlifts.

Anaerobic A process that takes place without oxygen. Anaerobic *metabolism* occurs during high-intensity, short-duration exercises, such as weightlifting and sprinting.

Antagonistic muscles Muscles that are arranged in pairs to carry out flexion and extension of a joint; for example, one muscle of the pair contracts to move a limb in one direction, and the other contracts to move it in the opposite direction.

Anterior The front part or surface, as opposed to *posterior*.

Barbell A type of *free weight* made up of a bar (usually metal) with weights at both ends, which is long enough for you to hold with at least a shoulder-width grip. The weights may be permanently fixed to the bar or may be removable disks (plates) that are fixed to the bar with a collar.

BER (Basic Energy Requirement) The number of *calories* expended by your body when you are at rest.

Biceps Any muscle that has two *heads* or origins, but commonly used as shorthand for the biceps brachii, which is located on your upper arm.

Blood sugar level The concentration of the sugar *glucose* in your blood.

BMR (Basic Metabolic Rate) The minimum amount of energy (in *calories*) that your body needs daily to stay alive. BMR accounts for approximately two-thirds of your total daily energy expenditure.

Body fat percentage The weight of your body fat expressed as a percentage of total body weight.

BMI (Body Mass Index) A measure of body fat based on height and weight that applies to adult men and women. It is a useful measure for "average" people, but should be interpreted with caution, especially when applied to athletes with considerable muscle bulk.

Bone density The amount of bone tissue in a given volume of bone.

Cable pulley machine A resistance training machine in which various attachments, such as a bar, handle, or rope, can be linked to weights by a metal cable. The force for moving the weight is transferred via a pulley or system of pulleys. These machines are designed to offer many exercise options while providing continual resistance throughout the full range of motion of the exercise.

Calorie A commonly used unit of energy taken in or expended.

Carbohydrates A group of organic compounds, including sugar, starch, and cellulose. An essential part of your diet, carbohydrates are the most common source of energy in living things.

Cardiac muscle A type of involuntary muscle found in the walls of your heart.

Circuit training A routine of several exercises performed in sequence, each for a specified number of *repetitions*. The exercises are separated by timed rest intervals, and circuits are separated by longer rest periods.

Clean and jerk A technical two-part lift that, with the *snatch*, is one of the two *Olympic weightlifting* disciplines. It involves lifting a *barbell* to shoulder height, then jerking it overhead to arm's length.

Cool-down A period after completion of your main training session that includes activities such as slow jogging, walking, and stretching of your major muscle groups. It is designed to help return your body to its pre-exercise state.

Conditioning A program of exercise designed to improve your performance or to prepare you for a sporting event.

Creatine A chemical compound made by the body or taken in from food (principally meat); it is used to store energy and supply it to muscle tissue.

Drop set A form of weight training in which you perform one *set* of a particular exercise to muscle failure, then immediately lower the weight and carry out a subsequent set to failure.

Dumbbell A type of *free weight* made up of a short bar with a weight at each end. It can be lifted with one hand.

Dynamic exercise Any activity in which your joints and muscles are moving.

Erector A muscle that raises a body part.

Extensor A muscle that works to increase the angle at a joint—for example, straightening your elbow. It usually works in tandem with a *flexor*.

Fats A group of organic compounds, including animal fats, such as butter and lard, and vegetable fats, such as vegetable and bean oils. Fats are a significant source of energy in the diet and many play essential roles in your body's chemistry.

Flexor A muscle that works to decrease the angle at a joint—for example, bending your elbow. It usually works in tandem with an *extensor*.

Free weight A weight—usually a *barbell*, *dumbbell*, or *kettlebell*—not tethered to a cable or machine.

GI (Glycaemic Index) A way of quantifying the effect that taking in a particular type of *carbohydrate* food has on your *blood sugar level* on a scale of 0–100. High GI foods are those that break down quickly, releasing energy soon after digestion; low GI foods break down more slowly and release their energy over a longer period.

Glucose A simple sugar used by the body's cells as their primary source of energy.

Glycogen A type of *carbohydrate* found in the muscles and liver that provides energy during strength training. Glycogen is made up of linked units of *glucose*; any glucose that is not used by the body is converted into glycogen for storage.

Head (of a muscle) The point of origin of a muscle.

Homeostasis The processes by which your body regulates its internal environment to keep conditions stable and constant.

Hypertrophy The increase in size of a body tissue or cell, particularly an increase in muscle bulk.

Interval training A form of training in which short periods of work at near maximal intensity are alternated with periods of rest or lighter exercise, such as brisk walking or jogging.

Isometric A form of training in which your muscles work but do not contract significantly, such as when pushing against an immovable object.

Isotonic A form of training in which your muscles work against a constant resistance, so that the muscles contract while the resistance remains the same.

ITB (Iliotibial Band) A tough group of fibers running along the outside of your thigh that primarily works as a stabilizer during running.

Kettlebell An iron weight resembling a ball with a handle.

Lactic acid A waste product of *anaerobic* respiration. It accumulates in your muscles during intense exercise and is involved in the chemical processes that cause muscular cramps.

Lateral Positioned toward the outside of your body or a part of your body. Movement in the lateral plane refers to a side-to-side movement.

Ligament A tough and fibrous connective tissue that connects your bones together at your joints.

Metabolism The sum of all your body's chemical processes; it comprises anabolism (building up compounds) and catabolism (breaking down compounds).

Mineral Any one of many inorganic (non-carbon-based) elements that are essential for normal body function and that must be included in your diet.

Neural adaptation The adaptation of your nervous system in response to *strength training*. Increasing the neural activity in your muscles can provide dramatic increases in strength with little change in muscle size, especially at the beginning of a training program.

Neutral spine The position of the spine that is considered to be good posture. In this posture, the spine is not completely straight, but has slight curves in its upper and lower regions. It is the strongest and most balanced position for the spine and needs to be maintained in many exercises.

Olympic weightlifting A sport in which the goal is to lift dynamically a *barbell* loaded with the heaviest possible weights. The sport includes two distinct movements—the *clean and jerk* and the *snatch*.

Overload The progressive increase in weight used for a particular exercise. It is designed to promote adaptation of the body in response to training.

Periodization An approach to training planning that involves alternating cycling activities, loads, and intensities over a defined period of time, usually to prepare for optimum fitness for an event. It is a preparation technique used by elite athletes for competition or the start of a season.

Posterior The back part or surface, as opposed to *anterior*.

Power The amount of force produced in a given time—a combination of strength and speed.

Powerlifting A sport in which the goal is to lift a *barbell* loaded with the heaviest possible weights; it consists of three events—the squat, the bench press, and the deadlift.

Pre-exhaustion A form of training in which you perform a single joint exercise before a heavy compound movement for that body part, so stressing the target muscle before you start to work it properly.

Protein One of the three main nutrients (along with *fats* and *carbohydrates*) that supply energy to your body. Protein is required for muscular growth and repair.

Quadriceps Any muscle with four heads, but commonly used to describe the large muscle of your thigh.

Regimen A regulated course of exercise and diet designed to produce a pre-determined result.

Repetition (rep) One complete movement of a particular exercise, from start to finish and back.

Resistance training Any type of training in which your muscles work against a resistance; the resistance may be provided by a weight, an elastic or rubber band, or your own bodyweight.

Rest interval The pause between *sets* of an exercise that allows muscle recovery.

Rotator cuff The four muscles—the supraspinatus, infraspinatus, teres minor, and subscapularis—and their associated *tendons* that hold your humerus (the long bone of your upper arm) in place in your shoulder joint and enable your arm to rotate. Rotator cuff injuries are common in sports that involve throwing motions.

Set A specific number of *repetitions*.

Shoulder girdle The ring of bones (actually an incomplete ring) at your shoulder that provides an attachment point for the many muscles that allow your shoulder and elbow joints to move.

Skeletal muscle Also called striated muscle, this type of muscle is attached to your skeleton and is under voluntary control. Contracting your skeletal muscle allows you to move your body under control.

Smith machine A common piece of gym equipment made up of a *barbell* constrained within sets of parallel steel rails that allow the motion of the bar only in a limited vertical direction.

Smooth muscle A type of muscle found in the walls of all the hollow organs of your body that is not under voluntary control.

Snatch A technical lift that, along with the *clean and jerk*, is one of the two *Olympic weightlifting* disciplines. It involves lifting a *barbell* in one continuous movement from the ground (or more usually from a lifting platform) to a position where it is held overhead on your locked arms.

Split routine A pattern of training in which you focus on working one part of your body (for example, your upper body) in one *strength training* session, and another part of your body (for example, your legs) in the next session, rather than working the whole body each time.

Spotter A training partner who assists you with a lift, providing encouragement and physical support if necessary—for example, intervening if you are about to fail the lift.

Static exercise An exercise in which you hold one position—for example, pushing against an immovable object.

Strength training A form of *resistance training* in which your goal is to build the strength of your *skeletal muscle*.

Superset A type of training in which you perform two exercises in a row with no rest in between; the exercises can target the same or different parts of your body.

Supplement Any preparation in the form of a pill, liquid, or powder that contains nutrients.

Tendon A type of connective tissue that joins your muscles to your bones, so transmitting the force of muscle contraction to your bones.

Training to failure Performing *repetitions* of a particular exercise until you cannot lift the weight without assistance.

Triceps Any muscle with three *heads*, but commonly used as shorthand for the triceps brachii, which extends your elbow.

Vitamin Any one of a group of chemical compounds that is required by your body in small amounts for healthy growth and development. Most vitamins are not made by your body, so must be taken in the diet.

Warm-up A series of low-intensity exercises that prepares your body for a workout by moderately stimulating your heart, lungs, and muscles.

INDEX

ACKNOWLEDGMENTS

ABOUT THE AUTHORS

Len Williams is an International Weightlifting Referee and a Senior Coach for the British Weight Lifters' Association. He tutors at colleges and universities on various training courses. Len is currently in the squad of officials preparing for the 2012 Olympic games in London.

Derek Groves is a professional sports coach and a staff coach with the British Weight Lifters' Association and a Consultant Staff Coach to the Saudi Arabian Federation of Sport for Disability Powerlifting. He has over 30 years' experience of strength training and conditioning for elite athletes and is currently an International Classifier for IPC Paralympic Powerlifting.

Glen Thurgood is a professional BWLA coach and Head of Strength and Conditioning at Northampton Town FC. With over 10 years' combined experience as an elite athlete and coach, he has worked with rugby union, football, and baseball teams at university, professional, and national levels.

PUBLISHER'S ACKNOWLEDGMENTS

Dorling Kindersley would like to thank Jillian Burr, Joanna Edwards, Michael Duffy, Conor Kilgallon, and Phil Gamble.

Cobalt id would like to thank the following individuals and organizations for their generous help in producing this book:

Chris Chea, Caroline Pearce, William Smith, Michelle Grey, Sam Bias Ferrar, Sean Newton, and Anouska Hipperson for modelling so gracefully and professionally.

Anouska and Roscoe Hipperson, Matt, Jon and all the brilliant staff at Fit Club, Wymondham in Norfolk for allowing us access to their fantastic facilities, and for all their kind support and guidance during the photoshoots. Jackie Waite and the staff at Woking Leisure Centre & Pool in the Park and Karen Pearce and the staff at Fenner's Fitness Suite at the University of Cambridge.

Many thanks also to all the illustrators who worked so hard throughout the project: Mark Walker, Mike Garland, Darren R. Awuah, Debajyoti Dutta, Richard Tibbitts (Antbits Illustration), Jon Rogers, and Phil Gamble. Many thanks to Patricia Hymans for indexing.

ABOUT BWLA (THE BRITISH WEIGHT LIFTERS' ASSOCIATION)

The British Weight Lifters' Association (BWLA), the national governing body for weightlifting and weight training, was formed 100 years ago. While it is now primarily recognized as the guardian of the Olympic sport of weightlifting in the UK, it remains deeply involved in weight training of all types, particularly as an aid to improved performance in other sports. As part of its aim to develop weightlifting and weight training, the BWLA has been involved in education for much of its history. In the late 1940s, its first professional coach, Al Murray, pioneered the application of resistance training to other sports, collaborating fruitfully with celebrated coaches like Bert Kinnear (swimming) and Geoff Dyson (athletics), and drawing on the advanced, research-based knowledge of Russian coaches. A body of knowledgeable coaches, nurtured through his courses, helped scientific weightlifting and weight training to flourish. The BWLA retains many expert coaches with a strong grounding in academic theory, and above all, an unrivaled level of practical skill in both performance and teaching.

SAFETY INFORMATION

All sport and physical activity involves some risk of injury. Participants must take all reasonable care to ensure that they are free from any medical condition that could contra-indicate participation in weightlifting, weight training, or any other form of resistance exercise.

The publishers of this book and its contributors are confident that, when properly performed, weightlifting and weight training are safe, and that the exercises described in this book, correctly executed, with gradual increases in resistance and proper supervision, are also safe.

However, it is incumbent upon users of weightlifting and weight training facilities to exercise sensible judgement, and to ensure that floors, equipment, ventilation, and hygiene are all fit for purpose.

Supervisors must all carry adequate insurance and have relevant up-to-date certifications, including emergency first aid. In the UK, the British Weight Lifters' Association (BWLA) is recognized by the governmental authorities and its agencies as the National Governing Body for Weightlifting and Weight Training. Participants should check that their supervisors are current members of this body; participants should check that adequate insurance is in place if the supervisors are members of another body.

Although sports scientists have worked to improve the knowledge underpinning the construction of training programs, the choice of resistance, and the many other variables considered when creating them, there remain very few absolutes. Different combinations of exercises, diverse ordering, and the variation of volumes and intensities, etc., may all work. The effectiveness of a schedule is markedly influenced by the individual using it, and the period of time before it is changed: coaches constantly observe athletes and vary programmes whenever they appear to be losing effectiveness. In training for sports other than Olympic weightlifting, it is clearly essential that a strength and conditioning coach works closely with well informed coaches of that sport.

All current research shows that weightlifting and weight training is safe for children, in comparison with traditional school sports, but, for obvious reasons, children should always be particularly well supervised.

The publishers and contributing authors of this book disclaim all responsibility for injury to persons or property consequent on embarking upon the exercises herein described.